Revising the Clinic

Revising the Clinic

*Vision and Representation in
Victorian Medical Narrative and the Novel*

∼

MEEGAN KENNEDY

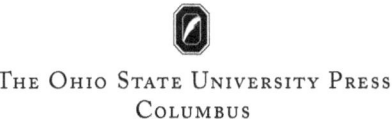

THE OHIO STATE UNIVERSITY PRESS
COLUMBUS

Copyright © 2010 by The Ohio State University.
All rights reserved.

Library of Congress Cataloging-in-Publication Data
Kennedy, Meegan, 1966–
Revising the clinic : vision and representation in Victorian medical narrative and the novel / Meegan Kennedy.
p. cm.
Includes bibliographical references and index.
ISBN-13: 978-0-8142-1116-8 (cloth : alk. paper)
ISBN-10: 0-8142-1116-X (cloth : alk. paper)
ISBN-13: 978-0-8142-9214-3 (cd-rom)
1. Literature and medicine—19th century. 2. Medicine in literature—19th century.
3. Medical writing—19th century—History and criticism.
4. Fiction—19th century—History and criticism. I. Title.
PN56.M38K46 2010
823'.8093561—dc22
2009025707

This book is available in the following editions:
Cloth (ISBN 978–0–8142–1116–8)
CD-ROM (ISBN 978–0–8142–9214–3)
Cover design by Mia Risberg
Text design by Juliet Williams
Type set in Adobe Caslon Pro

∞ The paper used in this publication meets the minimum requirements of the American National Standard for Information Sciences—Permanence of Paper for Printed Library Materials. ANSI Z39.48–1992.

9 8 7 6 5 4 3 4 3 2 1

CONTENTS

List of Figures / vii
Acknowledgments / ix

INTRODUCTION
Vision, Representation, and the Production of Knowledge / 1

CHAPTER ONE
Curious Observations, Curious Sights:
The Eighteenth-Century Case History / 30

CHAPTER TWO
Staging Clinical Realism in the Victorian Periodical / 54

CHAPTER THREE
The Sentimental Eye in Dickens and Gaskell / 87

CHAPTER FOUR
George Eliot's Realist Vision:
Mechanical Observation and the Production of Sympathy / 119

CHAPTER FIVE
Speculation and Insight:
Experimental Medicine and the Expansion of Realism / 148

CHAPTER SIX
Mapping an Unnavigable River:
Freud, Rider Haggard, and the Imperial Romance / 168

CONCLUSION / 203

Notes / 206
Works Cited / 230
Index / 247

List of Figures

Figure 1.
From William Chesselden,
"An Explication of the Instruments Used, in a New Operation on the Eyes,"
Philosophical Transactions 35, no. 402 (1728): 451–52.
49

Figure 2.
From George Cruikshank, "The Blue Devils_!!"
(London: G. Humphrey, 1823).
72

Figure 3.
Illustration of camera obscura.
From *The Museum of Science and Art,* ed. Dionysius Lardner (1855).
135

Figure 4.
Chevalier achromatic microscope, c. 1824.
From William B. Carpenter, *The Microscope and Its Revelations,*
7th ed., edited by W. H. Dallinger (Philadelphia: P. Blakiston, Son, 1891), 148.
153

Acknowledgments

Ars longa, vita brevis: this is as true in scholarship as in medicine. This book began as a dissertation under Robert Scholes, Nancy Armstrong, and Tamar Katz. They challenged me to find the thread of argument in what was a voluminous project; I hope they can recognize some of their work with me here.

I owe much of what is best here to discussions with colleagues at Brown, Trinity, Harvard, and Florida State University, as well as at conferences across the United States and the United Kingdom. I am deeply indebted to Julie Nelson Couch, Annette Van, Nina Markov, and Susie Castellanos for their provocative readings and a deep well of encouragement. Many colleagues in Victorian studies and the history of medicine, especially Geoffrey Sill, Jay Clayton, Jason Tougaw, Jane Thrailkill, Michele Martinez, John Mackey, and Jutta Schickore, offered productive discussions of the field and sound practical advice. I have enjoyed the intellectual vigor of the community at FSU, in English, History and Philosophy of Science, and Medical Humanities; especially Candace Ward, Nancy Warren, Leigh Edwards, Tomeiko Ashford, and Fritz Davis, for their thoughtful readings and support.

I am grateful for the financial and intellectual support of my department through its Faculty Research Series and its travel and research grants;

and the support of the university through travel grants, the First Year Assistant Professor grant, and the Committee on Faculty Research and Support grant. The College of Arts and Sciences provided critical small-grant support as well. Research for this book was also enabled by the Wood Fellowship, Francis C. Wood Institute, College of Physicians of Philadelphia.

A short segment of chapter 2 appears, slightly altered, in *Victorian Literature and Culture* 32, no. 2 (2004). A short segment of chapter 5 appears, slightly altered, in *Nineteenth-Century Literature* as "'A True Prophet': The Uses of Speculation in Victorian Sensory Physiology and George Eliot's 'The Lifted Veil.'" A portion of the introduction appears, slightly altered, in *RaVoN: Romanticism and Victorianism on the Net* as "Diagnosis or Detour? The Uses of Medical Realism in the Victorian Novel" (48 [February 2008]). My thanks to these journals for permission to reprint this material.

For assistance in obtaining the images appearing here, I would like to thank the John Hay and Rockefeller libraries at Brown University, and Alderman Library and the Claude Moore Health Sciences Library at the University of Virginia; and the Interlibrary Loan and Special Collections offices at Florida State University's Strozier Library, especially Velma Smith. For research assistance I am also grateful for the assistance of the staff at Harvard University's Widener Library and Countway Medical Library, especially Jack Eckert; the College of Physicians of Philadelphia, especially Richard Fraser; the National Library of Medicine, History of Medicine Reading Room; the Wellcome Library; Yale University Historical Medical Library, especially Toby Appel; and Trinity College (Connecticut), Watkinson Library.

I am deeply grateful to Richard and Gail Hanson for their unvarying support and for a "room of my own" to work in, summers. To Robert and Elizabeth Kennedy for another research haven, unswerving support, and, most important, for giving me life in a world of books and ideas. To Schooner and Skipper for their insistence that innumerable games of fetch would enable critical thinking. (They were right.) To Caty and Bay for their patience and some really good advice, and for their exuberant reminders of life beyond the book. And most of all to Scott for his enthusiasm and understanding, his cheerful support, and his faith in my work.

Introduction

Vision, Representation, and the Production of Knowledge

> Her relations with the world ... pressed so incessantly and so forcibly on the springs of interest and curiosity, that there seems to have been hardly a moment when she was not observing, speculating, or analyzing and recording the results.... Perhaps the most distinctive feature of her literary faculty is her power of seeing and stating brief problems of life, and so conveying in a sentence the result of a process of observation and thought.

In 1885 E. B. Hamley, writing in *Blackwood's Edinburgh Magazine,* characterized George Eliot as having lived at a constant pitch of awareness, stimulated incessantly to practice and refine the arts of seeing and representing.[1] Victorian medical and literary authors alike grounded their work in a serious attention to these arts, and to exploring and evaluating the range of modes of observation and representation available to them. George Eliot is of course a necessary figure for the study of literature and medicine in this period, given her complex and legendary fascination in working out these questions. But the modes of "interest" and "curiosity," and the proclivity for "observing" and "speculating," or "seeing and stating," are not exclusive to her; medical as well as literary communities intently examined and debated these. In particular, Victorian case histories usefully referenced a historically specific authority, based on a particular notion of truth, its collection, and its transmission. Clinical methods of observation and representation offered writers some useful and powerful strategies, conveying a sense of rigorous scrutiny, careful description and narration, and professional knowledge. It is evident how useful these could be for novelists facing what Peter Brooks has called the "descriptive imperative" of the nineteenth-century novel, since physicians used these methods to meet the same imperative in medicine.[2] Thus, this book is interested in pursuing not only the question Gillian Beer asks—"How much do the discursive strategies of scientists and poets have in common?"[3]—but how and why do physicians and novelists share these discursive strategies; and how and why do the same strategies play differently in different kinds of texts?

Nineteenth-century literary and medical genres—in particular the novel and the case history—shared a central concern over different modes of seeing and stating; but diverging disciplinary norms constrained their use of these practices. Previous analyses of "medicine and the novel" have examined a common realist ideal, usually by reading novels with medical content. But even a realist methodology shared by the novel and by medicine did not find identical expression in both genres.[4] Lawrence Rothfield identifies "medical realism" by its clinical or diagnostic voice, and he suggests that a medical discourse might "help to shape such formal features as point of view, characterization, description, diegesis, or closure, even in the absence of terminology." Indeed, "one should be able to find some of these same techniques at work in other realistic novels where doctors and patients do not appear as such or appear only at the margins of the story" (xiii, xvii). This book takes up Rothfield's suggestion, arguing in part that nineteenth-century novels may employ clinical observation and representation even where medicine is not strictly at issue. Although many of my readings focus on medicine and the body, others demonstrate how novels profitably use these strategies even when they portray neither doctors nor illness. Case histories model not just compelling characters and motifs but also a textual methodology for Victorian novels.

If novelists free these techniques of seeing and stating from their anchor in medical prose, both medical writers and novelists revise them in use, adopting them in a manner that contradicts medical authority or norms, or in the interests of literary aims such as sympathy, sentiment, sensation, irony, humor, or morality. The medical case history likewise borrows narrative forms and strategies from the novel, even after physicians establish a normative clinical genre for the case history, and especially in cases where professional knowledge or abilities fail.

Both genres—the novel and the case history—are crucially oriented around issues of vision and representation in this period. Critical interest in Victorian visuality has burgeoned, ranging from visual art to ideologies of perception to the science of optics, reflecting the consensus that it was a visual age.⁵ I am most interested in how literary and medical notions of seeing and stating changed over time, in relation with each other and with nineteenth-century historical developments and professional structures such as the rise of dissection, practical microscopy, psychoanalysis, literary periodicals, serialized fiction, and the like.

One foundational assumption of this project is that seeing and stating are crucially linked: changes in seeing made new forms of representation necessary, while new theories of representation codified and valorized particular kinds of seeing. Previous work on the medical narrative in relation to nineteenth-century literature often focuses on a binary model of reading—Romantic or materialist (Janis Caldwell), sympathetic or diagnostic (Jason Tougaw)—which critics offer as an alternative to the flawed binary of "literature or medicine."⁶ However, despite these critics' careful attention to how these modes are in fact interpolated rather than distinct, these vexed couplets can reimport an oppositional notion of genre. By parsing out the distinct stages of seeing and stating that novel and case history share, this book hopes to present another model of genre, one that can flexibly trace the changing relationship between medical and literary narratives.

Accordingly, I trace the development of three stages of the case history—curious, clinical, and psychoanalytic—and varieties of the novel—sentimental, realist, romantic—as they develop and deploy a range of modes of vision to suit specific and historically contingent disciplinary needs. My interest in charting and examining the types of vision that physicians and novelists employed owes much to Lorraine Daston and Peter Galison's work on objectivity, and to Martin Jay's thesis of competing scopic regimes within modern culture. He suggests a "contested terrain, rather than a harmoniously integrated complex of visual theories and practices." Similarly, Chris Otter argues that "reductive visual paradigms should be replaced by a multiplicity of overlapping, intersecting, and contrasting perceptual 'patterns.'"⁷ It should be evident, then, that this project not only builds on but also complicates Foucault's notion of the clinical gaze, both because the power relation of the gaze was not unambiguous, and because physicians themselves struggled to incorporate it. I analyze the development of each mode of vision out of a specific historical moment, defined in relation to the predominant concerns and tensions in that moment as writers differentiate themselves from the past; but "each new regimen of sight supplements rather than supplants the others," as Daston and Galison caution.⁸ Some modes of vision, like clinical observation, define themselves in reaction against the excesses of a previous mode; others, like speculation or Freud's imperialist mapping, incorporate aspects of their predecessors. My interest is not in how Victorian physicians and novelists actually saw, but in how they theorized seeing, and how those theories changed representation. Finally, none of these texts realizes its ideal of vision or representation. Each author brings a specific set of needs and interests to his work, so any individual ideal of vision, like clinical observation, can only be realized in a multiple and fragmentary way; that is, in its many partial textual instantiations. One of my aims is to explore how far a text can flirt with other modes of vision or incorporate other genres before it risks losing disciplinary identification.

I begin with the oscillation in many eighteenth-century case histories between "curious observations" and "curious sights." Curiosity was a favored attribute of eighteenth-century science, but the most authoritative way to pursue that curiosity was through a carefully managed observation: the unusual phenomenon would be exhibited for an assembled audience of disinterested experimentalists. This empiricist practice valorized the individual "matter of fact" in order to counter a proliferation of theories and systems. At times, however, as chapter 1 demonstrates, if the phenomenon becomes spectacular or the audience become voyeurs—linked to the scene more through affect (interest) than rational evaluation—then "curious observation" gives way to "curious sight." This brief survey of eighteenth-century case histories grounds later chapters examining how the clinical and psychoanalytic case histories respond to and rework curious observation.

Chapters 2 through 5 explore the Victorian development of a distanced observation associated with clinical realism. In this book, I use the term "clinical realism" (rather than "scientific realism" or "medical realism") to locate this theory of accurate mimesis historically, shaped by the clinical methods of observation and communication established during the long nineteenth century. Chapter 2 examines how clinical observation, such as the accurate examination, careful quantification, and dispassionate stance associated with the autopsy, developed into a theory of clinical realism marked predominantly by mechanical objectivity, the term Daston and Galison use to identify a nineteenth-century moral ideal for producing scientific knowledge.[9] This ideal valorizes accuracy and precision to the extent that the human observer should resist not only bias but judgment or any kind of mediation, so that natural phenomena might be (nearly) mechanically recorded through the incessant, selfless labor and attention to detail of the scientist. It specifically excludes any form of imagination, intuition, or insight—modes associated with literary writing instead. I adapt this notion as "mechanical observation" rather than "mechanical objectivity," to indicate my focus, and that of clinical realism, on modes of visual perception. Although Daston and Galison identify the mid-nineteenth century as the period when this construct became a dominant ideal for scientists, instances occur earlier in medical debates over the proper matter and means of producing case histories.[10] This model influences medical narrative throughout the century, despite requiring the physician to sacrifice his sensibility, even his visible authorial role, on the altar of objectivity.

The remaining chapters of the book trace what happens to mechanical observation—how it is revised, adapted, enlarged, and subverted in novels and case histories throughout the century. The ideal of clinical medicine emerged only through an uneven development and was never unchallenged, especially given the competing ideal of "medicine as an art," which championed a third mode of vision, insight. Versions of human insight appeared in case histories coded variously as sensibility, sentiment, sympathy, and even speculation. The movement toward experimental medicine at midcentury, influenced by the French pathologist Claude Bernard, helped make space in medicine for a kind of insight, hypothesis, or "speculation." This must be grounded in the clinical ideal of observation, even as it rehabilitates the notion of intuitive or imaginative judgment. Speculation and insight in nineteenth-century medicine, unlike mechanical observation, invite a sympathetic or humanist mode of investigation that acknowledges the subjective experiences of both narrators and their objects of study. The status of this subjective knowledge in medical narrative is ambiguous at best. It is explicitly disavowed at the peak of the early-nineteenth-century empirical backlash against theory but judiciously admitted, if under suspicion, from the midcentury.

Although Freud is not British, this discussion of the case history must conclude with his model of the genre. His cases, and his remarks on case-taking, proudly mark their difference from most clinical case histories, as is evident in the dismayed reactions of many of his contemporaries. These help demonstrate how far clinical ideals dominated Victorian medicine, in a formalization of the case history that would remain unquestioned until the work of late-twentieth-century medical humanists. Partly because Freud uniquely combines clinical observation with a curious sight and an intuitive, speculative insight, his narratives are no longer legible within the generic tradition associated with the discipline of clinical medicine. The overt discursive hybridity of the Freudian case history is one reason, I argue, for the contested role of psychoanalysis as "science," and its welcome within the literary community. Another is Freud's unique model of vision, a romantic vision that heroically explores, reads, and maps the resistant wilds of a labyrinthine hysteria. If speculation required an imaginative projection into the unknown, Freud's probing gaze goes even further in its active intervention and conflation of diagnosis with treatment.

Each of these modes of vision demands its proper method of representation. While the curious observations of experimental philosophers are certified by their record in "plain speech," their curious sights attract an exoticizing, sentimental, sensational, or romantic discourse—a curious discourse, which knits narrator to reader through the circulation of a shared affective response to a spectacular textual "sight."

The ideal of mechanical observation, in contrast, requires a particularizing, distanced representation in order to properly communicate and preserve its enlarged, objective knowledge. This new form of methodical, detailed representation helps construct a clinical realism for science. The term "science," describing "a precise and demonstrable knowledge," has existed in English since the Middle Ages and was clarified during the early seventeenth century. However, Sydney Ross argues that it was only after the publication of the astronomer Herschel's *Preliminary Discourse on the Study of Natural Philosophy* in 1830 that "science" approached our modern sense of the term, implying "scepticism of authority; dispassionate description of phenomena; the framing of hypotheses capable of being tested; and the measurement of the limits of reliability of data."[11] Mechanical observation idealizes the notion of an almost automatic representation, in which seeing and stating are collapsed, but its clinical realist narrators set out their authorizing markers as anxiously as any experimentalist. The scientific article thus accrued a constitutive written style, marked by its visual scrutiny, fetishization of detail, and impersonal tone.[12] Although compliance with these norms differs, the clinical case history references the new scientific norms more consistently than its predecessors had, to mark itself as new and modern. The positivist ideology of nineteenth-century science, rooted in a narrative of progress, required that the achievements of early empiricists like Bacon and Boyle be superseded by the efforts of the Victorians, who by midcentury had claimed the title of "scientist."[13]

Surprisingly, clinical case histories continue to draw from these non- or even antirealist subgenres, especially the sentimental. Speculative moments in nineteenth-century case histories are often flagged by hedging, signaling an anxious care to demonstrate a judicious balance between science and imagination. In contrast, the florid speculations and literary prose of Freud's psychoanalytic case histories dramatize, by their difference from clinical norms, how decisively medicine had rejected literature and its insights. Significantly, medical narratives continue to engage with literary forms and techniques throughout the century, even if under erasure. Given the frequency with which literary prose appears in failed medical cases, it is likely that retaining a range and variety of rhetorical strategies offered a distinct advantage in challenging cases.

In the story of the case history, then, eighteenth-century medical narrators authorize observation and plain speech but flirt with spectacle and curious discourse. Nineteenth-century physicians valorize (but do not entirely realize) mechanical observation and clinical realism, contracting the modes available to the author, and they experiment with speculation, expanding them again. And Freud forces a rupture between observation and insight, when his model of the physician as a visionary charting dark and treacherous depths fatally strains the capacity of the medical case history to contain his floridly romantic model of medical vision.

The changes in the nineteenth-century British novel are more complicated to survey, given the proliferation of generic types and subtypes throughout the century. The novel emerges from an eighteenth-century model of sensibility, in which virtue is attained and displayed through the visual circulation of suffering and sympathy, into a century marked by a remarkable array of generic models for the novel and its vision. These include five nodes in the history of the Victorian novel that I examine here: the staging of clinical medical realism in literary periodicals; the sentimental (mis)use of clinical observations in Dickens and Gaskell; the revision of mechanical observation to produce sympathetic realism in the early George Eliot; the experimentation with a speculative insight in the later Eliot; and the scientific mapping of a dark, exotic labyrinth, common to the imperial romance of both Freud and Rider Haggard. However, even when novelists borrow a methodology of clinical realism from medicine, their novels seek to convey insight about, as well as observation of, the world.

Of necessity, this study engages with the project of Victorian realism and the relation between literary and scientific forms of that project. Although there are almost as many definitions of realism as there are critics of realism, I focus here on the most salient characteristics for my study, predominantly its empiricist commitment to the details of experience; its overt concern with accuracy and reliability; its apparent desire for transparency and suspicion of mediation; its record of the quotidian rather than the extraordinary; its idealization of a dispassionate stance; and perhaps most important, its skeptical, deflationary approach. The protean term "romance" is useful to me here to describe primarily antirealist discourses, in particular the interest in "curious" people and events, and a florid solicitation of the circulation of affect through a sentimental, sensational, or melodramatic tone. A narrative with a pointed, exaggerated interest in historicity and documents (translation, transcription, editing) is likely to verge on the romantic in its overt attention to the mediation of representation.

INTRODUCTION

Medical and scientific narratives, I argue, theorized and (ideally) modeled a clinical realism that combined disinterested skepticism with a compensatory fetishization of description. The relation between these and literary texts encouraged an ingrained skepticism in realist novels about our ability to see and communicate reality, as well as a laborious collection of factual detail in an effort to make up for our inherent limitations. Thus, reading Victorian novels in company with case histories allows us to see the extent to which the realist novel is not, as some critics have claimed, either naïve or in bad faith about its relation to reality, with the caveat that a clinical realism is often necessary but not sufficient for the novelist's goals.[14]

This book also works to expand our sense of what kinds of novels find a medical narrative methodology relevant and useful, if only for a partial, momentary, or even critical adoption. It is no surprise that Gothic novels often draw upon medicine, given the nineteenth-century tradition of the scientific Gothic. But sentimental fiction and the imperial romance can also reference this realist methodology. That is, clinical medicine offered a useful cultural resource for a range of literary authors and audiences, even when they did not fully subscribe to its tenets, because clinical discourse usefully referenced a historically specific authority and technique for collecting and transmitting knowledge, even though novelists might differ from physicians on the ultimate truth that was being served.

Miriam Bailin has argued for a "marginalization of medical knowledge and discourse" in early and mid-Victorian fictional scenes of "illness and recovery," which she finds uninflected by clinical discursive norms.[15] It is possible, however, that Victorian novelists' clinical realism may be masked by being deployed strategically rather than universally, and often in settings outside that of the sickroom. Thus, despite the useful work by critics like Athena Vrettos, Peter Logan, Jane Wood, and Maria Frawley, I am not focusing on the "illness narrative" in fiction; nor (like Roy Porter, Bailin, or Frawley) telling the patient's side of the story.[16] Indeed, it is not necessary to focus on the "illness narrative" in fiction in order to examine the uses of medical discourse in the novel. Rather, this book studies the case history as a narrative genre in order to understand how clinical-realist observation and representation get used not only in, but outside the realist novel, and not only as part of, but also beyond the illness narrative.

At the most basic level, this book is a history of the engagement of two literary forms, the novel and the case history. It is grounded in the claim that the changes in the genre of the case history and that of the novel are fundamentally in relation with one another throughout the nineteenth century. If this book somewhat uneasily combines two narratives—the trajectory of the Victorian novel's revisions of medical observation and clinical discourse, and a literary history of the case history's flirtation with human insight—it is because, I contend, each of these stories cannot be fully told without the other.

MEDICAL OBSERVATION AND MEDICAL AUTHORITY

The physician's eye, trained to a clinical gaze, often represents in Victorian novels a dispassionate, accurate evaluation, a keener access to reality, like that of a reliable but not omniscient narrator. While the ne'er-do-well father of an injured child, in Margaret Oliphant's *The Rector and the Doctor's Family* (1863), panics so that "his trembling nervous fingers and bemused eyes could make nothing of the 'case,'" his brother, Dr. Rider, shifts into professional mode in the midst of his own frustration and anger. "Both father and mother thought [the boy] dead," the novel comments, "but the accustomed and cooler eyes of the doctor perceived the true state of affairs. Edward Rider forgot his disgust and rage [at the negligent father] as he devoted himself to the little patient—not that he loved the child more, but that the habits of his profession were strong upon him."[17]

Rider's authority here derives from his capability for distanced observation, combined with a medical knowledge born of experience (his "accustomed and cooler eyes") to enable an accurate evaluation of the situation and competent, engaged action. What characterizes the doctor qua doctor here is the training that enables him to overcome himself as character, to submerge his mere individuality, his love, and his rage, and to become a type. "The Doctor" of Oliphant's title has earned his distinctive social authority by virtue of this skill, innately associated with the clinical gaze that Michel Foucault has identified. It had become an axiom of medical professionalism (although a contested one, as I will show) that the physician's knowledge could only be gained by cultivating this distanced view, one that paradoxically also sees more closely. A disinterested medical vision, it was thought, can peer beyond surface impressions to perceive the innermost workings of the body, emulating the anatomical dissections that inaugurated the clinical era.

Dr. Rider's distanced gaze is not a Foucauldian one, however. His authority is not simply that of a "clinical gaze," because his diagnostic eye both marks the forced submersion of his inner man and, paradoxically, enhances his humanity. His ability to "forg[e]t his disgust and rage" by losing himself in clinical observation paradoxically suggests what the narrator must disavow—that "he loved the child more." Oliphant is typical of Victorian novelists in her interest in the relation between two modes of vision, clinical observation and human insight. While some physicians thought these incompatible, novelists like Oliphant consider whether one may in fact enable the other.

Nineteenth-century British medical narratives increasingly project a realist medical discourse that both invokes and enacts this cultural authority, that of the disembodied, knowledgeable, and professional eye. The theory and ideology of medicine change in the 1830s, with the medical reform movement and backlash against "heroic" medicine; but medical education and practice do not change greatly until the advent of germ theory and antibiotics decades later. As a result, much of the progress of professional Victorian medicine occurs through changes to the structure of medical practice, including the representation of that practice in narrative form (the case history). This moves away from the spectacular, curious cases of the eighteenth century toward the dispassionate scientific ideals of the nineteenth.

These newly disciplined narratives are central to the construction of professional medicine. If a physician engages with a case by observing the signs, evaluating them in the light of his previous knowledge (diagnosing the illness), and suggesting action (treating the illness), the clinical case history completes the cycle by returning the product—new clinical experience, whether real or vicarious—to a now-enlarged body of professional knowledge.[18] These narratives invoke the insights of clinical observation through a prescribed narrative form, ritualizing the process of professional practice and realizing medical knowledge in a new, distinctive way.

This book will explore the two aspects of this cycle that nineteenth-century physicians teaching or revising the genre of the case history tend to emphasize: vision and representation. By combining clinical observation with realist representation, physicians had access to a powerful new methodology for producing a professional knowledge and identity. The advantages of clinical realism proved portable beyond the bounds of the medical narratives for which it was developed.

Medical Observation and Representation in the Novel

Given that clinical observation and representation come to evoke an ideal of accuracy and discernment, and carry a measure of cultural authority, it is not surprising that novelists turn to it. It allows novels to describe and evaluate some object, or narrate and judge some process, whether it be a person, a landscape, a social system—or the efficacy of a particular style of housekeeping, the popularity of purchased pastries in a small town, or rumors of a bank failure.[19] The methodical, diagnostic gaze associated with the clinical close reading of an object facilitates a consideration of the moral, emotional, or spiritual, as well as physical, state of individual characters or of British society as a whole. However, even inanimate objects such as landscapes may resonate under diagnosis, and even authors who are ostensibly skeptical about scientific methods may adopt a clinical approach.

In Benjamin Disraeli's *Sybil* (1845), the narrator overtly takes on the role of a physician when diagnosing the town of Marney, which represents the sorry "condition of the People" of England.[20] The approach to the town appears "delightful" to the untutored traveler, who perceives only its situation "[i]n a spreading dale, contiguous to the margin of a clear and lively stream, surrounded by meadows and gardens, and backed by lofty hills, undulating and richly wooded." This pastoral scene is, however, a "[b]eautiful illusion," which the narrator rapidly dispels through authority gained from a kind of dissection, cutting through this superficially "merry prospect" to reveal the decay deep in the body of England. "[B]ehind that laughing landscape," the narrator warns, "penury and disease fed upon the vitals of a miserable population" (51).

Disraeli adopts the methodology of surgery and dissection for this description of a diseased England. His narrator searches deep to reveal the inner organs or "vitals" of England and the nation's hidden cancer, "full of pain." Despite the "traditional epithet of [the] country," this England is not so much merry as delirious, displaying a disordered and entirely symptomatic disconnect between face and flesh, appearance and reality, surface and depth. This is a pathological landscape, which to be cured must be opened to the fresh air and to the reformer's cleansing scalpel.[21] To provide that healing cut, the narrator records a series of details, from the general state of the "narrow and crowded lanes" and "cottages built of rubble," to a catalogue of the disorder in structures such as the "leaning chimneys" and "rotten rafters" (51–52).

Disraeli does refer to actual diseases, in a reference to the sanitary movement and Edwin Chadwick's 1842 *Report on the Sanitary Condition of the Labouring Population of Great Britain*. Disraeli's narrator returns again and again to the "open drains full of animal and vegetable refuse, decomposing into disease," the "foul pits," and "stagnant pools" of "dissolving filth" (52). The passage mentions typhus and malaria and describes "Fever, in every form, pale Consumption, exhausting Synochus,[22] and trembling Ague" (52–53). Disraeli's capitalization personifies these fevers as dread persons haunting the land—a literary touch at the deepest point of the narrator's surgical exploration, testifying to novelists' tendency to combine a clinical discursive methodology with more affecting techniques.

Disraeli's "case history" of a literally diseased landscape points to the metaphorical power of clinical narratives in the hands of a novelist. Like the physician-turned-social reformer James Phillips Kay, Disraeli argues here for "England's social problems as a kind of disease."[23] These diseases are not only literal threats but also potent signifiers of the failures of domestic policy: cancers on the body politic. Although the scene offers the opportunity to fulminate about a number of moral and social ills—national security, crime, the economy, industrialization and labor relations, and the like—the narrator uses its public health failures as a synecdoche for the economic and political health of the land, and the consequences for England's moral and spiritual health.

While individual persons in the scene suffer from particular diseases, this passage focuses its "diagnosis" on the landscape as a whole. It presents a clinical examination, not of any individual body, but of the landscape and the town, as synecdoches for the nation; and its reference to these fevers suggests how they sap life and health from the economic and social as well as the individual body. Disraeli, like other nonmedical novelists, demonstrates familiarity with medical observation and representation, and refocuses these to diagnose subjects other than characters. Rather than simply depicting and diagnosing the diseases of particular characters, the clinical perspective here examines and evaluates a social function. The narrative is structured by and oriented toward a clinical perspective, rather than merely recording some character's use of that perspective; and clinical observation and narration become a mode of representation rather than simply being represented.

A novel may thus strategically employ a technique drawn from medicine, even when the plot—or novelist—is not particularly invested in medical or scientific culture. Acknowledging the uses of clinical realism beyond direct experience usefully opens up the available field of analysis beyond George Eliot, Charles Dickens, Sarah Grand, and others with established personal connections to the medical or scientific community. Disraeli is not known for his interest in science and medicine. The "Young England" movement of which he was a member generally scorned the statisticians working on public health, arguing that statistics distance the reader from the true human cost of endemic poverty. Indeed, Mary Poovey argues for

Sybil as "a counter to [the] anatomical realism" that she associates with Chadwick and Kay (137).

The case history boasts a unique relation to scientific narrative because of the inherently subjective interest of its human subject. Some physicians asserted the role of medicine as an art every time medical statistics and clinical science crested a new wave of popularity. As this book will show, case histories are more likely than other kinds of scientific texts to attempt a balance, albeit an uneasy one, between science and art, observation and insight. Like many case histories, Disraeli's narrative juxtaposes medical practices such as diagnosis and dissection with more evocative descriptions of a pathology. This reformist approach links a critical observation of environment, as in public health treatises, to the human insight that must accompany any practice of the medical art.

Literary Representation and Insight in Medical Narratives

While novelists made use of medical techniques of observation and representation, Victorian physicians did not entirely eschew literary techniques in writing case histories, even as the genre became more formal and less elastic. Despite the demands of increased hospital training for students, literary reading remained central to physicians' reputation as men of letters. Edward Forbes argues in 1843 for the importance of literary and aesthetic subjects even in medical school. While the medical profession "must become more and more scientific every day," he warns, "[t]he air of a hospital is mentally unwholesome, unless mingled with a full proportion of collegiate atmosphere. The very neighbourhood of literary and scientific studies has a purifying and elevating effect on the mind of the student."[24] Thus, he concludes, the aim of a proper medical education must be to produce a physician who is at once "a scholar, a man of science, and a man of taste; and, above all, imbued with sound principles of religion and morality" (12). Forbes is echoing a widespread concern that physicians must continue to read literary texts, to retain not only their status as men of culture, but also their professional acumen.

The physician's elevated status over surgeons, apothecaries, and irregulars had traditionally been due in part to his university training, little of which was required to be scientific until a medical school entrance examination on physics, chemistry, and biology was instituted in the 1880s. Although the divisions between the ancient "corporations" (physician, surgeon, apothecary) diminished after the Medical Reform Act of 1858, which created a list of all licensed practitioners, new distinctions arose between provincials and their metropolitan colleagues, whose status as consultants and fellows of the professional societies were still supported by a liberal education.[25] Thus the author of an 1846 article in the *Dublin Medical Press*, referring to recently released statistics, decries the absence of bookshops in some areas of Ireland. He laments, "[T]here are many [towns] in which the medical practitioner can find neither book nor journal to enable him to keep his mind in a state of cultivation and his information equal to that of others more favourably circumstanced." The article examines "*medical bookselling*" separately," since "the fatal mental repose which the absence of literary food and stimulus induces extends to this department."[26]

Literary norms and strategies, even those of the devalued form of the novel, would have been familiar to most physicians as readers. Indeed, cases even late in the century testify to their continued influence. The physician Byrom Bramwell published as late as 1890 a "Case of So-called Perforating Tumour of the Skull" in which a large part of the history and examination are presented in dialogue with the patient's mother (the patient was a four-year-old boy). The boy presented with his left eye discolored and protruding from its orbit, and with an orange-sized lump on his head. Bramwell cross-examines the mother while instructing his students in the case.[27]

> DR. B. (to the patient's mother). How long is it since you noticed the lumps on the boy's head?
> PATIENT'S MOTHER. Three weeks yesterday.
> DR. B. How long has his eye been like that?
> PATIENT'S MOTHER. Six or seven weeks....
> DR. B. (to the Students). The head is large.
> PATIENT'S MOTHER. He always had a large head.
> DR. B. Did you notice anything wrong with his head before the lumps appeared?
> PATIENT'S MOTHER. No, there was nothing wrong with his head till three weeks ago.
> DR. B. Was he quite well till three weeks ago?
> PATIENT'S MOTHER. Yes. He was a strong healthy child. We noticed nothing the matter with him till three weeks ago. (250)

This interactive, inefficient manner of presenting the facts of the case is unusual, even in a book like this, reporting pedagogical lectures. In fact, dialogue had not been a normative part of medical representation since the eighteenth century, when it was derived from the philosophical genre of the Socratic dialogue. By 1890, when Bramwell is writing, a distanced, terse, third-person prose had long constituted the normative discourse of a medical case history. Educated and practicing in Edinburgh, a center of British medicine, Bramwell, who later was knighted for his contributions to medicine, was already a Fellow of the Royal College of Physicians of Edinburgh, an instructor of medical students at the Edinburgh Royal Infirmary, and the author of a textbook and other writings on medical diagnosis and "case-taking." His decision to present this case in dialogue is unlikely to follow from ignorance of the norms of medical representation.

Rather, this dialogue presents a striking pedagogical demonstration of how human emotion and error often obscure the true history of an individual case of disease, and how to elicit this history from a lay interlocutor. Further examination brings out what Bramwell calls "the confusion in the mother's statement" about the progress of the disease (250). He eventually ascertains that the boy's eye had become discolored six or seven weeks previously, he'd complained of headache a few weeks later, and then had become seriously ill with the appearance of the lumps. Bramwell's presentation in dialogue emphasizes the performative nature of the diagnostic process and cannot help but resonate with literary portrayals of the anxious, loving, ultimately helpless mother. Despite Bramwell's dispassionate reportage, her distress appears in her confusion over the dates, her denial of anything untoward about the child's swollen head ("He always had a large head"), and her insistence that he was a "strong, healthy child" despite evidence that he'd been sick for some months (in fact, the left eye had been more prominent since birth). As with many medical case histories that flirt with literary techniques, Bramwell's prose seems to tolerate the incursion of dialogue in part because this fatal case draws attention to the limits of medical knowledge and skill. It is this kind of fascinating juxtaposition of discourses that allows the genre of the case history to interrogate the development of "properly" literary and medical narratives.

As a result of this discursive hybridity, case histories can become porous to alternate methods of observation as well as representation. While the case above resists overt sentiment, a space for insight does sometimes open in Bramwell's cases when he comments on the human circumstances of his patients, as with this patient with aneurysm:

> This patient is very poor; he lives in lodgings with his wife; his rent is with difficulty paid; and yet he is not willing to come into hospital. He has not definitely told me so, but I suspect that his reason is this: he knows that

if he comes into hospital his house will be broken up, and his wife will have to go to the Workhouse. He wants, I suspect, to avoid that as long as possible. Now that is a plausible reason, and moreover, a reason which we can not only sympathise with, but also admire."[28]

The irony is strong here, for the patient will likely die without proper care. Although his professional knowledge argues that the patient is at risk outside the hospital, Bramwell voices his sympathy for him and his difficult choice. "I do not, under the circumstances, feel myself justified in pressing him too strongly to come into hospital," he concludes (119).

Bramwell's work suggests that, like many physicians, he cultivated an interest in the form and effect of medical representation. He sometimes notes the "beautiful" example a case presents of its particular diagnosis.[29] He is remarking, of course, on how perfectly these individual presentations exemplify the general type, but his choice of terms inevitably implies a kind of aesthetic of medical form. Bramwell also displays his awareness of literary concepts such as suspense and irony; he structures his cases to make the most of these. In one case, he tells the story of a servant girl who mysteriously died overnight, after a brief illness, and was thought to have been poisoned ("Stricture"). In the case of the impoverished young man, above, he describes the "peculiar and puzzling" pulse that the patient exhibited.[30] Using his skills, training, and tools, Bramwell takes on the role of medical detective in these cases, proving the servant girl to be suffering from perforated ulcer and the young man from aneurysm, distorting the true pulse sounds. He reports these histories in such a way that his readers must follow in his footsteps from perplexity and suspicion to certainty. He concludes by offering and confirming his diagnoses, bringing closure to these cases, with evidence provided by clinical technology (postmortem examination and the sphygmograph, respectively). Despite his reliance on clinical technology, the narrative structure of suspense and resolution promotes an appreciation of the physician's human insight as much as his clinical observation.

While these cases deftly manipulate a pattern of suspense and release familiar to readers of novels, another case displays Bramwell's acute sensitivity to irony. His "Remarkable Case of Euphoria" details the condition of a friend of his, an officer (physician) in the Indian Medical Service. This friend manages to remain cheerful and unaware of his fatal abdominal tumor even as it develops from "a small hard tumour about the size of an egg" to "a large tumour, fully the size of a child's head, of great hardness, and evidently malignant," one day before his death. Bramwell emphasizes both the irony and the unlikelihood of the situation, pointing out that "[b]oth the patient and his wife seemed amazed when the presence of the tumour was pointed out to them." "How it could possibly have escaped the attention of the patient, a most cultured and intelligent medical man, I am utterly unable to conceive," he continues, "for it was impossible to place the hand on the abdomen without at once recognizing the large tumour and its dense, hard character."[31] The irony here points to a human insight that drives this case history: the case is really not about the heavy tumor, which is unexceptional, but about this patient's "remarkable" evasion of the unbearable weight of his own mortality.[32]

Bramwell's subtitle for this collection identifies these cases as "some of the more interesting" ones in his experience. As I argue in the chapters to follow, it is not unusual for such curious cases to call forth a narrative that can escape the clinical norms set forth by nineteenth-century physicians. In fact, it is possible that the literary forms evoked here help to normalize or naturalize cases that otherwise disturb the case history—the narrative site of medical professionalism—particularly when these cases call attention to the boundedness of medical knowledge and practice.

The examples above open up numerous questions about the ways in which British novels and medical case histories share an interest in vision, representation, and genre, especially as the novel and the case history become professionalized over the course of the nineteenth century. The novels and cases I draw upon in this book testify to an influential rapprochement between these forms even while physicians were instructed to strive for a clinical discourse and novelists like George Eliot were chided for employing a "medical habit."[33] Furthermore, the novels and cases examined in this book demonstrate that, although professional literary and medical writing are conceived of as antipathetic, they are not infrequently combined and even used against the grain of their native ideology.

Complications of Discursive Hybridity

When novels import visual and representational norms from other disciplines, the resulting discursive hybridity complexly engages the ideologies underlying those norms. Thomas Hardy, in the short 1872 novel *Under the Greenwood Tree*, both deploys and ironizes a medical observation, in a scene of diagnosis early in the novel. This clinical way of seeing temporarily confers a discursive authority on Mr. Penny, the shoemaker, in a scene reminiscent of the demonstrations in a teaching hospital, where the physician instructor would lead the students through the basics of patient history, examination, and diagnosis. Hardy's shoemaker performs his clinical expertise on two telling, but unlikely, patients: a shoemaker's last and a boot, which—under his expert gaze—yield crucial information about the symptoms and traumas of their owners. "Now whose foot do ye suppose this last was made for?" he asks his audience of villagers rhetorically, before launching into a demonstration of what can only be deemed professional knowledge.

> "It was made for Geoffrey Day's father [Penny explains], over at Yalbury Wood. Ah, many's the pair o' boots he've had off the last! Well, when 'a died I used the last for Geoffrey, and have ever since, though a little doctoring was wanted to make it do. Yes, a very queer natured last it is now, 'a b'lieve," he continued, turning it over caressingly. "Now you notice that there"—(pointing to a lump of leather bradded to the toe), "that's a very bad bunion that he've had ever since 'a was a boy. Now this remarkable large piece" (pointing to a patch nailed to the side), "shows a' accident he received by the tread of a horse, that squashed his foot a'most to a pomace. The horseshoe came full-butt on this point you see."[34]

Penny offers here a particular kind of evaluation: a diagnosis. The shoe last is curious, "queer natured." It is symptomatic, with its bradded leather lump and nailed-on patch, of a history of pathology, whether the suffering be chronic and quotidian (the bunion) or extraordinary (horse accident). Penny expertly reads its symptoms, correlating each to its cause and commenting on the distinguishing marks in an almost pedagogical manner, with his audience circled around him respectfully, like medical students in an operating theater watching a surgeon discourse on a difficult case. The shoe last functions as a synecdoche for the foot and the patient; and Penny's dispassionate, informed gaze on it, his expert reading of its symptoms and their causes, confers a certain authority on him. As Peter Mere Latham explains to students, his role as a hospital lecturer is that of a "demonstrator of medical facts": "engaged to direct the student where to look for, and how to detect, the object which he ought to know; and, the object being known, to point out the value of it in itself and in all its relations." This is precisely what Penny does for his auditors.[35] A medical methodology is suggested throughout this scene by its atmosphere and tone, and in Hardy's specific word choices: by Penny's easy air of expertise and specialized knowledge of the trajectory of the lived-in body, his descriptive interest in physiological peculiarities marking that trajectory (a bunion, a "squashed" foot, and other "deformed" aspects of the body), and his activity in what Hardy terms "doctoring" and "operating" upon his subjects.

Medical observation and its authority are useful to Hardy because they enable the reading of less tangible realities, in an allegorical reading of character. When Penny turns to the boot of the new schoolmistress, Miss Fancy Day, his diagnostic gaze allows him to explicate the family "likeness between this boot and that last," between the "deformed" foot and the "pretty" one. The narrator, too, takes on this diagnostic mode of observation, in a delicate examination of character.

> There, between the cider-mug and the candle stood this interesting receptacle of the little unknown's foot—and a very pretty boot it was. A character, in fact—the flexible bend at the instep, the rounded localities of the small nestling toes—scratches from careless scampers now forgotten—all, as repeated in the tell-tale leather, evidencing a nature and a bias. (26)

Fancy may be at this point "the little unknown," but her character is both foreshadowed by her name and circumscribed by the ambivalent qualities evident in her boot: pretty, flexible, childlike, and "nestling"; "careless" or even thoughtless; energetic and not entirely demure (she "scampers"); and unreflective (her scampers are "now forgotten"). The boot is "light" of foot; not only nimble of foot but also, perhaps, footloose. Under the directed examination of the narrator, the boot reveals itself, and by extension its owner, as playful, unencumbered, easily influenced, and difficult to steady, perhaps even inconstant. The "tell-tale" leather records Fancy's "nature" and her "bias" as clearly as her father's shoe last reports on his hardworking life, although, as often occurred with physical symptoms in the era before germ theory, the definitive diagnosis must be deferred. The novel centrally pursues just this question of Fancy's possible lightness of character, asking its readers which of the two, Fancy or Geoffrey, is more truly "deformed." Hardy's novelistic process is founded upon, and requires of readers, this kind of diagnosis, in which disinterested, detailed observation of the world may ground a human insight into its reality.

Medical observation in the novel does not necessarily remain unchallenged. Not all Penny's listeners accept his diagnostic authority, although he asserts both its truth and its specificity to his informed experience. "To you, nothing," he modestly avers, "but 'tis father's voot and daughter's voot to me as plain as houses" (26). Penny's expert demonstration only momentarily allows him to assume that authority, and the suggestive diagnosis of Fancy is in question throughout the novel. However, Geoffrey's last and

Fancy's boot demonstrate the symbolic potential of medical practices in a narrative. They foreground questions of authority and expertise, observation and interpretation, even when they are ironized.

I do not mean to suggest that all instances of close examination in the novel should be understood as diagnostic readings. Hardy draws on a variety of descriptive modes to depict rural village life. He often sets the scene with recourse to a botanical vernacular, to use Amy King's term, as with the opening of the chapter "A Confession":[36]

> Fuchsias and dahlias were laden till eleven o'clock with small drops and dashes of water, changing the colour of their sparkle at every movement of the air; and elsewhere hanging on twigs like small silver fruit. The threads of garden-spiders appeared thick and polished. In the dry and sunny places dozens of long-legged crane-flies whizzed off the grass at every step the passer took. (128)

After this scene's record of natural history at high summer, Fancy is surrounded by early apples and butterflies, birds and hollyhocks, in a synecdochal enunciation of her bloom and a descriptive articulation of rural Wessex. This passage doesn't draw on clinical realism, but it helps establish the dominance of visual examination in the novel, and it works with clinical observation to ground and authenticate Hardy's imagined world.

Hardy's nuanced use of the trope of professional examination and diagnosis demonstrates how a novel's adaptation of medical discourse often resists simple reading. Even novels that adopt a clinical discourse do not spurn all affect or affect a disinterest in human character. On the contrary, as I will show, because the effect of genre differs depending on its context, novels often adopt a clinical discourse partially, momentarily, strategically. Esther Summerson's competent, experienced eye enables her to detail the symptoms of an ill-run household during her visit to the Jellybys in Dickens's *Bleak House:* the "tarnished" nameplate, "litter" in the rooms, "marshy" atmosphere, unkempt curtains, rumpled and torn stair-carpets, uncooked dinner, and above all the injured and filthy condition of little Peepy, who had fallen down the dark, ill-kept stairs and is superbly ignored by his mother (51, 52, 55). These symptoms would signify within the midcentury discourse on public health, or to any reader familiar with contemporary theories of domestic hygiene. However, Esther's enumeration does not register an emotional distance from the situation, as might be suggested by the act of diagnosis. Rather, it only intensifies her—and presumably the reader's—pity for Peepy. Ultimately, the focused, diagnostic, clinical detail of medical observation can be deployed to much greater range of effect in the more forgiving contexts of a novel than it can in a Victorian case history.

The "Case," Genre, Discipline, and Profession

The case is a peculiar genre, perched as it is—like the novel—between an individual and a more general knowledge. The modern "case," an anecdote or exemplar, collects details about an occurrence or person in order to come to some conclusion. The *Oxford English Dictionary* lists the earliest textual example in the 1400s, the "case of conscience," concerning theology and philosophy. The legal case appears in print in the 1500s; the medical case in the 1700s; and the police case in the 1800s. The philosophical case, like the curious medical cases of the eighteenth century, signifies the singular or the extreme, "the exception that proves the rule." An alternate tradition presents a case as typical or representative, an illustration of a general type.[37] Because it allows this mediation between the individual and the general, the phrase "a case of malaria" implies both a detailed narrative of an individual patient's unique history and the broader context of a disease type. It offers the interest of an anecdote within the rigor of a classificatory system. But the case attracts controversy, because it sits at the center of a debate over truth and disciplinary norms.

The authority of the case suffers from its association with casuistry, a method of ethical philosophy that argues through the individual case of conscience. The case seems to assert a general truth despite its basis on limited, individual experience, and because it deploys a possibly fictional narrative. Opponents of the case study argue that even if a case is true, it might not be relevant, representative, or significant.[38] Harvard Law School introduced the case method of instruction in the early 1870s to some debate, which also erupted when W. B. Cannon suggested in 1900 that American medical schools should also move to a case method.[39] Although the case lacks the authority of logic or the force of numbers, it strengthens an argument through its narrative appeal, which some critique as illogical and manipulative. This narrative force, with its ability to navigate between the individual and the universal, also makes it useful to novelists. Novels like Jane Austen's *Sense and Sensibility*, Wilkie Collins's *The Moonstone*, or Oscar Wilde's *The Picture of Dorian Gray* turn upon extended case histories.[40]

The narrativity of the case becomes explicit when it becomes a case history. In referencing "history," the case draws upon an ideal of linearity, of teleology, and of fact. The "true history" sets itself over and against the "romance" in the seventeenth and early eighteenth centuries;[41] it is in its role as "history" that the case dissembles its interest in the curious, that which is both anomalous and singular. Despite the changes in contemporary historiography, during the nineteenth century the narrative of "history" records the normative or symptomatic; anything else is "lost to history" or becomes myth. And the teleology of "history" narrates the destiny of the group—nation, clan, dynasty—rather than the individual. In the case history, the scope of history contracts to fit the singular fact.

This book will show that case histories work like novels or other genres: not monolithically, but realized through an accumulation of contingent instances. They adapt other genres or modes and develop in a historically specific cultural field in which other genres are also developing. Genre is inevitable but never sufficient; it cannot entirely direct its effects. If Frederic Jameson reads a text "as the coexistence, contradiction, structural hierarchy, or uneven development of a number of distinct narrative systems. . . . [as] a synchronic unity of structurally contradictory or heterogeneous elements, generic patterns and discourses," I am most interested in how a text works to manage, although not always contain, that heterogeneity in the interests of a particular knowledge and community.[42] I argue that genres allow authors to establish, as a normative frame, a discourse that may confer narrative and professional authority within their historical context—for nineteenth-century medicine, clinical discourse. However, to meet specific demands, their text may strategically incorporate or even discredit other discourses, as in sentimental medicine or Hardy's shoemaker scene. While Jameson argues that "genres are essentially literary *institutions,* or social contracts between a writer and a specific public, whose function is to specify the proper use of a particular cultural artifact" (106), genres also constitute disciplines as institutions. Beer argues that "genres establish their own conditions which alter the significance of ideas expressed within them."[43] Genres also attempt to establish their own readership, specifying the disciplinary codes that restrict what counts as knowledge; the difficulty of this task becomes especially clear in Freud.

Nineteenth-century novels and case histories are texts woven from diverse genres, each entailing particular professional and class benefits and disadvantages. Clinical scientific ideology and nineteenth-century literary criticism largely construe these genres as conflicting. Novels and cases must serve simultaneous discrete imperatives: the demand to show objectivity or transmit knowledge; a subjective demonstration of affect; a professional notion of rigor, value, or rectitude; and disciplinary notions of truth.

Disciplines name, access, and limit the cultural authorization of different kinds of knowledge. The archive, which Foucault calls "a complex volume, in which heterogeneous regions are differentiated or deployed, in accordance with specific rules and practices that cannot be superposed," gets revisioned when seen as a discipline: a cohesive and harmonious whole consistent with an internal logic and teleology.[44] Although, as he notes, the archive must "take account of statements in their dispersion, in all the flaws opened up by their noncoherence, in their overlapping and mutual replacement" (127), my project emphasizes instead how the end of "discipline" is order. Participants agree to ignore the dispersion and noncoherence of these constituent statements, condemn them as unruly, or read them as aligned in some crucial way with one another, to preserve the greatest possible sense of consistency, community, and common purpose. I do not examine unpublished case histories here; published narratives are more likely to project community norms of discourse. Discussions of professional methodology became especially acute just before and after midcentury for both medicine and the novel.[45] These often focus on techniques of visual observation (collection of knowledge) and representation (transmission of knowledge), two actions that ground generic distinctions in literary and medical narrative. In both, professional norms of seeing and stating help limit or control the relationship between author and audience, especially any "interested" visual and affective relation between text and reader.

Given the roots of "discipline" in teaching and discipleship, the concepts of history, lineage, and tradition anchor literature and medicine as disciplines, or knowledge projects, and the novel and the case history as disciplinary documents. Although few texts are generically "pure," the nineteenth-century case history faces a uniquely heterogeneous set of demands: it must produce both a fact and a story, represent both a disease and a person, display both the disinterested stance of the man of science and the physician's subjective insight. The struggle over disciplinarity is visible within the case history; it looks to literature even as it asserts medicine as an autonomous, scientific practice.

Debates over the pressures of science and professionalism markedly shape nineteenth-century medicine.[46] Before the Medical Act of 1858, the three branches of medicine (physicians, surgeons, apothecaries) were presided over by the London-based corporations.[47] Victorian physicians' membership in the traditional professions (Navy, the Church, law, and medicine) was transformed by the development of a broader, bourgeois professionalism. Despite the growing dominance of ideals of clinical medicine, Victorian physicians gained more cultural capital from their classical, liberal education than their scientific training. Even hospital consultants resisted privileging science over a classical (Oxbridge) education, good character, and experience.[48] M. Jeanne Peterson notes that "medical men themselves...shared with their lay patients...a belief in the superior virtues of liberal learning and gentlemanliness and the inferiority of technical training and skill. The struggle for the authoritativeness of medical knowledge had to be waged not only in the public arena but within the doctors themselves." Medical students did not have to pass a preliminary exam on physics, chemistry, and biology until the 1880s.[49]

This book focuses on the broad trends in nineteenth-century British medicine, at first toward increased visual discipline and textual restriction, then toward a freer, more speculative inquiry. But at every point many physicians resisted the dominant mode of inquiry (the hegemonic discourse, if you will), and others strayed ahead toward an emerging one. Even later in the century, some physicians declared that clinical practices destroyed the "art" of medicine; others, such as antivivisectionist physicians, accepted clinical medicine but decried experimental science.[50] Other physicians might "routinely invoke science as the foundation of medicine" but in practice emulate "the gentleman, broadly educated and soundly read in the classics."[51] Indeed, the *Lancet* endorsed polite letters by retaining "Literature" in its title until 1871; and in 1882 the Charter of the Royal College of Physicians—the most prestigious of the medical societies—listed as criteria to become a Fellow, "not only 'Professional Eminence' and 'Distinction in...Science' but also 'Distinction in Literature' and 'Social Position.'"[52] However, scientific professionalism offered other benefits: it allowed physicians to transform an occupation associated with messy bodies, personal service, and physical manipulation into one associated with precision, expertise, and rationality.

Nineteenth-century debates over "literature and science" indicate both the instability of disciplinary boundaries and their growing importance in regulating modern culture.[53] The Romantic era marked the "beginning of an anxiety" over disciplinary difference, with William Blake's fiery criticisms of Isaac Newton.[54] By the end of the century, T. H. Huxley's defense of science education met Matthew Arnold's refusal to acknowledge the educational value of science.[55] And Freud highlights the rigor of his prose to claim the status of the "man of science" instead of the "man of letters." Twentieth-century critics replayed both the debate and the divide. C. P. Snow's "two cultures" prompted F. R. Leavis's fierce defense of "literary intellectuals" against the increasing cultural authority of science.[56] The discussion erupted into controversy again with the science wars of the 1990s, contesting the authority of literary and cultural critics to examine scientific practice.

In the novel, disciplinary exchange is more easily tolerated, even after Blake and Coleridge had established and defended literature's purpose as an aesthetic, rather than simply moral, instructive, or pleasurable, text. The permeable discursive borders of the novel can embrace even irregular medicine. Dickens could reanimate the old medical controversy of human spontaneous combustion, in *Bleak House,* garnering scorn from G. H. Lewes, and George Eliot could explore animal magnetism in an experiment like *The Lifted Veil.* Many writers also drew on the sciences of the mind and body; novelists from Godwin, Austen, and Charlotte Brontë, through Walter Scott, to Stevenson and Du Maurier applied or anticipated medical theories of melancholy, hysteria, amnesia, paranoia, and the subconscious.[57] Nicholas Dames shows how the very theory of the Victorian novel develops from contemporary physiology.[58]

Why the Case History?

With the rich and variegated territory of the Victorian novel spread out like an intriguing landscape, why would any critic spend time pursuing a little-known genre like the case history? Reading novels and case histories against one another interrogates the history of the novel; it opens a new view onto Victorian culture; and it allows us to trace how disciplines develop in and through texts. The rich genre of the medical case history—which boasts an extensive, though little-known, archive—illuminates the history and context of the British novel in several ways. First, the novel borrows from the case history. Critics have identified various prose genres as models for the novel, but the medical case history remains a rich resource that too few readers consider.[59] Some early prose genres that critics have discussed include the newspaper, travel narrative, captivity narrative, spiritual autobiography, conduct book, and anthology.[60] The case history provides another compelling example of a developing narrative model. It illustrates how authors can construct genre and disciplinarity as difference, even while strategically deploying a heterogeneous text; and it offers a model of narrative in which fictional status and the attempt to represent historicity are crucial to the authority of the text.

Second, the case history foregrounds its status as a text, even a literary text, by sharing literary strategies with the novel. Medical authors develop a genre of the case history through a disciplinary anxiety arising from their incorporation of medical observations into a record shaped by the conventions of narrative. But Victorian physicians defined themselves as readers—"men of letters." Writing in and reading elite periodicals, living among and socializing with their literate peers, they were likely to be familiar with norms of the contemporary novel even if they were not themselves novel-readers. Their notions of narrative were accordingly likely to be informed by developments in the British novel.

Third, the case history shares one of the novel's major concerns: how to narrativize the self. If the novel is a textual mechanism for producing subjectivity, the case history similarly constructs the modern subject. Of course, the case history, by combining previous history, patient autobiography, and chronicle of observation, helps to constitute not a fictional but a real historical subject. But by corralling the experience of the body within particular categories of the self, the case history provides an alternative narrative structure that makes available the model of a coherent subjectivity accumulated through experience.

Finally, the formal and generic evolution of the case history roughly tracks, and illuminates, that of the novel. Like the novel, the case history traces a path from a curious sensibility of the eighteenth-century case history, through the realism of the clinical era, dedicated to the precise rendition of surfaces, and finally blossoms inward with Freud. And like the novel, the case history demonstrates two disjunct strands in its realist and romantic discursive traditions, with authors and contemporary critics defending one against the other in an oppositional model of genre. The tremendous archive of the case history, still relatively unexplored, offers a vast textual resource to critics of the novel.

The genre of the case history also localizes some of the most contentious questions shaping Victorian society. With the rapid developments in scientific knowledge and methodologies, some of the period's most prominent cultural critics mounted debates over the proper role of science in culture, a concern that underlay narrative choices in many nineteenth-century novels and case histories. Novelists from Dickens and Collins to Eliot and Hardy articulate a struggle to find the proper relationship of science to art. The medical case history usefully focuses nineteenth-century debates over the nature of truth, from the discussions of a mechanical objectivity common to realist novels and medical texts, to the question of distinct modes of truth, as when Gaskell reminds us that the novel, medicine, and religion differently consider the bodily transformation we call death.

The case history also allows us to study the Victorian period's particular interest in visuality, characterized, as critics like Jonathan Crary and Kate Flint have shown, by remarkable changes in aesthetic theory, in art itself, and in how visual images are narrativized in texts. Medical narratives channel and magnify this "visual turn." Physiologists debated the mechanism of perception, complicating simple tropes of vision. Medical instruments offered new possibilities for extending sight and for representing information visually, with not just the new achromatic microscope, but also instruments like the sphygmograph, which could graph the body's rhythms, rendering them visible for the first time. Visual "figures" like graphs and tables functioned magically in medical narratives by signifying rational, scientific work even as they allowed a continued focus on curious bodies.

The case history also illuminates the history of periodical publishing, as medical cases gradually disappear from general-circulation periodicals, like the *Gentleman's Quarterly*, to surface in new professional medical journals. In Thomas Wakley's reformist *Lancet*, "the case" enables the development of forensic medicine, paralleling the rise in juridical discourse during this period. Like the lurid police "Case-Book Fiction" of the 1850s and 1860s, forensic medical cases help introduce new literary genres like detective and sensation fiction. The links between police and forensic medical cases, both precursors of detective fiction, become especially clear in novels like Collins's *The Moonstone*. With the midcentury drive toward standardizing and professionalizing the case history, the new status of the case history as an analytic tool made it an important narrative model (and in novels, a trope) for the diagnosis of ills in what Poovey has termed the Victorian "social body."

The case history obviously tracks the rise of professionalism in the Victorian period. Science moves away from the natural history model of the amateur toward a centralized model of specialization and expertise. This trend affects medical authorship and authority, and the development of specialized journals.[61] In the early 1830s England of *Middlemarch*, the science of a Parisian-trained Lydgate can collaborate with that of the vicar Farebrother, whereas at midcentury, a self-trained scientist and popularizer like George Henry Lewes must work hard to become a respected member of the physiological community.

Rapid industrialization also becomes focalized in the rich archive of the case history, which increasingly details railway and factory accidents. Case histories in occupational medicine allow labor to define the body in new ways and revisit the vexed questions of class and environment. Old concerns about the decadent rich and the "criminal" poor gained scientific status with the use of statistics. The case also grounds public health initiatives once investigators like John Snow began tracking clusters of cases to understand the geography and, eventually, the etiology of diseases like cholera. The phenomenon of public health, and its incorporation into novels like *Sybil*, suggests that when narrative turns the attention from the individual to the aggregate, the narrator's voice negotiates a new kind of authority.

The case history is especially useful for studies of developing notions of gender and sexuality in the Victorian period. From debates over man-midwives and chloroform for childbirth, to nursing reports from the Crimean War, and from Weir Mitchell's hysterics to Havelock Ellis's inverts, the case history offers a newly authoritative unit of knowledge from which Victorians may build certainty in contested questions of gender and sexual identity. The work of Martha Stoddard Holmes demonstrates how usefully medical narrative testifies to Victorian cultures of disability as well.

Finally, Victorian case histories also allow us to track developments in fields that deserve focused investigation but range largely beyond the scope of this book. The case history also mediates vexing questions of empire by providing a textual site for medicalizing racial and cultural differences. And case histories chronicle the birth of a professional imperial medicine. Here a narrative structure native to British bourgeois professionalism attempts to tame a florid tropical environment and contain what was perceived as a foreign threat to the vulnerable, expanding British national body, whether domestically (as in cholera) or overseas (as in remittent fever). Overall, the case history, as a genre, offered Victorian novelists a powerful narrative instrument for the analysis and management of their world. Individual case histories, read closely and as a corollary to novels, help clarify some of the most significant questions agitating British Victorian culture.

Many scholars of literature and medicine focus on medical scenes in literary texts, reflecting the persistent perception that medical narratives are, as they claim to be, strictly functional. Critics who do acknowledge the importance of narrative in medicine often identify with the field of "narrative medicine," a pragmatic pedagogical or reformist project to improve the practice of medicine. Work in these fields, while valuable, can rely upon a notion of the text as a simple reproduction of reality that broadens the physician-reader's humane understanding of individual suffering. The value of reading would be its ability to prompt a vicarious experience of sickness through an illness narrative that reliably communicates the subjectivity of the patient. This practice draws upon a universalizing model of textuality, and it relegates literary texts to a strictly instrumentalist function. Because cultural studies of medicine is grounded in the history and theory of the novel and of medicine, it can more flexibly appreciate the historically contingent relation of writers to the larger culture. However, this approach does not always recognize the specificity of the text and its language. My work argues that the cultural studies of medicine should sustain a close formal reading of the text and a sensitivity to its language as well as its culture. This book pursues a rigorous analysis of textuality in order to illuminate how both form and culture shape the history of disciplines.

The chapters of this book lay out a general, but not necessarily chronological, cultural history of "the case history and the novel." My first two chapters briefly chart the historical shift from the eighteenth-century case history, which negotiates between the curious observations of the "New Science" and some less-admissible curious sights, to the nineteenth-century case history, which valorizes mechanical observation recorded with a clinical realism. Chapter 2 examines the growth of restrictions on clinical seeing and stating, with the development of mechanical observation; and demonstrates how lay Victorian readers and writers could share a discussion of clinical medical norms through their performance in the "literary commons" created by Victorian periodicals.

The following three chapters examine what happens to the restrictive ideal of mechanical observation as it is intensified, revised, and supplemented by literary and medical writers. These chapters track the complex relation between novel writing and case history writing during the mid-century surge of the Victorian novel. I examine the subversion of clinical observation by sentiment in Dickens and Gaskell and in medical cases; the reorientation of mechanical observation toward sympathy in George Eliot's early fiction; and the freeing of the speculative gaze in experimental medicine as well as in Eliot's later novel *Middlemarch*. I map the circulation of modes of vision and representation between disciplines and the genres that help to constitute them. These chapters argue for the traffic between disciplines of a shared constellation of visual and textual methodologies, which are always revised in use to align more completely with particular disciplinary aims.

The final chapter turns to Freud to understand what happens to the story of the case history in its relationship with the novel. As Freud explores, reads, and maps the knotted mind of the patient, his imperial romance does not disguise its debt to literary modes, however vexed that debt may be for Freud himself. It is at this point that, while novels may strategically tap various stages of clinical realism for its cultural authority and effect of precision and accuracy, medicine itself turns decisively away from the novel and its insights and rededicates the case history to clinical observation and the clinical voice.

CHAPTER ONE

Curious Observations, Curious Sights

The Eighteenth-Century Case History

In 1688 the Irish scientist William Molyneux proposed a question, quoted by John Locke six years later:

> Suppose a man born blind, and now adult, and taught by his touch to distinguish between a cube, and a sphere of the same metal, and nighly of the same bigness, so as to tell, when he felt one and t'other, which is the cube, which the sphere. Suppose then the cube and sphere placed on a table, and the blind man to be made to see. Quære, whether by his sight, before he touched them, he could now distinguish, and tell, which is the globe, which the cube.[1]

Locke and Molyneux agree that the answer to Molyneux's question was "no," and William Cheselden answers the question definitively in 1728 after restoring a boy's sight: "When he first saw, he ... thought no Objects so agreeable as those which were smooth and regular, tho' he could form no Judgment of their Shape."[2] Cheselden, a Fellow of the Royal College of Surgeons in England, published "An Account of some Observations made by a young Gentleman, who was born blind," after he had couched the eyes, removing the cataracts and incising the pupils to reopen them. He is clearly interested in Molyneux's famous philosophical question, focusing his report on the boy's need to learn or relearn color, shape, and distance.

The boy's "Observations" are foregrounded in the title, but the information he offers is disciplined by mediation through Cheselden's membership in the Royal Society for the Promotion of Natural Knowledge. This organization had been founded in 1660 to promote the "natural philosophy" or "experimental philosophy" inspired by Francis Bacon. The society developed an experimental methodology that helped shape the development of medicine and its narratives.[3]

Cheselden's case models many important aspects of experimentalist narratives. It is a curious case, foregrounding what is most unusual or striking about its subject. It combines the dispassionate "curious observation" of the experimental philosopher and the enthusiastic "curious sight" of the onlooker. It combines experimentalist and literary, even romantic narrative elements. And it demonstrates the attention early scientists gave to vision and visuality. By separating seeing from stating and knowing, it denaturalizes and inspects the process of vision itself, even as it acknowledges that its own knowledge practice, experimental philosophy, builds on a visual economy.

The historians Steven Shapin and Simon Schaffer, examining Robert Boyle's air-pump experiments, argue that the unit of knowledge for experimental philosophers was the "matter of fact" established through witnesses, the more the better.[4] The members of the Royal Society sought to multiply witnesses by meeting to observe each others' experiments; by publishing directions on how others might reproduce an experiment; and by publishing experimental reports in their journal *Philosophical Transactions of the Royal Society*. These could attract almost unlimited "virtual witnesses" by recording—that is, replicating—an experiment in print (60). For experimentalists, seeing and stating were linked and necessary stages of knowledge production.

Boyle considered how several rhetorical strategies could authenticate a textual replication of experiment, by presenting himself and his aims as modest; dissociating himself from rationalist philosophical "systems"; adopting a "functional" rather than "florid" prose style; speaking with confidence; and avoiding unnecessary citations of authorities. These strategies all help to certify the investigator's disinterested stance, one of the few guarantors of authority in the New Science.[5]

Thus in experimentalist medicine, narrative becomes crucial to producing and authorizing knowledge. It guarantees the production of the "matter of fact" by certifying the disinterestedness of the observer who writes, and the reliability and efficient utility of the text. Cheselden's narrative clearly references these norms. He pairs his case history with a detailed, disinterested "Explication" with a diagram of the surgical procedure.[6] The "Explication" foregrounds the plain speech and dispassionate stance that experimentalists prized.

In his "Account," however, Cheselden also turns to narrative strategies that would drive the powerful tradition of the novel. That is, he employs two different narratives that construct knowledge through vision: an experimentalist narrative deriving a disciplined knowledge out of a curious but distanced observation; and an affective narrative emphasizing the visual attraction of the boy as a "curious sight" and eliciting a subjective, empathetic understanding through the visual circulation of sensibility. These two strands of discourse in Cheselden's text align with the interpenetration of realist and romantic narrative vision in the eighteenth-century medical case history.

The complex imbrication of these narrative strands provokes later physicians' reaction against curious medicine. Nineteenth-century physicians narrowed the range of acceptable methods of seeing and stating. For them, "curious sight" and indeed even "curious observation" irreparably undercut empiricist methods of "clinical observation"; while romantic narratives soliciting an affective response were inappropriate for a clinical-realist representation. However, as later chapters will show, the nineteenth-century clinical case history cannot entirely eradicate curious medicine.

Plain Speech and Curious Discourse

The eighteenth-century case history is a disciplinary document. It establishes its authority and announces its membership in a broader medical community by foregrounding education and training, fellowship and patronage; by strategically deploying Latin as the language of learning; and by referencing other physicians.[7] Robert Whytt, in a 1767 treatise on hysteria, distinguishes himself as "M.D.[,] F.R.S.[,] Late Physician to his Majesty, President of the Royal College of Physicians, and Professor of Medicine in the University of Edinburgh." The letters and titles after an author's name proclaimed his training and certified his membership in the community of experimentalists; this practice continued into the nineteenth century. But medical reputations also relied on the favor of influential patients. Thus eighteenth-century prefaces strategically express gratitude to powerful benefactors, as when George Cheyne dedicates his *English*

Malady to Lord Bateman. Earlier physicians had augmented their image as well educated by writing in Latin, the language of scholarship and of the classical education that still dominated medical training. While Latin disappeared from the case-historical narrative during the eighteenth century as part of the drive toward a vernacular "plain speech," it remained in texts dealing with sexuality or other delicate matters. Latin helped constitute a medical community by implicitly differentiating lay or popular medicine and its readers from a properly medical text and its imagined readers, although in fact it excluded only those who could not read Latin: women, children, and the lower classes.[8] When nineteenth-century physicians formalized other textual indicators of professionalism, Latin disappeared from the case history, except in naming anatomy and disease.

Eighteenth-century case authors also invoked a medical community by frequently referring to other physicians. They often cited earlier authorities, drawing upon experience gained vicariously through reading. William Pargeter explains, "[I]f it was necessary, authorities upon authorities, both ancient and modern, might be cited, proving the efficacy of *friction,* as a deobstruent, &c. in all chronical complaints," and he references both Hippocrates and Galen. Some "authorities" were contemporaries; Cheyne references his colleagues Drs. Baynard, Taylor, and Cranstoun (whose letter of recommendation Cheyne reprints). And John Monro writes his 1758 *Remarks* in specific response to William Battie's *Treatise on Madness.*[9] Even when physicians disagree, the reference codifies their joint membership in a medical fraternity, despite differences in training, knowledge, theory, and practice.

Some physicians signaled their presence within the larger context of the New Science by adopting the epistemological and rhetorical strictures of the Royal Society. Although physicians associated with the New Science would be leery of the theories of ancient authorities, they do cite cases published by other physicians, an acceptable form of virtual witnessing.

Eighteenth-century physicians' central narrative strategy—the guarantor of their disinterested stance—is the Royal Society's principle of "plain speech." Experimentalists opposed "Rhetorick," a language of excess which is formally superfluous; untrue in that it is fanciful, fictional, dramatic, or insincere; and designed to elicit a subjective response or aesthetic pleasure.[10] This rejection of "Rhetorick" ironically subverts the society's stated focus. At first, the society—its motto *"Nullius in verba"* ("On no man's word") announcing their disdain for words—had resolved not to waste time on matters of language. Robert Hooke marked it out of bounds, since "[t]he business and design of the Royal Society is—To improve the knowledge of natural things, and all useful Arts, Manufactures, Mechanick practices, Engynes and Inventions by Experiments—(not meddling with Divinity, Metaphysics, Moralls, Politicks, Grammer, Rhetorick, or Logick)."[11] However, the society's members in fact worried frequently about the effects of language—especially an excess of language—on the "matter of fact." Hooke's statutes warn, "In all Reports of Experiments ... the Matter of Fact shall be barely stated, without any Prefaces, Apologies, or Rhetorical Flourishes."[12] Royal Society apologist Thomas Sprat similarly defines experimentalist discourse as an exclusion of linguistic excess. He warns that "the luxury and redundance of *speech* ... this superfluity of talking" threatens the society's collegial undertaking of experiments. "The only Remedy," he explains, "that can be found for this *extravagance*" is

> constant Resolution, to reject all the amplifications, digressions, and swellings of style: to return back to the primitive purity, and shortness, when men deliver'd so many *things*, almost in an equal number of *words*.... a close, naked, natural way of speaking; positive expressions; clear senses; a native easiness; bringing all things as near the Mathematical plainness, as they can: and preferring the language of Artizans, Countrymen, and Merchants, before that, of Wits, or Scholars.[13]

Sprat here discusses a rhetorical project—the eradication of "style"—powered by the dream of an originary language, one which in its "primitive purity" and "native easiness" shrugs off the cloak of a corrupting civilization to reveal the "naked, natural" truth. The Royal Society thus proselytized for a language marked only by its "Mathematical plainness," a linguistic style devoid of style, even of noticeable learning, in hopes of attaining a materialist empiricism that could collapse the gap between sign and signifier, word and thing.[14] This ideal of plain speech imagines a purely *functional* language, although functionalism itself is an aesthetic choice. These prohibitions of "style" do constitute a rhetoric—an empiricist rhetoric of opposition to "Rhetorick."[15] Despite Hooke's original suggestion that the society avoid "meddling with ... Grammer" or "Rhetorick," the ideal of plain speech became a cornerstone of experimentalist ideology, which in turn became central to British medicine. Thus, eighteenth-century physicians would strive to establish that—as one case history of "a bullet voided by urine" states—"This is the plain relation of the matter of fact."[16]

However, eighteenth-century physicians also employed what I call a curious discourse. In contrast to plain speech, this aims to recruit readers' interest in the case; it often appears in titles. It highlights a rhetoric of extremity, asserting the rarity, value, secrecy, difficulty, or oddity of the phenomenon under study. It typically uses an extravagant, exaggerated rhetoric, with exclamations of affective interest that punctuate the narrator's process of discovery. It may also use suspense and dramatic irony, delaying the moment of revelation and response and heightening narrative tension. It thus enrolls its audience by suturing the reader's interest with that of the narrator, demonstrating how an object elicits an observer's curiosity. A curious discourse is therefore as much about the narrator as a "subject," his subjective response, as it is about the natural "subject" of his investigation. Moreover, it implies fictitiousness by calling upon "Rhetorick." Lorraine Daston and Katherine Park suggest that one characteristic of the curious itself is its refusal of functionality, its affinity for superfluity.[17] Curious discourse, too, indulges superfluity in its excessive language; its focus on oddities reveals its fancifulness; and its affective expostulations speak to its subjective interest. In its affinity with these qualities of "Rhetorick," then, curious discourse vexes a strictly experimentalist narrative. Its extravagant lines solicit "interest" in a narrative that can be characterized as exoticizing, sentimental, sensational, or Gothic; that is, romantic.

The pressure toward plain speech in medicine continued through the eighteenth century but was never entirely successful, so that John Ferriar can complain in 1795 when "new applications of words are introduced, which, though desirable in the art of poetry, are very inconvenient in pathological books ... for between the ancient language, which practitioners cannot entirely reject, and the new dialect, which they cannot wholly adopt, the style of medical books is reduced to a kind of jargon ... which his readers find it very difficult to unriddle" (viii–ix). Indeed, the case history in this period works hard to reconcile the disinterested plain speech authorizing the experimentalists' work with the curious, fanciful "Rhetorick" they disdained.

Curious Observation

Despite the importance of narrative form in constituting the genre of the case history, physicians' experimentalism also grounds it in an empirical emphasis on perception, especially visual perception.[18] It is no accident that experimentalist treatises so often were titled "Observations on" their subject. The case history offers three possible narratives of the visual. The physician's curious but disinterested observation forms the first model of vision, one which proves nearly impossible to sustain consistently, if published cases are a reliable source. Eighteenth-century physicians were also encouraged to develop their human insight into patients' ailments, concomitant with their role as men of culture, judgment, and sensibility. Finally, the exotic, sentimental, sensational, or Gothic details of a curious case can prompt the affective charge of curious sight, placing the physician and reader in the role of a stealthy voyeur or vulgar (common) spectator.[19] Of these three narrative models, only the first two are authorized and authorizing in the experimentalist context; however, curious sight also suffuses the eighteenth-century case history.

The experimentalist project centered on "curious" matter, which includes the physiologically singular—the "monstrous"—as well as the psychologically odd. It comprises a number of other peculiarities as well, not all of them medical: the rare, the ornate, the exotic, the valuable, and the sexual. It marks off the secret, the unknown, or the unexplainable. Finally, it both expresses and solicits the subjective response of the observer and the reader. As Daston and Park have argued, unknown or curious phenomena were considered the proper matter of science in the early modern period. Although, they argue, the early eighteenth century "banished marvels" by valorizing skepticism over wonder (350), historians have shown that odd phenomena in fact remained central to eighteenth-century science and medicine.[20] Because the establishment of the "matter of fact" depended upon its dissemination in print, tales of the curious regularly appeared in the journals of the new experimentalist societies, building a convention of the curious within these texts.[21] The *Philosophical Transactions of the Royal Society*, for example, includes accounts of "An Extraordinary Rainbow," "A small Egg within another," "a Double Pear," and "a Shower of Fishes."[22]

Physicians also privileged investigation into what was unknown. The *Philosophical Transactions* regularly reported the unusual size or placement of a tumor, "polypus" (polyp), or stone; a patient's extraordinary size, shape, or physical ability; a birth through the anus or navel; and other unexpected physical findings. When Dr. Molineux says, "Among the many secret workings of Nature, none seems more to deserve our Observation, than the rise and progress of Epidemick Distempers," he implies that the experimentalist physician's task is to discern what is secret.[23] Cheyne also demonstrates the focus on what is strange when he notes that he "was obliged to lay aside all those whose Cases were pretty much alike, and to pick out such only, as seem'd to me to be more particular, or which were most proper . . . to direct the *Valetudinarian*, in the less obvious and uncommon Symptoms."[24]

Thus, although eighteenth-century cases do not necessarily focus on curious phenomena, experimentalist medicine does gravitate toward the secret, the strange, and the estranging.

In fact, Michael McKeon has argued for the formulation "strange, therefore true" as a guiding principle of early modern science. "The fact of 'strangeness' or 'newness,'" he points out, "ceases...to be a liability to empirical truth-telling, and becomes instead an attestation in its support."[25] Experimentalist medicine is thus centrally concerned with the unknown despite, or perhaps because of, the ever-present risk (or promise) of deception.[26]

A curious observation is close, careful, and intricate. Thus, as Starkey Myddelton says in reporting an extrauterine pregnancy, "I was not very curious in my Examination" until the unusual nature of the case became apparent.[27] Pargeter notes, "There is a very curious and just observation of Dr. [Richard] *Mead's*, which he illustrates with two cases...[which] are very remarkable." As this suggests, "curious" observations can readily be "just."

Sensibility and Insight

Eighteenth-century physicians, unlike pure experimentalists, could draw upon another visual stance besides curious observation. When a case excites a subjective response that might prompt Rhetorick and endanger the physician's authority, the narrator often recasts that response as insight—an individual sensitivity to the patient's condition, enhancing medical judgment—not unlike sensibility in the eighteenth-century novel.[28] For example, Misomedon, a patient in Bernard Mandeville's *Treatise of the Hypochondriack and Hysterick Diseases* (1730), asks if he has "tired" the physician Philopirio after telling "so tedious a Tale" of his illness. But Philopirio reassures him. "Your Story is so diverting," he says, "that I take abundance of delight in it, and your Ingenious way of telling it, gives me a greater insight into your Distemper, than you imagine."[29] Philopirio defuses his admission of "delight" in two ways. First, he deftly positions the "diverting" tale as symptomatic of the illness, in contrast to his own presumably disinterested narrative. And second, he couches his "delight" as a specifically medical "insight." Such insight was central to the physician's task; Cheyne attacks "systematick Writers in Physick" for lacking "the Perspicuity and natural Way of convincing the ingenious, sickly, and tender Sufferers, so necessary to make them chearfully and readily undergo such severe Restraints."[30]

Sensibility as medical insight persists throughout the eighteenth century. In 1792 Pargeter paints a picture of the ideal physician as not only "well acquainted with the *pathology* of the disease" but also "possess[ing] great acumen—a discerning and penetrating eye—much humanity and courtesy."[31] Clearly the context of medicine, with its human subjects, required the physician to own subjective responses, but the larger context of experimentalist science required that they be functional. As later chapters will show, nineteenth-century clinical medicine, especially the theory of mechanical observation, would go further and demand an utterly disinterested gaze; but many Victorian physicians made room for human sensibility in their practice, whether in a high-minded sentimental gaze, or in a judiciously acknowledged speculative insight.

Curious Sight

The curious case can complicate the physician's disinterested stance by emphasizing the degree of his affective interest. Other terms which substitute for "curious" in the eighteenth century—"wondrous," "remarkable," "surprising"—likewise foreground a strong emotion: the "wonder," "remark," and "surprise" evoked in the physician-observer by his object of study. The emotions roused by "the curious" range from amazement to ridicule, disgust to desire. If establishing a matter of fact rests upon the disinterested stance of the observer, curiosity undercuts it with a subjectivity born of the most exaggerated "interest." Amazement in the researcher endangers the experimentalist project. It might induce him to exaggerate what he sees; overlook fraud; or naïvely accept a suspicious phenomenon. In 1742 Benjamin Boddington worries, in the case of a young woman who eats, speaks, and sings perfectly without a tongue, that "many who shall hear this account will ... think he and his friends are all mistaken [in their observations] ... and that their ignorance is the only ground of their admiration."[32] The curious case thus testifies to the physician's intellectual quest but also displays and seeks to create an excessive interest. That interest emerges when the experimentalist "curious observation" shifts toward a "curious sight."

Although the term "curious observation" recurs frequently in the *Philosophical Transactions,* its ostensible synonym, "curious sight," occurs only rarely. It can be used as a synonym for observation, as in these remarks made by "Mr. C":

> In some Water which I took out of a Pit, I found a small *Water-Newte*, not an inch long.... This I kept by me (in lieu of Tadpoles) to shew the Circulation of the Blood in its Tayl. But that was not the only entertainment it gave me; for I found the course of the Blood in every part of its Body, and particularly in every digit of the Feet, it was a curious sight to observe the Stream come to the Extremity of the Toe in one Channel, and return by another.[33]

Here, curious sight and its "entertainment" remain entirely within the bounds of experimental practice.

However, a "curious sight" is more common in other contexts—in literature, popular works of instruction, or pornography—which is why I use this term to denote the onlooker's more interested visual stance. Here, the act of seeing is no longer confined to experimental investigation, but it peers into an undisciplined space, either a private (voyeuristic) or public (spectacular). The phrase a "curious sight" is useful because of its shifting valence, like the shifting focus and the circulation of affect in eighteenth-century medicine. In one instance of a "curious sight," the physician's gaze shows a curiosity beyond a dutiful attention; in another, the patient becomes a curiosity. In either case, the observer shifts away from the discipline that constitutes "seeing" as the proper and necessary, disinterested approach to knowing, and toward "seeing" as an approach to affective exchange instead.

Curious sight thus troubles the visual logic grounding the physician's observation of the patient in the eighteenth-century case history. An experimentalist's proper role can include a more private, even intimate investigation, as in Abraham Cowley's poem "To the Royal Society," where he compliments the experimentalists, "Y'have taught the curious sight to press / into the privatest recess / of [Nature's] imperceptible littleness!" But this curious sight, as Cowley's poem suggests, proves a delicate negotiation, especially in medicine. Even a common medical case history invades an intimate space, acknowledging and defying the borders of privacy. In a century intoxicated with the new pleasures of domestic privacy, the physician's advance into the bedchamber becomes a sign of medical privilege. And if, as Ian Watt argues, this period defined "virtue" primarily in sexual terms, as a determination to uphold the privacy of the body, then the physician's venture into that space must be carefully negotiated.[34] Like the novel, the case history chronicles an essentially private experience, limning the details of domestic life—sleep, food, sex—and how they mark the body. In eighteenth-century case histories, the physician usually appears in the

CHAPTER ONE

text, allowing the reader to identify with his privileged view of an often intimate scene. The case history's printed, first-person narration duplicates what Watt called "[Samuel] Richardson's 'keyhole view of life,'" suturing the reader's to the physician's curious eye (200).

Another danger of a curious case is its potential, as a secular marvel no longer carrying the elevating effect of traditional spiritual meaning, to slip into vulgar spectacle when the spectators are many. This changes the meaning of both the case and its observers, as in Stafford's discussion of "an untapped scientific literature wrestling with virtuoso dexterity, on one hand, and the master showman's compulsion for visualization and self-display on the other" (140). Mass spectatorship was actually encouraged. Sprat boasts that the Royal Society affirms only those matters of fact that "have the concurring Testimonies of *threescore or an hundred*" men (100). Thomas Dent's case of worms in the tongue demonstrates the importance of display and spectatorship. Having heard of "Worm-Doctresses," he visits a famous one at Leicester, Mrs. French, who

> picked out five or six Worms at a time, some of which I have here sent to you for your more Curious Observation. She plainly shewed them to the Spectators as they came out of the Flesh; they were all alive, and moved their Heads.... And to be short, though the Operation was very surprising, and so will (I suppose) seem to you Incredible, yet neither I, nor any one present could discover any Fallacy, but all the plain dealing that Ocular Demonstration can admit of to prove the reality of the Operation....[35]

Here the spectators are respectable witnesses, "two Aldermen of the Town, Mr. Gibbs, my Lord of Derby's Chaplain, and several others," standing in for the experimentalist readership (220). Both the physical and virtual witnesses employ a "Curious Observation" in examining Dent's unusual case of worms.

But many of the cases examined by the experimentalists involve spectacular exhibitions in which the audience is not carefully chosen. The elision between disciplined demonstration and public spectacle threatens to collapse the distinction between a dispassionate gaze and a vulgar interest.[36] Thus James Parsons, discussing a "Friench [*sic*] girl, now shewn at Ludgate as an hermaphrodite," writes to prevent "the generality of the world" from taking "the erroneous side of the question ... for want of having a proper knowledge of the parts." He explains that the girl is not a hermaphrodite, but that "[t]he *vagina* being ... cover'd, and the *clitoris* ... large, it is no great wonder, that she should at first sight be taken for a male by the vulgar: but it would seem a little too careless in any of the faculty to be so deceiv'd."[37] The distinction between "the vulgar" observers and "the faculty" requires not only prior knowledge but also properly curious (not "careless") observation.

While the experimentalist audience (real or virtual) is a necessary guarantor of authority, it must be distinguished from the gawking of the vulgar crowd. Examples of the spectacular line the pages of the *Philosophical Transactions* like sideshows at a fair, or like the "monsters" exhibited in public by "exhibitors" throughout the eighteenth century.[38] One account reports "A Negro Boy That is Dappel'd"; another a "White Negro Shewn Before the Royal Society." Another describes "the Posture-Master," a man who could disjoint his entire body. The skeptical audience and the vulgar crowd shared many objects and interests; the "uncommon Case of a Distempered Skin" known as the "porcupine man" had been exhibited as a popular attraction in London.[39] James Parsons compares the "White Negro" to a girl who had been "made a shew of" "about four years ago here in London." "I did not go to see her," Parsons concedes, "but I read an advertisement, concerning her, several times in the public papers, wherein she was called a white negro girl; and was informed by those that saw her, that she answered the description in the advertisement very truly. She was shewn in town for some months every day" (47). The experimentalist's curiosity is figured in these cases as little different from that of the viewer of a public spectacle. Parsons even cites the spectators, who are otherwise nobodies in the case, not the titled or influential witness usual in experimentalist cases. Ironically, the very "uncommon" quality of the curious case serves to attract a public audience, rendering it an experience "common" to all. A spectacular curiosity thus threatens to generate a dispersed rather than a specialized knowledge, and a commodified rather than disinterested "matter of fact." The spectacle, and the curious sight it inspires, should be set off from the project of experimentalism, but in fact they become undifferentiated.

The curious case can convert a respectable gathering of physician-witnesses, skeptically observing an experiment, into a pushing, shoving, curious crowd around a spectacle. The danger of precisely this kind of collapse of the experimentalist stance is demonstrated by a case published by J. Denis in the *Philosophical Transactions* of 1667 and cited repeatedly.[40] In what Pargeter calls "this most wonderful case," which he quotes "on account of its singularity," a young man disappointed in love goes mad and is cured by two transfusions of calf's blood into his veins (122, 117). Denis frames his case with an experimentalist's concern for accuracy and corroborating testimony, and little curious discourse. "I thought myself obliged," he says, "for the clearing up of what false rumours had darkened, to give you a faithful and exact account of the condition, to which this poor Man was reduced before the Transfusion; of what passed during that Operation; and the surprising effects that have followed upon it hitherto." Where he must describe the transfusion, he carefully reports the witnesses. "Many persons of quality were present," he notes, "together with several Physitians and Chirurgeons, too intelligent to suspect them of being capable of the least surprise."[41] Such narrative precautions were necessary, since, as Stafford notes, "Any fine art that purported to demonstrate something ... and any scientific experiment sustained by machinery—no matter how obvious the technique—was liable to the accusation of *trompe-l'oeil* and pandering to spectatorial desire" (134).

Denis's retrospective textual caution may reflect his chagrin at the outcome of the experiment. The transfusion had to be stopped "by reason that [the patient's] constrained posture, and the crowd of the spectators interrupted very much this operation."[42] The experiment fails when the skeptical crowd collapses into a curious one. Here the curious case—and the crowd it attracts—first heralds and attests to the advance of medical knowledge, and then impedes (or stampedes) that advance. And here the curiosity of the avid spectator merges uneasily with that of the physician, who attends ostensibly to witness and to learn. The spectators attend for the dual attraction of the experimental and the monstrous (the young man is both patient and man-calf). Denis proleptically invokes this troublesome crowd in a defensive maneuver early in the case. He acknowledges that

> [s]ome spread a rumour, that [the patient] died soon after the operation; others bore the people in hand, that he was relapsed into a greater madness than that before; and in short, it hath been so diversly discoursed of up and down, and with such differing reflections thereon, that I thought my self obliged, for the clearing up of what false rumours had darken'd, to give you a faithful and exact account. (618)

Denis works hard to differentiate his account from the interested and distorted accounts spread by the many. Victorian physicians' suspicion of marvelous tales is here foreshadowed in the slippage between "able physicians," who testify to the progress toward cure and medical knowledge, and "spectators," who obstruct that progress.

A discursive incoherence in a curious case by Thomas Stack dramatizes that this slippage can also occur in an individual viewer. Stack published the "Account of a Woman Sixty-Eight Years of Age, Who Gave Suck to

Two of Her Grand-Children," in the *Philosophical Transactions* in 1739, commenting:

> A Gentleman of Credit having lately inform'd me of a Woman near seventy Years old, who actually suckles one of her Grand-children, and courteously offering to accompany me to her, excited my Curiosity to see so uncommon a Sight; and the more, in order to try if I could not discover some Fallacy in the Affair.[43]

The "Gentleman of Credit" and Stack's own skeptical desire to "discover some Fallacy in the Affair" here testify to an experimental disinterest, which (despite the hint of amazement in "actually suckles") is initially sufficient to code Stack's "curiosity" as a proper one. Likewise, his focus on her breasts as "full, fair, and void of Wrinkles" is only to be expected (140). He seals his role by conducting a brief "Experiment." The old woman, "upon pressing her right Breast," he reports,

> fairly squeez'd out Milk, which gather'd in small Drops at three of the Lacteal Ducts terminating in the Nipple. This Experiment I made her repeat a second time, having myself carefully dry'd the End of the Nipple with my Handkerchief, as I had done before her first Trial. (141)

Here, too, by judicious use of medical terminology, Stack maintains his distanced discursive pose even while, physically, he leans forward to "carefully" dry the milk from the woman's breast. The repetition of the "Trial," too, serves as a symbol of experimentalist caution, after which he declares himself "[c]onvinced of the Truth of the Fact" (141).

However, a curious discourse also breaks through the integrity of the experimentalist project. Stack attends to the peculiarities of the woman's situation: how her grown son first noticed his baby niece seeming to swallow at her grandmother's breast; how "The Youth [himself] drew Milk from that same breast from which he had been wean'd above twenty Years"; and how the baby's mother, the old woman's daughter, "seeing she was provided with such an extraordinary and tender Nurse," promptly had another child for her old mother to nurse (141). Once Stack admits these "extraordinary" interpersonal relations, his narrative lurches between distanced observation (the second child "plainly perform'd the Actions of Suction and Deglutination") and enthusiastic amazement ("the two Children, both Girls, are, as to Constitution, such as I could wish to the dearest Friend") (142). His professed role of disinterested observer shares its privileged narrative space with his obvious enjoyment of the scene and imagined identification with the family.

The individual observer's slippage between curious observation and curious sight is underscored by her neighbors' presence among the observers. "When this good Woman came to Town," Stack explains, "her Milk abounded to that Degree in both Breasts, that, to convince the Unbelieving, she would frequently spout it above a Yard from her: A Particular which, among others, the good Man and Woman of the House, and others of the Neighbourhood, likewise assured me of" (142). Because they enter the scene as "the Unbelieving," the skeptical role of these onlookers is functionally the same as that of the experimentalist physician. Ideologically, of course, they are worlds apart; they are "others of the Neighbourhood," not trained observers. Their curious sight, however, recontextualizes Stack among the vulgar spectators. The "small Drops" of milk that the grandmother "fairly squeez'd" from her breast for Stack proves to be one in a spectacular continuum of demonstrations that finds its extreme in the stream of milk "she would frequently spout ... above a Yard from her" (no mean feat). The presence of the vulgar crowd, by coding the woman's performances as spectacular, retrospectively calls into doubt the disinterested nature both of Stack's "excited ... Curiosity" and his handkerchief's careful strokes.

To the physician unable to comprehend (to understand and contain) curious phenomena through an experimentalist narrative, a narrative of the curious offers both explanatory and rhetorical power. Francis Manginot turns to it repeatedly, in his 1701 "Account of an Unusual Medical Case." He writes,

> I was surprised yesterday with a very extraordinary case. Madam R——'s daughter fell into violent convulsion fits, and while she was in them voided a large quantity of blood by the mouth, the nose, the ears, and the eyes. All these symptoms were over in half an hour's time, and the girl ... was well presently. ... I am apt to believe they are epileptic fits; but the sudden relief and cessation of them by bleeding through all these parts, I must confess is wonderful to me.[44]

Not only does Manginot employ a curious rhetoric—"unusual," "very extraordinary"—but he also provides a model for curious readers in his own textualized interest: "I was surprised," "I must confess is wonderful to me." He admits to the limits of his medical knowledge. Although he cannot explain the case, curious discourse provides a rhetoric that holds the place of an ultimate explanatory cause.

However, the features that make curious discourse useful also render it unreliable, producing a discursive incoherence in the experimentalist text. Its logic calls for subjective expression; in its cries of sympathy, wonder, horror, and the like, curious discourse draws attention to the precariousness of experimentalist disinterest. For instance, although Denis keeps his narrative voice dispassionate, and although he vows that as a narrator, "I have confined my self to the Experiment alone," elements of curious discourse point to his troubles.[45] His "outrageous" patient, with his "Extravagance" (madness), exemplifies what defines the curious case: he elicits a strong interest from all who observe him; he "mov'd to compassion all good people that saw him." In a detail that recalls the virtuous circulation of affect in the novel of sensibility, it was a benevolent observer, a M. de Montmor ("the person most touched with" the patient's condition) who first urged the transfusion (619). This sentimental portrayal of the patient looses a flood of affective energy derailing a properly disinterested "curious observation." Curious discourse—as when Denis describes his patient as "this poor creature ... tormented with Medicines" (619)—often inaugurates a series of oscillations between it and the authorizing discourse of experimentalism. This discursive heterogeneity clearly departs from the experimentalist ideal of a steady, plain speech.

Eighteenth-century novels also combined curious topics, and curious discourse, with the claim to historicity. Defoe (in *Robinson Crusoe* or *Moll Flanders*), Jonathan Swift (in *Gulliver's Travels*), and John Cleland's "Fanny Hill" (in *Memoirs of a Woman of Pleasure*) fabulate similarly curious scenarios under the sign of fact. Some, at least, of the masquerade is nominal only. Swift's satire relies on his readers apprehending his journals as not "really" the record of his travels, but a commentary on British society. The possibility of "playing at" fact remains; and while the [false] claim to historicity develops new rhetorical strategies for the novel, it undermines the "matter of fact" in experimentalist narratives.

The eighteenth-century case history carves out a space explicitly dedicated to curious observation while still fostering curious sight; it builds a genre opposed to romance while indulging the affective exchange associated with it. Curious cases call forth the genre's most contested elements: the struggle to enact a disinterested interest; the heightened "Rhetorick" in the face of plain speech; the dispassionate observation of what is simultaneously sexualized voyeurism and dramatic spectacle. This discursive hybridity is a constitutive aspect of the eighteenth-century case history, despite the experimentalists' proscriptive stylistics; it will present even greater problems for the increasingly professionalized clinical case history of the nineteenth century.

"A curious sight" thus vexes the experimentalist case history in several ways. The physician becomes voyeur, as he records an intimate history, or common spectator, as he goggles at a surprising scene. The reader, complicit, doubles his vision. And the patient becomes spectacular in her singularity: an index of both the individual and the marvelous. All these aspects of "curious sight" carry an affective charge, soliciting or revealing the emotional investment in watching. It is not surprising, then, that the term "curious," with its excessive interest, suffers a rapid decline in the nineteenth century, when the intensified drive to professionalize medicine did not eradicate the electrified looking of the physician, but rendered it impossible to express in the language of the clinic.

Cheselden and "a New Kind of Seeing"

The shifting line between curious observation and curious sight in eighteenth-century case histories helps locate the beginnings of generic difference between scientific and literary writing. The early case history is discursively hybrid and the effects of that hybridity resonate with a quintessentially literary form of the period, the novel of sensibility. This becomes especially evident in Cheselden's case of the blind boy restored to sight.

Modes of seeing are clearly at issue here. Cheselden delights in evidence of how the boy's vision is educated, as when "[a] Year after first seeing, being carried upon Epsom Downs, and observing a large Prospect, [the boy] was exceedingly delighted with it, and call'd it a new Kind of Seeing." Similarly, the boy, "[h]aving often forgot which was the Cat, and which the Dog . . . was ashamed to ask; but catching the Cat (which he knew by feeling) he was observed to look at her stedfastly, and then setting her down, said, So Puss! I shall know you another Time."[46] The boy here adopts a mode of vision associated more with the surgeon than the patient, his "stedfast" gaze engaged in cataloguing the cat's visual detail. The case distinguishes this new kind of seeing from the boy's original, curious notions of sight, infused with affective value: he had imagined "that those Things which he lik'd best" would also "appear most agreeable to his Eyes," so that "those Persons would appear most beautiful whom he lov'd most"

(448–49). That original vision, in which beauty, morality, and love combine, reaches an apogee in the sentimental novel.

The boy's original, curious sight is figured here as naïve, undisciplined, and in need of correction, but it forms an important anchor for this case history. The boy's encounter with the cat produces an affecting scene that is also "agreeable" to the eyes. Cheselden draws upon novelistic techniques, suggesting rather than explaining the changes wrought in the boy's world, and humanizing the boy as thoroughly as the boy anthropomorphizes the cat in addressing her. Finally, Cheselden problematizes the observer's stance by allowing a kind of voyeurism to overlap the investigative gaze. The surgeon almost stealthily ("he was observed") duplicates the boy's "stedfast" gaze at the cat, and "knows him" in turn. The case history's treatment of this scene allows the reader, as well, to vicariously observe unobserved. Here the pressure which vision lends to the process of "knowing" ("I shall know you another time") is made explicit.

This eighteenth-century case history thus presents a curious sight, in a discourse bound to the unknown and unexplainable, evoking a voyeuristic or spectacular visuality, and both expressing and soliciting a subjective response. The boy's emotion stands in for and calls forth the emotion of the medical observer and the reader:

> He said, every new Object was a new Delight, and the Pleasure was so great, that he wanted Ways to express it; but his Gratitude to his Operator he could not conceal, never seeing him for some Time without Tears of Joy in his Eyes, and other Marks of Affection: and if he did not happen to come at any Time when he was expected, he would be so grieved, that he could not forbear crying at his Disappointment. (450)

Here Cheselden egregiously offers a curious glimpse of the boy, with information that adds little or nothing to the medical knowledge of the case but amplifies audience interest and knits sight to emotion. The transformative surgery prompts a rhetoric of the curious, in particular the claim to express the inexpressible ("he wanted ways to express it"). It looses a flood of emotion within the text, which veers between "Delight" and "Disappointment." Here the text produces not medical knowledge but sentimental affect as the boy's "Tears," both "of Joy" and from being "so grieved," blur those miraculously seeing eyes and displace the medical feat of vision. Eighteenth-century medical theories of perception underwrote the culture of sensibility; and the circulation of affect here produces the same tears that saturate the novel of sensibility some years later, signifying benevolence, discernment, and empathy.[47] This affective economy, where sensibility circulates as evidence of moral virtue, lends power and authority to the sentimental novel. And, given the relative lack of disciplinary distinctions in the eighteenth century, this affective economy authorizes Cheselden's report as well. But Cheselden's text registers a pronounced syntactical confusion at the point of circulation.

As in the novel of sensibility, the powerful emotional valence of the boy's tears threatens to disrupt the observer's (Cheselden's) own composure. These tears blur the distinction between observer and observed. Cheselden's distanced, third-person representation of himself as the boy's "Operator" breaks down in the pronominal confusion that overtakes the narrative when it attempts to detail the emotional interplay between one "he" and another: "[I]f he did not happen to come at any Time when he was expected, he would be so grieved, that he could not forbear crying at his Disappointment." The boy's overflowing emotion, and Cheselden's implied response, cannot be recognized within a disinterested, experimentalist medical narrative, but Cheselden's sentimental discourse manages and mediates the affective power of the scene.

In the eighteenth century, "disciplinary difference" as we know it had not yet been constructed. Cheselden's text registers a pressure to distinguish between kinds of prose, hinting at a process of differentiation between the case history and what would become the novel of sensibility. Cheselden's "Account" reports the history of the case in terms very different from his "Explication," detailing the surgery itself. In the disinterested "Explication," the boy's eyes are portrayed in isolation from his other features, and from the emotions which move them; in one illustration, indeed, the very pupil of the eye is punctured in a graphic illustration of surgical technique (Fig. 1). The plate distances and dehumanizes the patient who must painfully stare up at his "Operator" throughout this delicate surgery. Likewise, the prose of the surgical report—"C is a Sort of Needle with an Edge on one Side, which being pass'd thro' the *Tunica Sclerotis*, is then brought forwards thro' the *Iris* a little farther than E" (452)—consistently demonstrates a serious tone, specialized diction, and distant narrative voice that could not be more different from that of the novel of sensibility. Cheselden here shows his awareness that, in a surgical report, the ideally disinterested stance of the experimenter should be made evident in his distanced, plain, and clear discourse. This simplicity can produce miraculous results.

The fact that Cheselden presents both an experimental report, explicating his surgical procedure, and a more descriptive narrative pressured by the

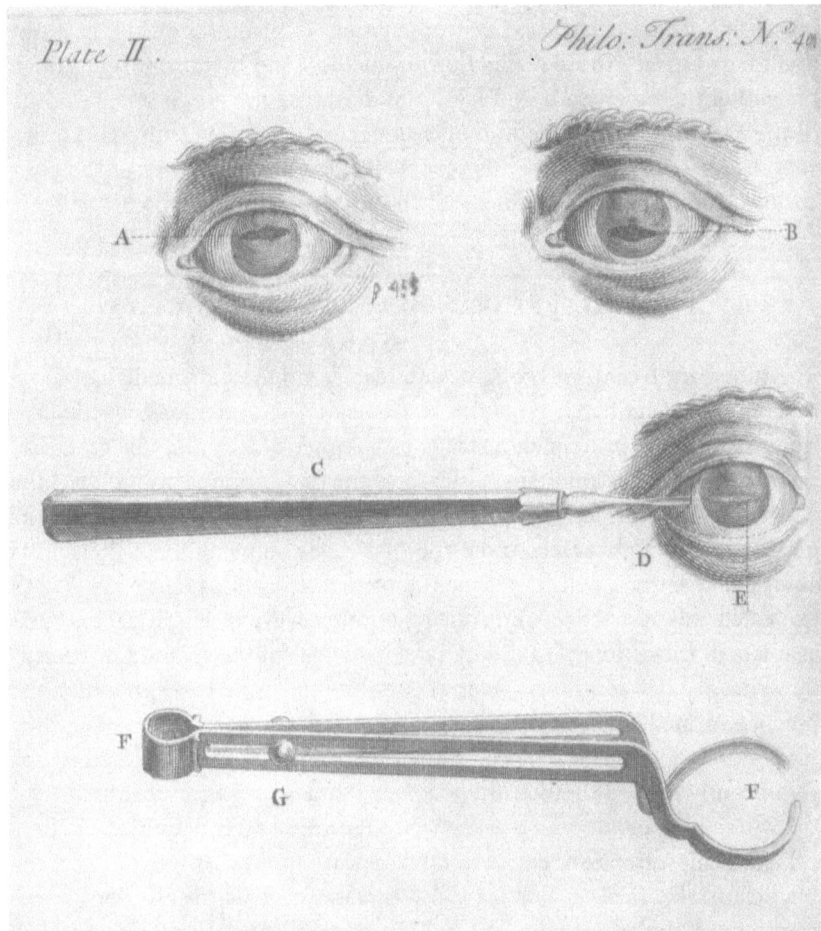

FIGURE 1. From William Chesselden, "An Explication of the Instruments Used, in a New Operation on the Eyes," *Philosophical Transactions* 35, no. 402 (1728): 451–52.

emotional freight this operation carried for the patient (and implicitly for his surgeon as well), underscores the extent to which his prose narrative, and others like it, interrogate the beginnings of the narrative genres we now recognize as the medical case history and the novel.

The case of the blind boy oscillates between the distanced perspective of an experimentalist observation and the affective closeness of a curious sight. Both produce knowledge, if different sorts. This case suggests how the powerful charge of the distanced view also provides a "new Kind of Seeing," the productive force of the experimentalist perspective driving generic change. Most important, Cheselden's case opens up the moment of perception. It dissociates seeing from stating and from knowing, in a way that helps us trace those distinctions in medical and literary prose through the end of the nineteenth century. It demonstrates the power and authority of the experimentalists' method of making, and recording, curious "Observations," even as it overlays this model with the affective force of the boy's curious "sight," and the curious sight he elicits from the reader.

THE DISAPPEARANCE OF CURIOUS SIGHT

The nineteenth century brought a retreat from "heroic" medicine and a repudiation of its harsh remedies like bleeding and mercury; a rededication to empirical principles; a struggle to regulate "irregular" or "sectarian" medicine; and a concomitant backlash against medicine's curious past. The effect was to contract the range of possible techniques available to the physician, although a freer, more speculative vision would become acceptable at midcentury, with experimental medicine. Philip Henry Pye-Smith expressed this restrictive spirit during another wave of empirical enthusiasm late in the century. "Our only safeguard against the spirit of quackery," he writes, "... is continued recurrence to the scientific basis on which the practice of medicine rests. Our art is most satisfactory and efficient when most closely resting on science."[48] The nineteenth-century case history was significantly shaped by this struggle over standard medical practice.

When nineteenth-century physicians narrowed their definition of clinical, scientific discourse, curious sight appears more disruptive. Even the physician's skeptical, exploratory, and precise "curious observation" began to disappear from the case history. The battle against sectarian medicine stood in for and amplified clinical medicine's embarrassed rejection of its past fascination with curious cases. Clinical medicine worked hard to define norms of practice, purportedly to discourage fraudulent or inept practitioners and increase public confidence in medicine.[49] This professionalizing movement (figured as a "reform") strove to exile any curious practices from its armamentarium, and curious practitioners from its ranks. Reformers attacked speculative or deceptive treatments like those linked to popular belief rather than to formal medical training, which was itself haphazard in content, uneven in quality, and largely unregulated.[50]

The *Lancet*, a radical medical journal supporting the newly emerging professional class, led the reforms movement. It was known for attacking homeopathy, hydropathy, mesmerism, and other sectarian approaches considered unreliable by regular (allopathic) practitioners. The *Lancet*'s editor, the surgeon and general gadfly Thomas Wakley, positioned the journal, which he founded in 1823, as an alternative to establishment medicine; but it rapidly became both powerful and influential in its own right. Driven by the ideal that medicine could be a science unswayed by personal interests or unfounded beliefs, the *Lancet* published case histories informed by the new clinical norms and (despite Wakley's radical politics) broadly representative of the practice of regular medicine in Britain.[51]

Because the borders of professional medicine remained unclear well into the nineteenth century, the case history, as the public face of medicine, became a crucial site where authors could construct an ideal of clinical medicine. The historian John Harley Warner comments, "In order to set themselves apart from sectarians, regular physicians continually had to reaffirm their regularity.... [Thus] the appearance of unity was an essential goal that demanded carefully guarded conduct in therapeutic discourse, [with criticism limited to] proper ... forums ..., [chiefly] medical journals and society meetings."[52] If, as Warner claims, physicians constructed a professional identity by policing medical discourse, then the changes in the case history underwrote the credentials of clinical medicine.

Nineteenth-century researchers re-centered science around the normative, so that the study of strange experiences and unlikely theories became in itself suspect, requiring vigilant policing and careful rhetorical management.[53] Physicians still investigated curious cases but now naturalized them as abnormal, bringing the oddity back within the system.[54] In founding the science of teratology with the publication of *Traité de tératologie* in 1836, Isodore Geoffroy Saint-Hilaire redefined hermaphrodites not as "monsters" but as errors of embryology. The collections of medical curiosities published in the nineteenth century, such as J. G. Millingen's in 1838, were generally not presented as serious medical monographs. Thus when George Gould and Walter Pyle compile their exhaustive collection of *Anomalies and Curiosities of Medicine* as late as 1897, they struggle to position their work (itself anomalous in its emphasis on "the most curious, bizarre, and abnormal cases") as a normative part of clinical medicine. Their "Prefatory and Introductory" essay argues for the text's "function far beyond the satisfaction of mere curiosity," and their cases exhibit a heightened awareness of the possibility of fraudulent or mistaken reports. But they also begin the essay with an acknowledgment of the power of "exceptional and pertinent fascination" in the curious case.[55] The existence of their compilation, however tenuously part of the clinical medical project, reminds us that singular cases still force a reformulation of the rules of medical knowledge, and provoke an interested human response.

CHAPTER ONE

While the term "curious" diminishes in case histories, increasingly it comes to denote the carnivalesque or miraculous. A vulgar, "curious sight," fascinated with spectacle, comes to dominate the curious case, crowding out other meanings of "curious" (skillfully crafted, rare, of medical interest, or worthy of study) that could have remained coherent within a clinical project. Among the last to advertise cases as curiosities are Thomas Barnes, in his "Account of William Dempster, Who Swallowed a Table-Knife Nine Inches Long" (1824) and William Reid Clanny, in "A Faithful Record of the Miraculous Case of Mary Jobson" (1841). The term "curious" itself became a rarity in medical discourse by the mid-nineteenth century.

The proponents of clinical science, who believed themselves more objective and more skeptical than their eighteenth-century predecessors, measured their progress in part by the attacks on such curious claims, a skirmish conducted through a series of case histories. In 1863, for instance, Lewis Albert Sayre offered a "Remarkable Case of Deception: A Woman Professing to Secrete Nothing but Charcoal and Stones for a Number of Years, All the Natural Functions Being Arrested, and the Deception Unmasked."[56] This back-and-forth of claimants and debunkers was not new to the nineteenth century—it recalls the debates over the Mary Toft case of 1726, for example—but it throve upon the nineteenth-century fervor of skepticism that helped to solidify an incipient scientific community.[57]

Physicians with unusual cases thus sought to balance the interest and value of the case with a moderate tone. For example, the *Lancet* in 1850 published a "Case of Concussion of the Brain, with Displacement of the Vertebrae." The patient, "Mary K——, aged twenty-five ... fell from a window thirty feet high, alighting on her head" but "recovered without a bad symptom" other than an unusual "tumour" on the back of her neck, caused apparently by displaced vertebrae. The author, a Mr. H. M. Greenhow, emphasizes how unusual this case is by reciting his patient's nonexistent symptoms:

> There is no pain, or paralysis, or other symptoms of compression of the cord. She uses her limbs with perfect ease, and has the proper control over them. Her mind is quite unimpaired. She has completely recovered from her other injuries. This case is worthy of observation, from the absence of all the symptoms which usually accompany any injury to the spinal cord.[58]

In other words, what makes this case extraordinary is the patient's utter absence of symptoms. The case of Mary K—— might a century earlier have been called "curious," since this term often included unexpected survivals after major trauma (drownings, falls, wounds). But Greenhow, while enunciating how Mary K——'s course is "worthy of observation," refuses to label, with the term "curious," what his presentation otherwise foregrounds: her *difference* from the normative case of concussion.

However, nineteenth-century physicians did not eradicate as much as obscure their fascination with "the curious."[59] Explaining away "the curious" could be another form of spectacle, as in Sayre's debunking of the charcoal-secreting woman. Ambiguously titling his pamphlet a "remarkable case of deception," Sayre both touts the "remarkable" and "unmask[s]" it as "deception." He retains the rhetorical pull of curiosity upon the reader—calling upon an avidity for the unusual and the scandalous—while portraying himself as a skeptical, objective observer. Sayre performs a verbal sleight-of-hand not unlike the carnival trick he debunks, drawing the reader's attention with a "remarkable case" only to substitute for it a "deception." Greenhow likewise deploys the force of curiosity while dissociating himself from its vulgar implications: he chooses to downplay the oddities of his case but still publishes it. Clearly, the current of interest in curious cases has been deflected into other channels rather than dammed up altogether.

Chapter Two

Staging Clinical Realism in the Victorian Periodical

As the nineteenth century opened, physicians marked their departure from the past by increasingly regularizing their modes of seeing and stating. "Taking cases" became a process to be learned, both discursive and methodical. "[I]n taking the case," Peter Latham advises, "I desire always to proceed after a certain method.... [But the student should for] the first three or four months record nothing; use your observation to the utmost.... [T]he student should allow his curiosity to range discursively over every variety of disease.... When I say discursively, I still mean diligently, and with an earnest purpose of improvement." Once the student has surveyed the landscape "you may begin to take cases."[1] The clinical case history with the "earnest purpose" of a newly professionalizing medical community articulates a vexed distinction between the physician's "curiosity" and his "observation." That community replaced the curious sight and even curious observation of the experimentalists with a clinical observation that peaked in an unattainable, mechanical ideal and eventually (as a later chapter will show) was supplemented with speculation and insight. Curious cases—the narratives of extraordinary bodies, and of the ingenious men who explored Nature's secrets and spectacles—were revised into merely "interesting" versions of the norm. Finally, the curious discourses common in eighteenth-century case histories—exoticizing, sentimental, sensational, Gothic—were repudiated in favor of a clinical realist discourse that promised to record observations with more objectivity, accuracy, precision, and reliability. The clinical case history deploys all these elements in order to authorize its ideology of objectivity; its aesthetic, a mechanical observation marked by the absent presence of the physician and communicated through a realist discourse; and its product, the medical fact.

This chronology is not surprising. Historians of medicine agree that nineteenth-century medical narratives became increasingly modern: clinical, empirical, and restricted to a professional readership.[2] While this is essentially true, I wish to trouble this history in a few ways. First, as my readings emphasize, the transition from curious to clinical medical writing was not a consistent, universal evolution, nor a sharp, distinct paradigm shift, but rather a vexed and partial shift, contingent upon the particular case and its context. Physicians were ambivalent about whether clinical practice and prose represented the "improvement" they sought. I include here not only commentaries on the case history, which articulate clinical ideals, but also a sampling of cases, which suggest how the narrative might approach but not entirely achieve the clinical ideal. Second, Victorian medical discourse is not as secluded within professional pages as the conventional history suggests. Indeed, recent scholarship has demonstrated the cultural work of science in the general-audience periodical. This chapter will demonstrate the extent to which clinical medical norms are also staged for lay audiences in some literary periodicals, providing a crucial link between Victorian literature and medicine. A later chapter will examine the extent to which another mode of vision, "speculation," condemned in the early 1800s as antithetical to clinical methods, became not only possible but necessary in the experimental medicine of the 1850s. Finally, the clinical case history, like the clinical gaze, is an ideal, not a reality. It is an aspirational genre toward which physicians could write, but it cannot be fully realized in any text.

The Autopsy and the Clinical Case History

During the late eighteenth and early nineteenth centuries, a new kind of medicine arose around the clinic.[3] Patients received a standard daily ritual examination, and patients with similar diseases could be observed over time and compared. Historians since Foucault have chronicled the effects rippling outward from Paris: the rise of hospital medicine; the burgeoning spirit of research bringing new medical treatments, instruments, and statistics; the formalization of medical training; and, most important, the birth of a science of pathology based on the cold gaze of the autopsy, regularly confirming or denying diagnosis after death.[4] While nineteenth-century British physicians were notoriously slow to adopt continental medical innovations, from autopsies to stethoscopes, hospital physicians were more likely to try out new methods on their (usually lower-class) patients.

Clinical medicine promptly appears in medical texts, due to the newsworthiness of the new methods, the evangelism of the early adopters, and the reformist influence of the *Lancet*, Thomas Wakley's influential medical journal. Case histories unevenly reflect the changes brought by the clinic. Physicians had been advocating a more rigorous narrative method for decades. Julia Epstein notes that they "did not become systematic . . . until physicians such as [John] Bellers and [Francis] Clifton began calling for a more formal approach to record-keeping in the first half of the eighteenth century. . . . At around the same time the case record became a fundamental text in the teaching of clinical medicine in Western Europe."[5] With the rise of the clinic, physicians—relying on hospital clerks and medical students to note down the details of increasing numbers of patients—redoubled calls to standardize the case history. However, the order and relative prominence of the elements of a case presentation did not settle into a standard form until late in the nineteenth century. "Three factors enter the discourse of a case report as it has been taught to medical students since the 1890s," notes Epstein. "[F]irst, *symptoms*, or complaints—the patient's own subjective perception of deviations from normal health; second, *signs*—the objective manifestations of disease located by the physician during a physical examination; and third (and historically most recent), laboratory and other *findings*" (31). Caldwell similarly finds a regularized format—in this case, the bipartite "history and physical"—developing in clinical medicine as it differentiated between the patient's and the physician's stories.[6] The case history gradually privileges the physician's observations, perceived as more reliable, although, as Caldwell points out, the patient's experience persists in the "history" even when reworded by the physician. Indeed, as late as 1878, James Finlayson argues for keeping the patient's "history of the illness" in the narrative: "The subsequent course of the case has often much light thrown upon it by this record of these early indications, for the patient may feel the importance of certain things which may be overshadowed in our minds by considerations based on our theoretical view of the disease."[7] The new genre gave disproportionate credence to the physical examination, which attempted to scrutinize patients with the same meticulous detail and dispassionate stance of the autopsy. This helped to establish clinical observation as a favored mode of investigation and clinical realism as a privileged discourse. Curious observation, curious sight, and human insight were not ceded any formal locus in the genre.

A standardized set of textual elements made it easier for physicians to compare different points in a patient's illness and different patients' illnesses, which (along with the rise of statistical analysis) facilitated the study of public health and of disease norms. John Ferriar decries "the method, so fashionable at present, of publishing single cases," because this "appears not well calculated to enlarge our knowledge, either of the nature or cure of diseases."[8] By locating the individual patient within a population and in relation to a norm, the clinic de-emphasizes the "singular" case and distances the physician from the patient's experience as a feeling human subject. Analogy recedes in medical argument, along with the almost obsessive citation of other physicians.[9] Characteristics of a liberal education, like the abstract mathematical debates of eighteenth-century physician Bernard Mandeville, were deemed irrelevant, no longer recognizable as medical data. Latin largely disappeared from medical narrative, both as the language of scholarly discourse and as quotations from the classical poets. However, Latin tags remained as a ritualistic nod to tradition on the title pages of medical monographs, and a Latin diagnostic language anchored the professional discourse.[10] Until about 1830, Latin also persisted as the proper language for sexual topics in the case history, implicitly excluding the vulgar reader; but the textual marks of a rigorous clinical observation supplanted it as a professional marker.

A proliferation of professional journals and societies expanded both the need and the audience for the case history, targeting not just clinicians in the metropole but also provincial physicians and other practitioners—even as this wider discursive space was increasingly marked off-limits to lay readers. New medical instruments exploded the amount of information to be recorded, forcing an increase in figural techniques like tables and charts.

The autopsy report provided a new model for medical seeing and representing. It became a standard text for medical training and research, and refocused the case history on a narrative of causality instead of analogy. As Latham insists, "[H]owever hard the task may be, we must still try to know the true relation of . . . things" (75–76). Despite the real influence of medicine's public narrative, which Maria Frawley calls "medicine's narrative of promise, a trajectory marked by diagnosis, treatment, and cure,"[11] it fails to acknowledge the centrality of another narrative. That narrative leads inexorably toward death, in a teleology in which the autopsy (not the cure) serves as the apex of truth and disclosure by generating clinical medicine's most valuable product, knowledge.

Almost all of these changes—standardization of the genre, the shift from a personal to a public medicine, the professionalization of the physician-author, the visual narratives of new medical technologies, and the assured voice of the autopsy—work to reify the relation between physician and patient as an objective, distanced seeing; that is, they attempt to banish the curious sight of the eighteenth-century case history, or the insight of the nineteenth-century novel. Foucault comments, "The clinic was probably the first attempt to order a science on the exercise and decisions of the gaze."[12] The voyeuristic or spectacular "curious sight" of the eighteenth-century case history, and even its curious observation, must be suppressed in favor of a clinical observation: a severely methodical visual analysis of the surfaces of the body that is close in attention but affectively distanced.[13]

Clinical physicians had to renegotiate the relationship between the case history and its curious past. The eighteenth-century valorization of plain speech becomes the nineteenth century's investment in a clinical voice that is still steadfastly down-to-earth and studiously unemotional but no longer necessarily simple in syntax or vocabulary. The clinical physician's affective relationship with the patient is obscured. The patient becomes an object of study primarily. The physician renegotiates his role, not as a character but as a director of the case—measuring, observing, listening, prescribing, and recording, all to new and exacting standards. As Foucault explains, "Descriptive *rigour* will be the result of *precision* in the statement and of *regularity* in the designation."[14] As a succession of "guides to case-taking" attests, however, such rigor was easier to assert than to achieve fully.

The physician Giovanni Morgagni, a transitional figure, helped introduce these clinical precepts. His *De Sedibus et Causis Morborum per Anatomen Indagatis* (*The Seats and Causes of Disease Investigated by Anatomy*, 1760) was translated into English by 1769. This massive, influential text stockpiles seven hundred cases, most with a clinical history and operative or autopsy report, a method still standard in academic medicine. Morgagni's case histories accord the autopsy both textual prominence and epistemological primacy. His case histories are brief, a mere frame for the autopsy reports, which anchor the work of diagnosis and education. In contrast, famed eighteenth-century physician George Cheyne rarely includes an autopsy report. When he does—as in the case of Colonel Townshend, who died and came back to life before dying again—he devotes much more space to the history of the man (three pages) than to the history of the autopsy (twenty-three lines), even though the autopsy should explain (it cannot) the mysterious event.[15]

Only three decades later, Morgagni's case history of a Venetian woman taken by a paroxysm in her carriage demonstrates a pronounced shift toward clinical medicine. He offers a scant paragraph to her living history (one sentence to her previous illness and one sentence to her fatal one) but directs three times as much attention to the autopsy. He even organizes his case histories by the autopsy results. Whereas Cheyne set out to chronicle the uncommon, or curious, presentations of disease, Morgagni declares that "observations of the common diseases are far more profitable than those of the unusual ones."[16] He thus navigates in constant reference to an ideal case, a "working object," an object deemed "typical" of its kind. Lorraine Daston and Peter Galison position this as a transitional stage between the typically Enlightenment aim of "truth to nature" and a nineteenth-century ideal of "mechanical objectivity."[17] However subjective the process of identifying a "working object," the clinical case history uses it to objectify, as a screen through which to assess the patient and her disease. Like the autopsy, the "working object" certifies the authenticity and accuracy of the physician's findings.

However, the transition between curious and clinical medicine was vexed and uneven. Morgagni's case history demonstrates many of the features of clinical narrative, especially the interest in typicality, the formal deployment of observation described with specialized terms, and the production of a medical fact; but his clinical voice and objective stance are distinctly provisional. His case opens with a scene worthy of any curious case history:

> The mother of a family, who was two-and-forty years of age, had liv'd long in a state of infirm health, and had long been subject to a kind of paroxysm, which appear'd in the following manner: on using pretty quick exercise of body, a kind of violent uneasiness came on, within the upper part of the thorax, on the left side, join'd with a difficulty of breathing, and a stupor of the left arm: all which symptoms soon remitted when these motions ceas'd. This woman then, having set out about the middle of October, in the year 1707, from Venice, to go up the continent in a wheel-carriage, and being chearful in her mind, behold the same paroxysm return'd: with which being seiz'd, and saying that she should die, she actually died on the spot.[18]

CHAPTER TWO

Like its eighteenth-century contemporaries, this case history's interest in the details of illness is measured in qualitative more than quantifiable terms ("pretty quick exercise," "a kind of violent uneasiness"). Its details provide information useful to the physician but also sketch the patient as a character: an optimistic woman, active, of some means, with insight into her illness. It presents a curious sight; the narrator, in a tone of incredulity, highlights the dramatic co-incidence of the woman's prophecy and her death, her proclamation "she should die" and the fact that she then "actually died on the spot." This offers the spectacle of an actor and a drama worthy of Cheyne's Colonel Townshend.

But the narrator quickly, in only his third sentence, turns to the autopsy report. Here Morgagni shifts his prose to the clinical voice, with its interest in method, detail, quantification, specialized terminology, and visuality, and its ostentatious disinterest in the physician's and patient's human relation. He explains,

> The body, being brought back into the city, was examin'd by me on the following day: the face of it was somewhat livid; the other parts appear'd to be quite of a good colour and habit; but the upper parts were somewhat lank and wrinkled.... I had a suspicion of an aneurism at the curvature of the aorta, the dissection was begun from the thorax. (819)

Already the patient has become "the body"; her face, "the face." That which lies before the clinical physician is a body, with a physical presence (he notes a "disagreeable smell" [820]), but it is no longer a person. Morgagni supplements this distancing, objectifying rhetoric with a specialized terminology, in which the sudden, dramatic, but nonspecific "kind of paroxysm" is reduced to its probable cause: "an aneurism at the curvature of the aorta." By the conclusion of his text, this "mother of a family" has been replaced by her fragmented body—the "bony scales" and "marks of ossification" in her vessels, the "osculum uteri ... dilated, and subsiding" (820). The personal, everyday description of the opening has been so thoroughly displaced by a clinical, impersonal observation that we are hardly prepared for the glimpse of the woman's humanity that Morgagni yields us as he closes: "The head I did not touch," he remarks, "for it was already late at night, and the woman died while she was speaking, as I said before" (820). Morgagni's sudden shift from "the head" to "the woman" and "she" juxtaposes not just two different addresses to the same patient, but two different registers of discourse and two different modes of apprehending the physical world. The discontinuity between Morgagni's first paragraph and his succeeding ones demonstrates the difference between curious sight and clinical observation. These distinct modes of vision produce entirely different images of this patient, as a woman or as a cadaver. Tellingly, Morgagni cannot achieve a truly clinical tone until he begins his autopsy; he does not display the formal signs of the clinic until his patient is not a live subject but a dead object.[19]

What the autopsy achieves for Morgagni, then, is to impel the physician into a clinically objective tone. The clinical case history of the nineteenth century attempts to accomplish that tone while the patient is alive. The clinical patient must be a "live object"—she must not appear as a subject or elicit the physician's own subjective interest.

"The Mechanical Labour of Observation" and the Empiricist Backlash against Theory

As physicians became professionalized during the early nineteenth century, they refined the clinical observation that had developed from the autopsy and hospital medicine. In an empiricist reaction against theorists, medical writers began considering how to anchor medicine in fact by removing or mitigating variable narratives and replacing them with a standardized, impersonal, and unmediated process of report. This revises the physician's earlier pose of empirical disinterest into an aesthetic of "mechanical" observation; his authority now derives from his emulation of the incessant, unguided labors of a selfless observing machine. While the clinical case history is still a narrative, it now works to realize an objective and scientific knowledge through the absent presence of the physician.

Although eighteenth-century physicians made sporadic attempts to formalize the case history, the genre did not change significantly until the nineteenth century. The clinical case history allowed the physician to transform individual patient experience through mechanical observation to produce a medical fact. John Hughes Bennett, an important early physiologist, acknowledges the increased importance of the medical record when he remarks, "I have endeavoured throughout, by reference to indisputable facts, to demonstrate the correctness of the principles which have guided my practice, and have, therefore, authenticated every case with the name of its reporter in the hospital books."[20] Physicians urged ever more dedicated observation and ever more careful organization and communication in their struggle to improve everyday medical practice and education. More than ever before, clinical physicians centered their practice on visual inspection.[21] Byrom Bramwell emphasizes the visual grounding of the case history, when he comments, "In recording cases, the object should be to make, as it were, a word-picture, or word-diagram, to include all the facts, bringing prominently into the foreground those of most importance." Language was also important; in an echo of the "plain speech" of earlier medicine, Bramwell warns, "The language in which the case is recorded should be as simple, precise, and intelligible as possible. The observer should record simply ... the bare facts."[22] The case history grounded medical research, although Peterson comments that "[m]uch of what was published and presented to professional audiences had limited scientific value, even by the standards of the day."[23] As a result of the pressure put on medical narrative to regularize medical practice, the "curious" case becomes rarer; it does not entirely disappear, but rather was renamed "interesting" in a curtsey to the precepts of clinical medicine, as a later chapter will show.

Many physicians thought empiricist ideals could reform the many theories, systems, and authorities that governed British medicine. Henry Holland, writing in 1852, notes wearily, "During the last thirty years ... I have known the rise and decline of six or eight fashions of medical doctrine or treatment."[24] Actually, as with Frederic Jameson's nostalgic escalator, such complaints had been voiced for decades. In 1774 James Sims disparages theory as

> ... boldly parading in all the tinsel dress of fancy; varying her charms to suit the taste of every beholder; promising to her votaries the giddy admiration of all the young, thoughtless, and inexperienced; offering us present fame without laborious study, and powerful support in all the errors of our judgment, or most excentric [*sic*] wanderings of our imagination.... View on the other hand empiricism, with her slow and modest step, scarcely obtruding herself to our eyes, much less to our admiration; using no meretricious caresses to entice us ... proposing to us a life of application, care, and pains, without reward or glory.[25]

In both the vehemence of his dedication to an empirical ideal, and the (ironically) florid enthusiasm of his rhetoric, Sims represents the evangelical tone of many of his contemporaries in promoting "facts" over "theories." Latham promotes a similar ideal when he counsels students, "You may adopt this mode of case-taking, or any other ... but no method of recording the particular facts will be of any use to you, unless you have right notions concerning the *facts* themselves. The facts, in truth, *are* the case."[26] While early-nineteenth-century physicians did cultivate a sensitivity to their patients as fellow humans, treatises of this period parade an empiricism that valorizes fact and observation over sensibility and insight.[27]

Alfred Stillé, a French physician practicing in Philadelphia, usefully articulates the precepts of this medical empiricism, which he, like others, had developed during study in Paris. His emphasis on the need to professionalize medical practice through objective observation marks him as an early advocate of clinical medicine and its textual product, the clinical case history. In his classic textbook *Elements of General Pathology* (1848), he provides a clear example of the skepticism, the compensatory precision, and the ultimately ethical telos demonstrated by practitioners of mechanical objectivity as Daston and Galison have identified it—"mechanical observation," rather, given its proponents' emphasis on observation. Although he is not British, Stillé discusses this concept in terms entirely congruent with British usage. He is particularly concerned with how physicians should take cases; that is, how they should observe and record the particulars for each patient. He argues that mechanical observation is the best and most authoritative technique for the kind of writing physicians do: transcribing people's messy lives into functional, realist narratives that enable the production of scientific knowledge.

Stillé dedicates his first chapter to case-taking. He defines ideal clinical discourse as "a system of close and methodical observation, by [a] series of cases reduced to writing, and analyzed, as nearly as possible, with mathematical rigor."[28] He emphasizes the need for an almost impossible "exactness" in observing and recording the progress of disease. He stipulates a precision and comprehensiveness achieved only by enumerating absolutely everything that is present, and by refusing to record anything that is not, by banning any principle of selection and requiring the physician to suppress any subjective response—by requiring the utter abstraction of the physician from the text. He associates this exactness with mathematics and the "numerical method" (statistics). He repeatedly uses the term "mechanical" to describe this kind of objective exactness and to capture exactly the evacuation of subjective, interpretive intent that he argues is necessary to achieve truth. He suggests, in fact, that the text become a representation machine: precisely, almost automatically reproducing reality in all its details, in a direct, unmediated relation to the patient.

Stillé thus directs physicians toward the self-evacuation that Daston and Galison term "mechanical objectivity," where scientists sought to produce a text or image that was exact in every detail and free of bias, understatement, hyperbole, editing, correction, ornament, interpretation, or frame—free (if such a thing were possible) of intent. Mechanical objectivity requires an immense amount of labor. They explain, "In its negative sense, this ideal of objectivity attempts to eliminate the mediating presence of the observer.... In its positive sense, mechanical objectivity rewards painstaking care and exactitude, infinite patience, unflagging perseverance, preternatural sensory acuity, and an insatiable appetite for work."[29] What is "mechanical" about "mechanical objectivity" is not just its valorization of dispassion and automaticity but also its tolerance for drudgery; the observer should strive for the virtues of a machine, "patient, indefatigable, ever-alert." It valorizes the subjective passivity and mechanical labor of the observer, his almost automatic recording of observations, his use of instruments to ensure this automatism when possible, and the increased accuracy and plenitude of his results.[30]

Stillé champions a "mechanical ... observation" based on labor, explicitly excluding intuition or invention. His is a methodological and ethical stance, in which the physician resists exercising "an inventive or creative faculty, of a natural and inherent power of seizing truth intuitively, without the intervention of the mechanical processes which have been described" (46). To counteract readers' faith in "the vigorous sallies of speculative genius," championed in 1827 by the American physician Nathaniel Chapman, Stillé attacks those who "decry and ridicule the mechanical labour of observation" (35). He argues,

> [I wish] to contrast the results of industry and method, with those attributed to genius.... [I]n the sense of an inventive or creative faculty, of a natural and inherent power of seizing truth intuitively, without the intervention of the mechanical processes which have been described.... But [there is in medicine] a genius, not a speculative, not a poetical, not a mere fantastic faculty, but a practical genius.... It creates nothing ... it only *sees things as they are,* and discovers truth in what it sees. For the truth ... is in things and not in our minds, and the less of ourselves we introduce into our judgments, the nearer we shall approach to truth.[31]

Stillé opposes the subjective response of the man—his inventive, creative, intuitive, poetical sensibility—to a mechanical, objective observation that is passively communicated. In his rejection of invention and his endorsement of "mechanical processes" as producing "truth," Stillé depicts the ideal physician as a mere registering device, less an author than a recorder, producing "a diligent and patient description of all such things as the learned observer *has marked down* ... and *committed to writing ... without adding anything of his own*" (36).[32] By "practical genius" Stillé suggests that, as

Daston and Galison assert, at midcentury "scientific genius was nothing more than a magnification of" contemporary epistemic virtues like patience and industry.[33]

Stillé combines his extreme skepticism about the role of human subjectivity with a positivist idealism about the possibilities of a truly mechanical observation through labor. This ideal of labor resonates throughout midcentury medicine when Latham dismisses "genius, and fancy, and eloquence" in contrast to "the labour of getting possession of knowledge in the hardest possible way, by sifting every particular, and by patiently observing at the bedside" (47). Or when Stillé recommends "the labour, the humiliation of intellectual pride, the length of time, the weariness of a pursuit so nearly mechanical" in this process as a moral scourge for what he perceived as his colleagues' intellectual arrogance. The ideal of labor persists as late as 1890, when Bramwell argues that "cultivating ... the power, the habit, the method, and the love of work" is "far more important" in medical training than acquiring "mere fact-knowledge." As George Levine puts it, "This is the scientist's trope. What constitutes scientific success is not some rarefied quality of genius but sheer moral self-discipline."[34]

Despite its rhetoric of visual mastery, an ideally mechanical observation could not be more distinct from the authority and power of the Foucauldian "clinical gaze." Mechanical observation produces its scientific and moral authority from self-abnegation and laborious abasement. "[T]here is no royal road to truth!" Stillé exclaims, voicing the keynote of early-nineteenth-century empiricism: enthusiastic evangelism, paradoxically employed in the service of a dispassionate ideal, made up of equal parts painstaking observation, unceasing labor, and self-mortification. The true scientist is but a passive vehicle channeling the facts of nature to the page. This incessant labor of the scientist should, paradoxically, establish his absence, emptying out his subjectivity from his relation to the world, so that he may be inhabited by and transmit the other as nearly as possible uninflected by the self, in a version of realism's aspiration toward transparent, ideally unmediated access.[35] If, as W. J. Mitchell argues, "illusionism" is contrasted to "realism" in that illusionism allows images to master the viewer, and realism allows viewers to master the represented real, the ideal of mechanical observation offers a distinct, paradoxical version of realism in which the power or authority of the observer is created only insofar as the observer renounces will and agency in the visual field.[36]

Consistent with this ideal, midcentury medical texts praise the virtues of patience, self-restraint, and an affinity for minute detail. John Elliotson valorizes precision and accuracy in 1844 when he exclaims, "How patient and searching an eye is required to note all the phenomena of a disease!" or warns students, "[I]t is in making an accurate, careful diagnosis, that the medical practitioner chiefly shines.... It is impossible to be too minute in making a diagnosis." Charles Williams boasts that *"clinical observation* has lately done much for the advancement of the science of medicine ... because ... it is carried on with the minuteness and precision which are essential to science." And Henry Hartshorne explains, *"[S]cientific* empiricism constitutes the most rational practice attainable.... What is most wanted now, is ... more *exact observation* of clinical and therapeutic facts." This ideal of exactitude cast a long shadow; in 1890, physicians were still, like Bramwell, exhorting students, "I cannot too strongly impress upon you the necessity of cultivating your powers of observation, and of getting into the habit of noting the most minute details." It is no surprise that Bramwell titles this essay, "Cultivating the Habit of Minute Observation."[37]

Some physicians doubted the practicality of mechanical observation, although most agreed that the process would produce more accurate representations. The American physicians Jacob Bigelow and Oliver Wendell Holmes acknowledge in 1839 that "[a] perfect medical history is ... an impossibility ... [because] the act of observation is not, and never can be, reduced to a purely mechanical process." Although H. M. Bullitt, writing in 1845, insists that "clinical observation [is] an *art,"* he also acknowledges a scientific methodology in that "the signs and symptoms of disease manifest themselves in obedience to fixed and invariable laws; and that when completely observed and properly understood, they are capable of yielding uniform results." Physicians must study "the proper method of observing and appreciating them."[38] This precarious balance of competing ideals—the "science" of mechanical observation and the "art" of old-fashioned medicine—distinguishes the medical version of mechanical observation from its analogue in science. This ideal had a good deal of staying power, perhaps because it could never be realized. John Southey Warter, in 1865, chides his colleagues for their disorganized practice, noting that "[n]othing can be more vague than many notes I have seen taken,—the clerk rushes wildly from sleep to the state of the bowels; and notes the character of the pulse, in connection with the patient's history."[39] This vexed movement toward regularization and routine in scientific medicine lasted through midcentury, when experimentalist physicians like Bernard revised the strictures of pure mechanical observation to introduce a complementary speculative gaze, although the structure of the case history continued to be formalized. Stillé represented an early peak of empiricism in the 1830s, reflecting increased professionalization and the debates over Louis and statistical medicine (the "numerical method"). Indeed, the American physician Elisha Bartlett dedicated his 1844 *Essay on the Philosophy of Medical Science,* an "empiricist manifesto," to Louis.[40]

Ironically, the clinic's very obsession with detail and precision leads to an effect of excess like that the experimentalists had condemned as "Rhetorick." Replication becomes a central goal: both textual replication, a holdover of the experimentalist "virtual witnessing," and its nineteenth-century scientific analogue, reproducible results, since the imperative to record and report, under mechanical observation, cannot be lifted for later trials. The repetition compulsion inadvertently multiplies inauthenticity; the copy can neither become nor replace the original. A mechanical reproduction, that is, becomes perceived as "false because [it is] so exact." Walter Benjamin refers to something like this phenomenon when he explains that "[t]he whole sphere of authenticity is outside technical . . . reproducibility" (220).[41]

Thus it is not surprising that mechanical observation, despite its tremendous influence, remains unrealized in the case history due to an internal logical contradiction. As Stillé's vision of an immediacy of knowledge—in which the physician "sees things as they are"—bears out, mechanical observation is an ideal of visual exactitude as well as of perfect objectivity. This nineteenth-century ideal of a perfect visual relation between the real and the represented reaches its apex with the photograph, although it is never realized.[42] The ideal of objectivity is made necessary by the ultimate goal of exactitude. Stillé and his peers seek to remove the "I" behind the eye precisely because the fallibility of human subjectivity interferes with an exact mirroring of reality. But the very process of documenting visual exactitude invariably reinscribes the observer as an "absent presence" in the text. That is, the case history cannot really be a representation machine because it cannot do without the intervention of a mediating observer to produce the representation. Unlike the "truth to nature" which an eighteenth-century case history produces by constructing an image of the observer as a reliable narrator,[43] the clinical case history wants to produce truth by absenting the observer altogether. But in order to demonstrate its clinical exactitude, it must inscribe innumerable traces of his assiduous, careful work: his aptitude for detail, his collection of measurements, his meticulous comparison of minute observations. In the clinical case history, the physician must be both nowhere and everywhere at once.

The weight of fact and detail becomes a hallmark of realism more generally, and illuminates nineteenth-century literary realism. Catherine Gallagher has argued, in the context of the eighteenth-century novel, that

> [t]hose techniques that make up what Ian Watt called the novel's 'formal realism'—its wealth of circumstantial and physical detail, its delineation of characters by specific class, gender, and regional characteristics, and so forth—are all overtly illusionistic confessions that the particulars of the novel character have no extra-textual existence.... [T]he particularities had to be fully specified to ensure the felt fictionality of the character.[44]

However, at least in the nineteenth century, formal realism does not always serve as a confession of fictionality in this way. The characteristics of formal realism that Gallagher cites here are also all central to the modern case history, especially early in the clinical era, when physicians tried to record everything observed—climate, occupation, clothing—although they did not yet know what details might be relevant. This comprehensive impulse in the medical case history compels us to nuance Gallagher's insight that "realism is the code of the fictional" (174) in order to acknowledge that eighteenth-century experimentalist reports establish a long-standing association of formal realism, especially the laborious collection of detail, with the production of fact.

The clinical physician's aptitude for excruciating precision also betrays a sensibility—an individual sensitivity and perceptiveness—as marked as that of his opposite, the "speculative genius" Stillé rebuffs. It is perhaps due to this irreducible trace of subjectivity that human insight proves similarly difficult to distinguish from clinical observation, or to eradicate from the case history, as the next few chapters will show.

Clinical Discourse and the Disappearance of Sensibility

Mechanical observation's advance upon impossible objectivity becomes clear in the medical community's enthusiastic adoption of it. Henry Blanc exemplifies the physician-author's attempts to meet the standards of this ideal, in his article on "The Cold-Water and Antiseptic Treatment of Typhoid Fever" in the *Lancet* in 1875. He begins,

> [T]he following case can give rise to no objection concerning the real nature of the disease; pulse, temperature, rose spots, bronchial râles, &c., all proclaim it to be a case of typhoid fever. On the 8th of April last I was called upon to attend a Mr. P——, an American gentleman staying at the Grand Hotel, Paris. For four or five days he had considerable fever, had

kept to his room, but had not taken any medicine beyond a few aperient pills.... I found him in the following condition: skin warm, pulse frequent, tongue coated in the centre, the point and margin red and dryish; slight cough; sibilant and a few moist râles; increased dulness in splenic region; no gurgling in iliac fossa, but great tenderness on pressure; stools somewhat frequent, loose and scanty; urine high-coloured; faeces pale; no head symptoms beyond a feeling of lassitude and drowsiness.[45] (191)

This report of typhoid fever prominently exhibits many textual characteristics of a clinical narrative, including an interest in typicality; attention to detail and a visual analysis of surfaces (consider Blanc's careful assessment of the various parts of the man's tongue); and a flat clinical voice marked by specialized terminology and an implicit reference to method.[46] There are only hints of the physician's presence ("I found him"), and these are separated syntactically from the observations themselves. His staccato prose style references the antecedents of scientific prose style, in the plain speech movement of earlier centuries. However, as Blanc's use of specialized terminology (râles, iliac fossa, five grains of calomel) makes clear, the clinical voice revises the ideal of plain speech in order to accommodate the difficult language which indicates a specialized medical knowledge. The case history dramatizes the process of mechanical observation, as the uninflected prose mimics an impersonal, methodical scan of the body. In fact, this physician-author shapes his narrative to foreground his meticulous attention to detail (he reviews each of the patient's symptoms in soporific detail daily) and punctilious detachment.

Such a prose style develops an almost entirely objectifying—ostensibly more objective—view of the patient. Unlike Morgagni, Blanc tells us little about the patient as a person. In order to achieve a truly mechanical observation, the case history must set aside not only the physician's human subjectivity but also that of the patient. Blanc quickly moves from depicting the patient as an actor ("He had ... fever, had kept to his room") to those fragmenting the patient into passive, inert parts, reporting his symptoms through a decapitated syntax lacking a subject or even a verb ("skin warm, pulse frequent") and with descriptive rather than possessive phrases ("the point and margin," not "his" tongue). When Blanc describes the man's "feeling" of lassitude and drowsiness, it is clear that such details enter the case history as symptoms rather than an acknowledgment of the patient's interiority. Furthermore, Blanc presents this patient as a type; he recodes the suffering individuality of the visiting American into a mere placeholder for a norm of typhoid.[47] Blanc's commitment to clinical discourse enables him to produce this patient as a medical fact, grounded not in a broad humanity but in a formalized and rigorously policed structure of knowledge imposed upon the messy stuff of human interaction.

Evacuating the physician's sensibility or even subjectivity in this way was not greeted without controversy. The American physician David Cheever warns in 1861 of the "fallacy of statistics" in medicine due to their tendency "to ignore the subjective, and to study only the objective phenomena of disease." Bennett offers as the first of thirteen "hints" for clinical examination, "It should never be forgotten that you are examining a fellow-creature, who possesses the same sensitiveness to pain, and the same feelings as you do, and that everything that can increase the one or wound the other should be most carefully avoided. Prudence, kindness, and delicacy, are especially enjoined upon those who treat the sick." Late in the century, instructing students in "case-taking and case-recording," Bramwell praises "the man ... who acts with courtesy and kindness tempered with firmness and decision, who takes a sympathetic interest in ... his patients ... as fellow-creatures." And Pye-Smith moralizes that a physician needed not only "vast knowledge, profound learning, and the best scientific training" but also "personal qualities" such as "the sympathy which puts one in the patient's place."[48]

But if physicians themselves were theoretically permitted to indulge their subjective responses in the patient's interests, in practice their texts were not. Case history after case history records not the physician's sensibility or sympathetic bond with his patient, but the effort to achieve mechanical observation. Traces of sensibility do persist, in isolated sentimental passages, generally when the text is pressured by medical error, limited knowledge, or sensitive subject matter, as chapter 3 will show. Clinical realism's success as the normative mode of medical narrative is apparent in Blanc's haste to move away from depicting the patient as a man, toward reporting the case as an objective catalogue of symptoms. It is only such textual restraint that can adequately discipline the narrative and mark it as "science."

Literary Medical Knowledge in the *Athenaeum*

Roy Porter points to the common inclusion of medical content in a popular eighteenth-century periodical to show that educated lay readers could deploy general medical knowledge to make decisions jointly with their medical practitioners.[49] Most scholars, like Porter, had long concurred that, with the rise of the scientific profession and its journals, medical and scientific articles disappeared from general-circulation periodicals. Lawrence Rothfield, for example, comments on "the disintegration of scientific culture" in the 1860s due to the rise of specialized periodicals and the decline of the amateur scientist. However, recent research initiatives have revised this conclusion, examining science in nineteenth-century periodicals. These projects recognize that scientific content does continue in general-circulation Victorian periodicals, even when article topics are not overtly scientific.[50]

Even outside periodical publication, the literate British public was well informed of advances and controversies in Victorian medicine. Indeed, the physician Peter Latham decries the trend for medical books to find a popular readership. "Mind that you are not betrayed to commit yourselves unwarily to books (especially of modern date) upon diet and digestion, upon the liver, and the stomach," he warns students. "Unfortunately, the public is well understood to have such a relish for reading upon these subjects, that new motives have been thus let in for medical authorship, which are not very creditable. There is a demand for books of the kind; . . . and a certain kind of reputation is gained by them."[51] A century and a half later, Rothfield also notes the emergence of "popularizers and philosophers of science," commenting that medicine—due to its "long-standing association with the issues of mimesis and knowledge"—is a science well suited to travel across the border between professional and literary periodicals (10, 12).

Some major literary figures, such as Dickens and George Eliot, had personal connections with the world of science and medicine. But even among those lay readers and authors who did not, many did have access to popular medical publications, as is evident in this caricature of "The Blue Devils" (depression) by George Cruikshank (Fig. 2). The melancholy man in the picture is resisting the attacks of little devils representing suicide, alcoholism, ennui, and the like—with his copy of *Buchan's Domestic Medicine* nearby on the shelf, ironically unopened (and weighed down by another volume called *The Miseries of Human Life*). In an illustration for Wilkie Collins's "Laid Up in Lodgings," similarly, the invalid keeps Buchan and the *Medical Gazette* close at hand. Popular illustrations like these remind us that such volumes of "domestic medicine" were very popular. William Buchan's *Domestic Medicine* required a reprinting or new edition in 83 of the 102 years from its first publication in 1769 to its last in 1871.

While some popular texts might not have used clinical terms or descriptions, others did instruct lay readers in the norms of medical observation

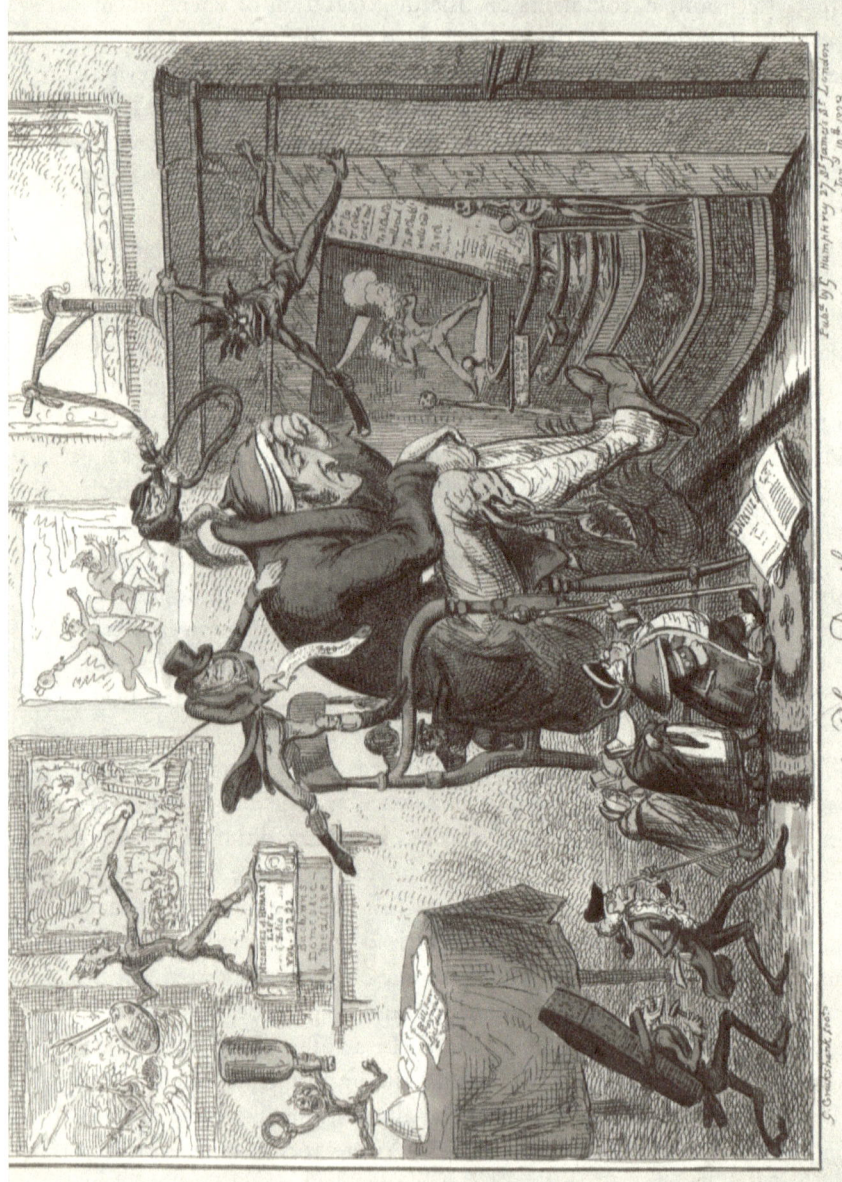

FIGURE 2. From George Cruikshank, "The Blue Devils_!!" (London: G. Humphrey, 1823).

and narrative. Maria Frawley comments on the extent to which an invalid culture encouraged immersion in the details, even clinical details, of illness.[52] Indeed, as late as 1870, the American physician Alfred K. Hills published "Instructions to Patients, How to Communicate Their Cases to a Physician by Letter," which shifts between folk and professional medical discourse, commenting both on ulcers "overgrown with what is called proud flesh," and on "particular cutaneous diseases." Hills's catalogue of symptoms illuminates for the patient the range and variety of details needed by the clinical physician for an accurate diagnosis, such as this too-vivid catechism for patients with digestive disorders:

> Is the taste natural or absent, slimy, salt, bitter, sour, foul? ... Is the patient troubled with frequent belching of wind, with or without taste,—or does it taste of the food just eaten, or of what? Is there regurgitation of fluids from the stomach, or a confluence of saliva in the mouth? ... Is there vomiting of water, saliva or mucus, of an acrimonious, acrid or bitter taste, or of a putrid taste and smell, or of a yellow, green or bloody aspect? Does the patient vomit coagulated blood, or food? ... Is the abdomen TENSE, FULL, HARD, or EMPTY and RETRACTED?

He also canvasses the range of descriptive terms for pain:

> Whether the pains are obtuse, and may be denominated dull or pressing, or whether they are sticking or piercing, rending, throbbing, perforating, pulling or drawing, pinching, scratching, gnawing, cutting, griping, burning, obtusely prickling or crawling, itching, tickling, numb or as if the part were asleep, as if from a sprain or contusion, or whether they consist of several of these sensations combined, or may be more accurately represented by other terms....[53]

Clearly, popularizing medical texts could initiate their readers into the kind of meticulous, detailed observation necessary in a medical examination.

Victorian literary periodicals can in fact be relatively authoritative sources of medical and scientific knowledge. Some periodicals were known for their scientific content. The *Athenaeum, Cornhill Magazine,* and *Macmillan's Magazine* published authors who were physicians or scientists, not "just popularizers." Accordingly, their discussions of medical science can "stage" the norms of medical observation and representation in a way that still conveys the lineaments of professional discourse. Dickens's two periodicals, *Household Words* and *All the Year Round,* were not overtly scientific, although he did regularly include popularizations of scientific material. But if some lay periodicals—generally the more intellectual ones—model and discuss the norms of medical observation and representation, they provide a crucial literary "commons" for novelists and physicians, and they enable an important relation between medical narratives and the British novel. Peterson comments, "[T]he medical profession in these years was working to monitor and limit patients' access to medical knowledge by prosecuting doctors from ... seeming to address their works too directly to lay readers. Thus the journals of home medicine, especially those produced by licensed doctors, have a potentially dubious status.... But the boundaries are uncertain."[54] Indeed, the evidence in the literary monthlies suggests that physicians seeking to augment their income through science journalism regularly published guides to the etiology of diseases and on medical procedures, even addressing matters of professional controversy. Articles might examine the problem of conflict of interest in physician researchers and expert witnesses, decry practitioners' decreased efficiency after long shifts, or lay out the differences in medical training by gender and nationality.

The *Athenaeum* (1828–1921) was one publication where nonmedical Victorian readers might encounter medical and scientific subject matter. The *Athenaeum*, a "literary" weekly, ran dozens of book reviews in each issue, including usually about half a dozen on medical or scientific books. Its reviews are brief—rarely more than a paragraph—although it also ran essays on scientific topics, especially in the regular section on "Popular Science." Its range of articles can be imagined from the title it adopted in 1830 under its most influential editor, Charles Wentworth Dilke: *The Athenaeum Journal of English and Foreign Literature, Science, the Fine Arts, Music and the Drama*. Other periodicals also reviewed scientific books—Jonathan Topham estimates that journals published over 120 reviews of the Bridgewater Treatises in the 1830s—but the *Athenaeum* demonstrates a particular commitment to the genre.[55] Like other periodicals, the *Athenaeum* also reported on meetings of medical and scientific societies and added to public discussions of the problems of professionalization and quackery, to name just two examples. It achieved a good reputation and wide circulation, up to 18,000 copies per week. The *Athenaeum* allowed general readers to develop a rich awareness of medical debates on, for example, the nature of vision, the treatment for consumption, the use of the microscope, climatological theories of disease, and the scientific method. One of its physician contributors, Edwin Lankester, reviewed over nine hundred books, largely on scientific or medical topics, for the periodical. While these reviews were generally short notices, they did reference norms of medical writing and practice.

The *Athenaeum* demonstrates that scientific knowledge was increasingly perceived as a necessary part of general knowledge. In fact, many of its reviews seem to argue for a general popular scientific education, thirty years before Arnold's and Huxley's famous exchange about "literature and science" in the university curriculum. The *Athenaeum* did differentiate between specialist and nonspecialist texts, although introductory texts might be of interest to a popular audience as well as beginning professionals. For instance, Lankester recommends John Hughes Bennett's *Outlines of Physiology* for a wide audience, since

> [t]he old practitioner of medicine, who has no time to wade through Carpenter's elaborate treatise, will find Dr. Bennett's little book a good refresher of his memory and guide to what is doing in science; whilst the general reader, anxious to get a bird's-eye view of the great facts of human physiology, will not find in our language a work at once so brief and perspicuous as this by Dr. Bennett.

Lankester's review thus indicates that the *Athenaeum* considered both a professional and a popular audience.[56]

Reviewers would distinguish more advanced texts, as when Lankester warns possible readers of A. B. Johnson's *The Physiology of the Senses*, "The work is not intended for popular readings, and is written in a condensed style, and perhaps is thus better adapted for the purpose of the student."[57] Another reviewer commented that a book on William Cullen "is of interest to the medical profession exclusively. It is, throughout, professional and technical. It is no more addressed to ordinary readers than a treatise on the possibility of asthenic inflammation or a discourse on the phrenic centre. We have, therefore, little to do beyond announcing the appearance, at length, of a second volume."[58] However, this reviewer, possibly Horace Stebbing Roscoe St. John, was not himself a physician. St. John reviewed copiously for the *Athenaeum*, but it was rare for him to review medical texts. The pattern of authorship in the reviews suggests that Lankester and another physician reviewer, Daniel Noble, were considered more accurate judges of the level of medical discourse and medical detail, that could be tolerated by the general reader.

Sometimes the medical information in the *Athenaeum* might not appear "scientific" to the twenty-first-century reader. Books on the climate of Madeira, Pau, and other destinations regularly appeared in its pages.

Lankester's review of C. Radclyffe Hall's book on Torquay reveals the medical purpose of these reviews. "Torquay will not cure consumption," he warns, "but its climate seems favourable to the alleviation of its symptoms, and prolonging the existence of those attacked by this terrible disease." Medical climatology was still an important part of the efforts to curb "that most incurable of all diseases."[59]

Readers of the *Athenaeum* would have learned, even from these brief reviews, elements of acceptable scientific method and discourse. Lankester castigates J. Francis Churchill for his theory that consumption "arises from deficient phosphorus in the blood" and his treatment with hypophosphite of lime. Churchill's cases, comments Lankester, "carry conviction to the popular mind, but unfortunately...are worth nothing to the scientific investigator of disease," since Churchill's theory is "founded on the relation of favourable cases alone."[60] Similarly, Lankester blasts Henry Lobb for writing on galvanism when "he must know that [his theory] rests on mere assertion, and that he has nowhere in his book given his readers an opportunity of judging of its correctness.... [L]et him record his cases, fairly and honestly, and his professional brethren will be able to judge of the value of his assertions."[61] Readers could learn much about normative Victorian medical methodology from a careful reading of the standards by which books are judged.

Lankester also teaches readers the value of statistics, if properly used, in a long review of George Johnson's book *On Epidemic Diarrhea and Cholera*, challenging his unusual "cure" for the disease, which was to administer a purgative like castor oil. The review approvingly cites a study performed by the Royal College of Physicians, saying that "after they collected the particulars of five thousand cases they proceeded to analyze them; and the result was, that the old rational condemned system of treating cholera by opium and astringents turned out to be by far the most successful, whilst the system of treating by castor-oil appeared to be a precursor of death." In contrast, "with regard to [Dr. Johnson's opposing] cases, we would remark [says Lankester] that they are only fifty-four in number, and quite insufficient to establish any general position with regard to treatment." Since 25 percent of Johnson's patients died, the review concludes, his cases are "worthless for establishing a sound generalization."[62] Similarly, Lankester warns seekers after a healthful climate who might buy Alexander Taylor's book on *The Climate of Pau*:

> Statistics much more copious and more accurate than any hitherto published must be obtained before we can say with certainty that the winds

and rain in one place are more propitious to health than in another.... Nor are the limited statistics published in such a work as this of much assistance. It is of little value to say that one person in every forty-five dies at Pau, whilst one only in twenty-eight dies at Naples. We must know the nature of the occupation, and all the other causes that may influence the life and health of individuals, before we can conclude from such data that the climate of Pau is more favourable to health and longevity than that of Naples.[63]

Clearly he considers that general readers should also understand exactly how its statistics fall short, and what would be required to make this epidemiological study sound.

The reviews register the growing influence of experiment in medicine. Lankester chastises John Ferguson for having written a book on the microscope when "we very much question whether he ever looked into a microscope." Homeopathy, in another review, proves "the unsoundness of any theory of medicine that will not bear the test of experiment and sound induction."[64]

Reviewers also judged books on their conformation to the contemporary norms for scientific observation and representation. Lankester briskly dismisses a "sentimental volume" titled *Stray Leaves of a Naturalist* with the comment, "[S]cience is not satisfied with admiration; it demands close observation and a rigid adherence to the true nature of things." Similarly, in a scathing critique of William Neilson's *Mesmerism in Its Relation to Health and Disease,* Noble comments,

> This work—like most of its kind—denounces doctors, exultingly proclaims the imperfections of medical science, and holds up mesmerism as the veritable panacea for nearly all our bodily ... ills. The author gives us the usual collection of wonderful cures.... To those whose perverted tastes give them a relish for such material, we may say that ... they will probably like it for its ready and rather pleasing style.

Similarly, Lankester faults Joseph Ridge's biography of John Hunter for its "assumed quaint style ... disfigured with peculiar and unusual expressions." In contrast, Noble praises *The Present State of the Theory and Practice of Medicine,* by the well-known physician John Hughes Bennett, as "eminently scientific and philosophical in its tone."[65]

Readers were occasionally treated to lengthier scientific explications. W. Desborough Cooley (whose books on geometry and ethnology had been reviewed by the *Athenaeum*) wrote a stand-alone article on the "Mystery of Inverted Vision." Cooley instructs his readers in recent theories on inverted vision, or the curious fact that we perceive images right-side-up when the retina receives them upside-down, complicated by the fact of our binocular vision, and proposes a solution:

> [I]t is evident that the images must differ [in binocular vision], inasmuch as they represent the same object or field of view, as seen from different points in the plane of the horizon; and, consequently, simple inversion, which reverses their horizontal relations, renders them quite irreconcilable.... [But] the rectification of the incongruity pointed out, and the change of the diverging into converging images, is effected by means of a peculiar though very simple arrangement. The optic nerves on leaving the orbits converge and cross each other or decussate, being perfectly united at the decussation, and then continue on till they join the brain.... [T]he images which are inverted and diverging on the retina are made to change sides, and so become converging images, before they reach the sensorium.[66]

Cooley works through this complex question, using specialized terms such as binocular vision or sensorium; his only seeming concession to a general readership is the appositive phrase that defines the term "decussate" as "cross each other."

While the articles in the *Athenaeum* were not generally written in great detail, they spanned most scientific fields. The *Athenaeum* reviews conveyed important contemporary medical conventions, discussing medical controversies or new discoveries such as the differences of opinion between legal and medical authorities on "moral insanity" and the legal status of insanity; the claims of mesmerism, homeopathy, and other forms of "quackery"; new forms of treatment with electricity or oxygen gas; anesthesia through ether, chloroform, and mesmerism; anesthesia through nitrous oxide; and the chemistry of the stomach. Optics and the use of the microscope were popular topics.

Readers of the *Athenaeum* thus participated in the expansion of "general knowledge" to include newly scientific fields of knowledge like medicine and physiology, even as those fields and their journals were becoming specialized and professionalized. This policy may have reflected the perceived need for better public awareness of science, especially sciences that, like medicine, affected everyday family life. As Lankester warns, in a review of

Francis Ramsbotham's *Suggestions in Reference to the Means of Advancing Medical Science,*

> [T]he public is unable to decide the question of what is true or false in a medical theory. As long as bishops, members of the legislature, judges, professors in our universities, are incapable of distinguishing between truth and falsehood in such systems as homeopathy, hydropathy, and a hundred other shams, the earnest and truthful medical man must be satisfied with having served his day and generation even if he has not filled his pockets. The better education of the upper classes of society is the only hope of the intelligent medical man.

The book reviews in a literary weekly like the *Athenaeum* are, it seems, necessary to preserve the integrity of professional medicine. Similarly, in a review of a book *On the Hygienic Management of Infants and Children,* Lankester decries "the almost helpless ignorance in which people live of the laws of life." He recommends William Fermer's popular *Atlas of Human Anatomy and Physiology* because "[t]he importance of raising the standard of public health is now everywhere acknowledged; and we know of no means by which this can be done so effectually as by instructing the public in the nature of those functions which, when deranged and stopped, cause disease and death."[67]

CORNHILL MAGAZINE AND *MACMILLAN'S MAGAZINE*: STAGING MEDICINE IN THE LITERARY PERIODICAL

Susan Holland states that the *Athenaeum* "devote[s]" a "far greater proportion" of its pages to medical or scientific topics than most other periodicals did.[68] It is true that the *Athenaeum* was known for its interest in scientific topics from the 1830s through the early 1850s. However, the Science in the Nineteenth-Century Periodical index demonstrates that the *Athenaeum* was far from unique in its range of content. In a volume of the *Boys' Own Paper,* relevant articles might be fanciful, like a story of a hippopotamus hunt, a cartoon mocking theories of human evolution, or a story in which the hero falls ill. Others, however, are more serious; they instruct readers in dissection and natural history or in simple chemical demonstrations. Even the *Englishwoman's Domestic Magazine* included a regular feature educating its readers on medical topics, referencing some medical authority, whether on lumbago or the medicinal properties of tomatoes. This periodical also reviewed scientific and medical texts and called, in 1856, for a college to train nurses, joining the national debate over the professionalization of medicine. At the very least, the SciPer index succeeds in demonstrating the availability of science as a topic and a discourse among lay British readers.

Cornhill Magazine (1860–1975) and *Macmillan's Magazine* (1859–1907) offer a literary diet particularly rich in medical and scientific matter. *Cornhill Magazine*, while edited by the novelist William Makepeace Thackeray from 1860–62, sought out "familiar reports of scientific discovery."[69] These were inaugurated by a series of articles on physiology by the physiologist, science writer, and literary critic George Henry Lewes, partner of the novelist George Eliot. Lewes helped edit the *Cornhill* from 1862–64. Similarly, *Macmillan's Magazine* included eminent scientists as contributors, including Francis Galton on hereditary character and an 1898 account of the infamous confrontation between Samuel Wilberforce and T. H. Huxley over evolution. Both periodicals included physicians among their contributors, such as Francis Anstie, James Sully, and Andrew Wynter writing for the *Cornhill*, and Douglas Spalding for *Macmillan's*.

The articles in the *Cornhill* and *Macmillan's*, more extensive than the *Athenaeum*'s brief reviews, are notable for the way in which they stage rigorous medical norms for a general audience. These articles combine accurate clinical observation and professional debate with a popularizing framework that made scientific medicine interesting and relevant to a lay reader. The *Cornhill* and *Macmillan's* were well-respected "shilling monthly" literary periodicals, market rivals for an educated middle-class audience, with a readership in the tens of thousands.[70] They earned a reputation for broad-ranging inquiry and openness to scientific topics, publishing favorable reviews of *Origin of Species;* indeed, *Macmillan's* first number featured Huxley on Darwin. Many of their articles were republished in other periodicals, such as *Littell's Living Age* or *The Eclectic Magazine*, demonstrating a broader interest in science among generalist Victorian periodicals.

A survey of these periodicals for 1859–1870 (roughly the first decade of publication) shows that scientific articles appear frequently. Medical articles appear at least once or twice per volume (half year). Occasionally, such as the period 1861–62 in the *Cornhill*, articles with medical or physiological content appear in almost every issue. *Macmillan's* demonstrates more consistent scientific content but less that is specifically medical, although 1862–63 saw a succession of medical articles. These periodicals demonstrate a detailed exposure to, and knowledge of, professional medical practices among the educated British middle class. It is clear, however, that the *Cornhill* and *Macmillan's* undertook their roles to popularize medicine and science, not disseminate new research. Excepting July 1862 to March 1863, when Lewes shepherded a feature called "Notes on Science," covering science news, these periodicals did not claim to cover the news of medical or scientific breakthroughs.

Many of the articles in the *Cornhill* and *Macmillan's* explicitly reference ideals of scientific discourse, even before and after the period in the early 1860s, while Lewes was most influential, that Gowan Dawson has identified as most characterized by scientific "rigour."[71] The very first issue of the *Cornhill* in 1860 features an article by the renowned surgeon Henry Thompson that tackles this issue. "Under Chloroform" acknowledges the public appetite for the sensational details of an "appalling accident" when "some unfortunate workman ... has fallen from a scaffold, or been mutilated by a railway train." Thompson also notes the "interest in any authentic account" of the operation on the victim. He decries the "remarkable combination of technical phrases culled from the brief remarks of the surgeon" quoted in the paper the next day, as they are usually erroneous ("the carotid artery was pronounced ... to be fractured"). He acknowledges not only the public interest in the details of medical practice but also the pitfalls of that interest, since "few people make more mistakes than our medical amateur who, on the strength of a weekly perusal of *The Lancet* at his club, sets up as an authority." Thompson also pokes fun at the naïveté of some physicians, as when "some very young gentleman" newly graduated from medical training, "astonishes his elderly associates" at the dinner table "with a highly-tinted sketch of some operative achievement, in which perchance he assisted." The neophyte medico holds forth on Medicine as he "complacently witnesses the admiration" of his listeners and displays his "familiarity with harrowing scenes, and ... his apparent absence of emotion," although Thompson suggests the young physician might hew closer to the truth if he were farther from the port (499).[72]

Thompson writes, then, to correct the public's "very erroneous ... notions about the nature of a surgical operation" (500). Indeed, his report of an amputation of the thigh offers a fastidiously detailed description of the operating theater, the surgical tools, and the procedure itself. Thompson reports the operation in terms that are nonspecialized yet precise: "[T]he operator, grasping firmly with his left hand the flesh which forms the front part of the patient's thigh, thrusts quietly and deliberately the sharp blade horizontally through the limb, from its outer to its inner side, so that the thigh is transfixed a little above its central axis, and in front of the bone" (503). Other articles, such as an 1863 *Macmillan's* article "On Physical Pain," by Anstie, do not sound substantially different than they might in a medical journal. Austie alludes to Sir W. Hamilton's theory that if "[p]leasure is a reflex of the spontaneous and unimpeded exertion of a power of whose energy we are conscious; [then] pain [is] a reflex of the overstrained or repressed exertion of such a power." Anstie proposes to "test the value of this theory by examining as to how far it applies to the phenomena of physical pain, as they are seen with the eyes of modern physiology and bed-side observation." His diction throughout is almost entirely in the now-well-established clinical voice, distanced, rational, expert in its statements that, for example, "neuralgia (e.g. tic douloureux, sciatica)" displays "the minimum of organic change in the affected part." In the careful delineation of referents, in his use of specialized terminology, and in his distanced, passive presentation, Anstie models the proper mode of discourse for an up-to-date, scientific practitioner. He is, of course, aware that his audience is mixed; he reaches out to his professional readers, noting at one point, "Medical readers will be at once reminded of the case of subfascial suppuration, of pleurisy and peritonitis, and of gout, respectively."[73] Physicians, as members of the professional middle classes, would of course have been likely readers of the shilling monthlies.

Although articles like these were written by professionals for a mixed audience, much of the medical science here is carefully staged: framed in a setting readily associated with the public interest, and poised or oscillating between specialist and popular discourse.[74] Thompson's piece on amputation even presents the operation in its natural setting of an ampitheater, an "operating theatre." He describes the audience waiting for the procedure to begin, the first entrants on stage, and the elements of the set ("A small table, covered with instruments, occupies a place on one side of the area; water, sponges, towels, and lint, are placed on the opposite") (502). Despite his care in describing the procedure accurately, he strategically employs melodramatic phrases: the "marvelously bright and sharp" surgical knife; the sense that "[a]ll is silence profound" before the first cut; the tourniquet that "holds life's current" (503–4). Most important, he repeatedly reminds readers that this is not only a surgical procedure that reframes a physical body but also a performance that grips an audience: after the leg has been severed, one onlooker "is heard to whisper to his neighbor, 'Five and thirty seconds: not bad, by Jove!'" and another "was observed to become very—very pale, and then slowly disappear" (503, 504). Clearly Thompson did not feel that the realities of surgery were incompatible with the imperative to attract readers' interest, although he displays some anxiety about combining surgery and spectacle when he argues, "There is no need . . . to question the taste which exhibits the details of a surgical operation to the vulgar eye" (501).

Similarly, Archibald MacLaren combines scientific and friendly commentary in a *Macmillan's* article on the makeup of the atmosphere and its effects on the lungs. He explains:

> Atmospheric air may briefly be said to consist of three gases in very unequal proportions. In 100 parts 79 will be nitrogen and 21 oxygen, with a very small quantity of carbonic acid—not more than about 5 parts in 10,000. . . . [N]othing can counteract the influence of impure air. The organs of mastication, digestion, and assimilation will all have an influence on the conversion of food into blood; but air passes through no intermediate channel.[75]

But this exposition, with its blend of chemistry and anatomy, quantitative reasoning and specialized vocabulary, appears not in an article on pulmonary anatomy but in one on "The Management of the Nursery." Typically, MacLaren balances such passages with down-to-earth language in a dramatic summary that is both memorable and accessible: "at once from lip to lung [the air] passes, and the union for good or for evil is final" (516). After the passage of dry explicatory prose, the melodramatic phrasing is welcome, and re-presents science as spectacle for the popular audience.

Other articles instruct on unlikely or even unsavory topics that seem more suited to the physician needing a survey of possible diagnoses than to the casual reader; yet they carefully frame this material so as to leaven the raw matter of knowledge with metaphor and classical allusion. An 1862 article in *Macmillan's* by the Reverend Hugh Macmillan offers a guide to the varieties of human "vegetation" (fungi and parasites). However, like the other authors here, Macmillan oscillates between scientific discourse and ordinary prose. He ventures into the intricacies of the various molds, fungi, and parasites that live upon the human body, soon plunging his readers deep in an exposition on the affliction variously known as porrigo, herpes, alopecia, tinea, scald-head, and ringworm. He veers immediately from the homely familiarity of a quotation from the thirteenth chapter of Leviticus—"if there be in it a yellow thin hair; then the priest shall pronounce him unclean"—to that symbol of medical science, the microscope: "Examined under the microscope," Macmillan notes, "the hairs are found to be considerably swollen, with nodosities here and there produced by masses of sporules or seeds embedded between the longitudinal fibres . . . the medullary portion, or the pith of the hair, is quite disorganized."[76] The disjunct styles of these contiguous sentences would be comical if it were not so typical of these periodicals' heterogeneity.

At times, the shifting perspective and tone recall the curious case history of the eighteenth century. In an article on "Corpulence," Anstie does include a fair amount of physiological fact; for instance, fat is "composed of a congeries of closed cells of large size, the walls of which are formed of a transparent structureless membrane, and among which ramify numerous capillary blood-vessels."[77] But he also brings forward the most spectacular aspects of the cases that he cites, beginning with Dr. Williams's case of "a girl who from her childhood was fat, and at the age of twenty weighed 450 lbs.; but who possessed an extraordinary degree of muscular strength, so much that at the age of six she was able to carry her own mother in her arms" (457). He also humorously includes "for the benefit of [his] stouter friends, a list of the principal measures which might have been adopted for the reduction of their bulk had they lived some fifty or sixty years ago." He warns "obese readers who may happen to be nervous to take a glass or two of sherry before reading the following list of remedies" (463). The remedies include

> bleeding from the arm; ... prolonged blistering; vegetable diet, with vinegar; ... hot baths; ... occasional starvation (to prevent apoplexy); decoction of guaiacum and sassafras, instead of wine (!); scarifications; purgatives (including the *dew collected at night*); pricking the flesh with needles during sleep; walking about with naked feet; the artificial production of grief and anxiety (if it could not be procured by natural means); and, finally, removal of the exuberant tissue with the *scalpel!* (463; his emphasis)

Anstie clearly expects this "queer therapeutical armament" (punctuated by the occasional exclamation point) to provide amusement as much as instruction to his readers. He also paces the list for greatest rhetorical effect, beginning with the more familiar remedies such as bleeding, a remnant of the old "heroic" medicine, and triumphantly concluding with the surgery, which he mocks as a "bright idea" (463).

These articles were entertaining, but readers of the shilling monthlies would also gain knowledge not only about diseases, but also about the medical profession and its norms. Anstie's article on "Medical Etiquette" for the *Cornhill*, for example, begins with a lecture on empiricism before launching into a detailed consideration of the proper behavior of "medical men" to one another and to the patient. Anstie is not entirely disinterested; he concludes that Victorian physicians do not demonstrate "any extraordinary tendency to humbug and quackery" despite "temptations... such as lawyers and divines have no idea of." Readers would doubtless have been reassured to know that, in his view, physicians are "honest, steady-going, genuine men."[78]

In fact, canny marketing is not uncommon here—even evangelizing for a particular practice, such as the new, rational medical knowledge associated with statistics. The two articles by the Rev. H. Whitehead on the Broad Street Pump ("an episode in the cholera epidemic of 1854"), for example, garner public interest through, first, their appeal to a perennial concern of British readers—cholera reached England four times from 1832–65—and second, its humanization of an intransigent public health problem. Like clinical physicians, and in the tradition of public health reform, Whitehead uses statistics to localize and quantify the threat of infection around the sources of impure water. Thus he offers evidence like the following:

> nearly 700 persons having been fatally seized, in that short time, within a circuit of 250 yards radius from the point of junction between Broad Street and Cambridge Street. Such was the intensity of the outbreak, that of 45 contiguous houses... only 4 escaped without a death; and at an average distance of 15 yards... were 4 houses which collectively lost 33 inhabitants.

He also attends to the development of disease over time, noting that

> though the *deaths* were as numerous on the 3d and 4th of September as on the 1st, yet the greatest number of fatal *attacks* occurred on the 1st, after which there were fewer fatal attacks on each succeeding day, the number positively decreasing 50 per cent. on the 3d as compared with the 2d, and 10 per cent. on the 2d as compared with the 1st.[79]

Referencing both Edwin Lankester and John Snow, both well-known public health reformers intimately involved in responding to the outbreak, Whitehead, although not a physician, clearly delineates what *counts* and what *doesn't count* as evidence in the nascent field of epidemiology and public health. In particular, he rebels against a piece of folk wisdom—still accepted by traditionalist physicians for puerperal fever—that "whilst pestilence slays its thousands, fear slays its tens of thousands" (114). In a rhetorical move worthy of the best clinical medical writing of the century,

Whitehead puts this notion in its place by reference to a case study, with all its facts and statistics:

> apart from all question of expediency, is this notion true? In St. James's Workhouse, situated within the fatal area, and filled with the old, the infirm, and the idle, the very class of persons likely to be afraid, the deaths in 1854 were only 1 per cent. of the inmates, instead of 10 per cent. as in the neighbouring streets. (114)

Indeed, Whitehead interviews one old inmate who testifies to his fear, and yet he survived. This kind of anecdotal reference not only serves as evidence but also humanizes and sensationalizes the elements of clinical prose—the facts and statistics, the specialist language, and the meticulous, impersonal logic—that he also offers.

Like the *Athenaeum*, the *Cornhill* and *Macmillan's* offer the literate public a rich and detailed awareness of medical practice and debates. While the articles strive for an authoritative tone and inform the public about the increased importance of science in medicine, their lively writing also argues for the relevance of science to everyday life. Other periodicals may not have offered as much medical content. But the circulation and status of *Cornhill* and *Macmillan's* ensured that educated lay readers, including most Victorian novelists, could be well-informed about the sometimes controversial shift toward scientific medical practice, including the textual characteristics produced by clinical observation and representation; while the memorable staging of the writing suggests the availability of such topics for more literary uses.

Moreover, because these periodicals asked physicians to write and review for them, they created a space where physicians' and novelists' texts circulated equally. Physicians and novelists were not just reading the same pages, as literate "men of letters," but some were actually writing in the same pages, for the same audience. Victorian periodical publishing makes evident how readily, then, physicians and novelists might share some of the same writerly resources, some of the same modes of seeing and stating.

CHAPTER THREE

The Sentimental Eye in Dickens and Gaskell

In Charles Dickens's novel *Dombey and Son,* Captain Cuttle gustily admires his friend, Sol Gill, who sells scientific instruments. Cuttle comments, "He's chockfull of science ... it's a fine thing to understand 'em. And yet it's a fine thing not to understand 'em. I hardly know which is best. It's so comfortable to sit here and feel that you might be weighed, measured, magnified, electrified, polarized, played the very devil with; and never know how."[1] Actually, Sol Gill, this "man of science," is hardly a master at reading and knowing his world, and Dickens's affectionate skepticism for the capabilities of Cuttle and Gill alike rests on a greater suspicion of "science" as a hermeneutic. Indeed, Dickens's portrayals of illness and death are noted for their sentimentality more than any scientific expertise.[2]

Despite the critical *donné* that sentimentality is "in fundamental, purposeful opposition" to the mimetic tradition of realism,[3] a sentimental circulation of affect persists between clinical physician and sufferer in particular cases. That is, clinical medicine occasionally adopts a sentimental stance, whether melodramatically, to substitute for "curious sights" of an earlier period; nostalgically, in pursuit of the old ideal of sensibility and insight; or—as I will argue—strategically, to provide a familiar explanatory narrative when clinical medicine falters. Interestingly, sentiment in the case history does not seem to disrupt the convention that these are generically realist texts. These cases do not seem anxious over their occasional lapse into sentimental language, despite evidence that these authors were well aware of the clinical paradigm. Rather, the sentimental narrative usefully compensates for and supplements the inevitable failures of medical practice, so that they become ubiquitous, normative, and in a sense necessary. Sentimentalism also provides a respectable harbor in the clinical case history for the affective energy of the curious. Although ostensibly rejected by clinical ideals of observation and representation, sentimentalism remains influential in the case history.

At the same time, novelists like Charles Dickens and Elizabeth Gaskell redirect the visual techniques of clinical realism selectively, to heighten ultimately sentimental insights. They adapt clinical observation provisionally, in the service of a decidedly nonclinical end; their narratives suggest that, in fiction at any rate, clinical observation and a more sentimental gaze cannot coincide but may have a symbiotic relationship. Dickens in particular could have been familiar with the norms of both "regular" and curious medicine. He was friendly with John Elliotson, a renowned professor of clinical medicine; and Dickens was interested in and even practiced mesmerism, an alternative medicine Elliotson championed at great cost to his career. In these novels, then, it is "a fine thing" to borrow the representational instruments of the clinic—to "understand them"—but the narrator ultimately renounces them for an emphatically nonscientific understanding.

It is possible to say of both Dickens and Gaskell that, as Miriam Bailin says, "Illness in Dickens's fiction is the *sine qua non* both of restored or reconstructed identity, and of narrative structure and closure."[4] Both rely overtly on the sentimental eye, and less obviously on clinical observation, to effect this aim. Dickens also makes reference to the curious sight of the eighteenth-century physician: individualized, saturated with sensibility, in which a patient's pathological body readily indexes his/her spiritual state of health or disease. While Dickens does rehabilitate the curious in his memorable grotesques, he uses sentimental sights as much as spectacular ones to accomplish the forceful solicitation of affect. As this chapter will argue through a reading of Dickens's two most famous sentimental deathbeds (in *The Old Curiosity Shop* and *Dombey and Son*), he frames these scenes carefully, alternating between clinical observation and sentimental sights, and combining the logical force and material detail of the suffering body with the dramatic emotional energy of grief and regret. The sentimental scene functions as a curious sight; it spectacularly solicits the visual and affective participation of the reader, allowing Dickens to marry a sentimental aesthetic with the social reformist ideals we associate with Victorian realism.

Similarly, Gaskell's *Ruth* uses medical discourse to drive home an ethos so spiritual it threatens to bypass the very world it painstakingly registers. The clinical representation of Ruth's fever ironically becomes a means by which to transcend realism and affirm another narrative altogether, powered by sympathy and producing insight into moral virtue. Gaskell's narrative and its concerns make use of a clinical observation to surpass medicine and the body, to make its modes of knowledge only a transparent medium to the spiritual view beyond, to make the invisible visible. While Gaskell's sentimental scenes are less spectacular than Dickens's, perhaps because her work is less influenced by Victorian melodrama, both novelists strikingly abandon clinical observation at the deathbed. Clinical medicine serves in these novels as a means only, and to a very different end.

Sympathy and Sentiment

Nineteenth-century sentimental fiction takes as its ostensible aim the production of the reader's sympathy for others, although the narrator's own paraded sympathy can also take center stage. Similarly, much of the criticism on sentiment traces "sentiment" to its eighteenth-century roots in sensibility and the virtuous circulation of sympathy.[5] Fred Kaplan and others have discussed the importance of eighteenth-century theories of the moral sentiments to Victorian sentimentality.[6] However, a distinction between sympathy and sentiment remains useful. Sentiment is usually associated with the ungrounded excesses of romance or melodrama; it is a bad copy of sincere affect, a hyperbolic version of emotion that verges on the spectacular in its active solicitation of the reader's or viewer's response.[7] Sympathy, in contrast, can be aligned with either romance or realism; indeed, it is fundamental to the work of an exemplary realist like George Eliot. If Laurence Lerner defines sentiment as a delightful sadness, sympathy might be usefully considered as a *not*-delightful sadness: the circulation of affect in cases where that circulation might in fact be uncomfortable or unpleasant.[8] Such a distinction allows us to distinguish between the kind of easy, pathetic melancholy of Paul's death, in Dickens's *Dombey and Son,* and the painful realization of Adam's despair, in George Eliot's *Adam Bede.* While novelists' attempts to elicit a romantic sympathy often slide into sentimentalism, Gaskell combines realist and romantic techniques, flirting with sentiment but not entirely succumbing, to draw from readers an unwilling sympathy for the fallen woman, Ruth. This chapter argues that what is sometimes termed "the sentimental eye" is not entirely antipathetic to the clinical one: that physicians use it strategically; and that novelists produce the romanticized image of the sentimental body by combining sentimental and clinical observation.

The phrase "the sentimental eye" suggests the centrality of vision to the production and communication of sentiment. Sympathy has long been theorized as a visual process, from its early exposition in Adam Smith and David Hume to more recent examinations in literary criticism. In his *Treatise of Human Nature* (1739–40), Hume emphasizes the visual transmission of affect in the sympathetic relation. He explains,

> When I see the *effects* of passion in the voice and gesture of any person, my mind immediately passes from these effects to their causes, and forms such a lively idea of the passion, as is presently converted into the passion itself. In like manner, when I perceive the *causes* of any emotion, my mind is convey'd to the effects, and is actuated with a like emotion.[9]

He here considers sympathy a mechanical visual process: in which particular visual stimuli automatically trigger particular affective responses.

Discussions of sympathy also often turn to perspectival analogies. The visual basis of Hume's ethics drives his discussion of the "common point of view," in his 1751 treatise, *Enquiry Concerning the Principles of Morals* (IX. i.272). Similarly, Adam Smith, in the *Theory of Moral Sentiments* (1759), argues, "We endeavour to examine our own conduct as we imagine any other fair and impartial spectator would examine it."[10] He makes an analogy between the limitations of physical and moral sight, explaining,

> As to the eye of the body, objects appear great or small, not so much according to their real dimensions as according to the nearness or distance of their situation; so do they likewise to what may be called the natural eye of the mind.... [T]o the selfish and original passions of human nature, the loss or gain of a very small interest of our own, appears to be of vastly more importance ... than the greatest concern of another with whom we have no particular connexion.... Before we can make any proper comparison of those opposite interests, we must change our position. We must view them, neither from our own place nor yet from his, neither with our own eyes nor yet with his, but from the place and with the eyes of a third person, who has no particular connexion with either, and who judges with impartiality between us. (191–92; III.iii)

A shift in vision crucially produces a shift in understanding, in passion, and thus in sympathy. Morality in this tradition is the affective knowledge produced by the visual relation between seer and seen.

That relation is not evenly distributed between subject and object; in this sense, the "sentimental eye" shares more than it acknowledges with clinical observation. Audrey Jaffe considers sympathy as the visual relation between spectator and spectacle, arguing that "[s]pectacle depends upon a distinction between vision and participation, a distance that produces desire in a spectator."[11] Although affect circulates freely (according to Hume, almost automatically) in the relation between sufferer and sympathizer, vision operates unidirectionally, in a spectacular relation of scopic mastery and distance that counters and to some extent undoes the commonality asserted by the exchange of affect. (The sufferer may indeed see the narrator, but that perspective is usually passive and unrepresented, except in expressions of gratitude.) Sympathy, argues Jaffe, "denies its object agency and intention" (92).[12]

The clinical and sentimental modes also share a topos; for if sympathy is constitutively produced by vision, it is triggered by a particular vision, that of the suffering body. Hume explains,

> Were I present at any of the more terrible operations of surgery, 'tis certain, that even before it begun, the preparation of the instruments, the laying of the bandages in order, the heating of the irons, with all the signs of anxiety and concern in the patient and assistants, would have a great effect upon my mind, and excite the strongest sentiments of pity and terror.[13]

For Hume, seeing even the anticipatory suffering of the waiting patient sparks a sympathetic response. Smith echoes him, "That pain which is occasioned by an evident cause, such as the cutting or tearing of the flesh, is, perhaps, the affection of the body with which the spectator feels the most lively sympathy."[14] Again, the notional "spectator" is construed as an observer of specifically surgical experience—perhaps sitting in the operating theater of a teaching hospital. Ironically, Smith calls upon this sympathy to replace the bridge of feeling that does not naturally exist between bodies:

> As we have no immediate experience of what other men feel, we can form no idea of the manner in which they are affected, but by conceiving what we ourselves should feel in the like situation. Though our brother is upon the rack, as long as we ourselves are at our ease, our senses will

never inform us of what he suffers. They never did, and never can, carry us beyond our own person, and it is by the imagination only that we can form any conception of what are his sensations.... By the imagination we place ourselves in his situation, we conceive ourselves enduring all the same torments, we enter as it were into his body.... His agonies, when they are thus brought home to ourselves, when we have thus adopted and made them our own, begin at last to affect us, and we then tremble and shudder at the thought of what he feels.... When we see a stroke aimed and just ready to fall upon the leg or arm of another person, we naturally shrink and draw back our own leg or our own arm; and when it does fall, we feel it in some measure, and are hurt by it as well as the sufferer. (3–4, I. i.1)

This sympathetic response to viewing a suffering body, it was thought, can extend to create not only affect but actual sickness in the observer. Hume notes, "[T]is certain we may feel sickness and pain from the mere force of imagination, and make a malady real by often thinking of it."[15] Smith examines this at length, commenting,

> Persons of delicate fibres and a weak constitution of body complain, that in looking on the sores and ulcers which are exposed by beggars in the streets, they are apt to feel an itching or uneasy sensation in the corresponding part of their own bodies.... Men of the most robust make, observe that in looking upon sore eyes they often feel a very sensible soreness in their own, which proceeds from the same reason; that organ being in the strongest man more delicate than any other part of the body is in the weakest.[16]

Seeing suffering underscores the affinity between bodies by affirming both the connection and the essential distinction between feeling and observing pain. The visual character of sympathy and sentiment thus facilitates the shifting perspective, in the texts I examine, between a clinical observation and a sentimental eye.

Much of the criticism on sympathy and sentiment focuses on the relation between text and reader: how the text produces a certain kind of reader.[17] The tradition of sympathy as a visual process has encouraged literary critics to examine the relation of reader to text as a visual relation between spectator and spectacle.[18] I, am, however, more interested in the relation between the author or narrator and the text: how authors produce a text and, implicitly, a particular kind of knowledge, through the circulation of affect (suffering and sympathy), prompted by the visual spectacle of the pathetic object. Both novels and medical texts posit that knowledge as insight, in an implicit reference to the product of an eighteenth-century notion of sensibility, but they also both rely on a structure of spectacle and sentiment allied to the curious sights of eighteenth-century medicine, that suggests a more invasive relation to the object than the unalloyed benevolence claimed by sensibility and insight.

My focus on the author-text relation does not deny, however, that the text often solicits a reader's affective response and that securing the reader's supposedly enlarged vision of sympathy is often ostensibly the reason for sentimental narrative. James Fitzjames Stephen, writing in 1864 with a legal interest in the validity of evidence, castigates this strategy as unfair. He condemns "the influence which novels exercise, not in their proper and natural sphere as amusements and works of art, but as irregular and informal arguments" based on "an appeal to feelings, and to feelings for their own sake." Because "[a] novelist never lays down a proposition properly limited and supported," the putative arguments of novels "can hardly ever be ... distinctly attacked or defended." Thus, he explains, "the sting of the imputation of being a sentimental writer. It is a way of charging people with being either weak, or dishonest, or both. It implies that a man tries to gain his ends not by legitimate means, but by appeals to the passions."[19] Despite Stephen's pronounced skepticism, the texts examined in this chapter demonstrate that the sentimental appeal to the passions was considered not only an admissible but even a compatible corollary to the more rational arguments of realism.

Dilatation of the Heart: The Professional Insights of Sentimental Medicine

Sentimentality is said to be "the discourse of the heart." It is thought to be "a natural, emotional response, a reflex of universal human nature instead of a particular form of cultural competence."[20] It isn't, of course; it's cultural, a learned response. And because of its constitutive link to sympathy, conventionally grounded in the suffering body, sentiment has a cultural—in fact a generic—relation to medicine. The sentimental eye can thus serve in the nineteenth century as a workable stand-in for the eighteenth-century physician's sensibility and insight, although it appears only sporadically and often strategically.

When nineteenth-century physicians campaigned for clinical observation and the formal, objective, and professional discourse that serves as their realist aesthetic, they explicitly rejected eighteenth-century medicine's curious sights and their affective pull on the spectator. Although case histories still invoke a curious sight to describe rare or spectacular cases, the nineteenth-century physician often turns to the euphemism "interesting" to mask his interest in what earlier he would have termed "curious."

"Interest" could also be suspect, however. Although clinical physicians surely use the term "interesting" to mean "worthy of further study," the alternate meaning, in which "interest" connotes prejudicial influence rather than scholarly attention, endangers its currency. "Interesting" suggests not only "of interest" but also "calling forth the emotion (especially the pity and sympathy) of observers." It descends from the eighteenth-century tradition of sensibility, in which virtue could be indexed by an observer's susceptibility to being moved by the sufferings of another. In particular, the term is a staple of the sentimental novel, where it is closely linked with emotion, especially the painful emotions of distress. A scene described as "interesting" aims to evoke sympathetic identification, exactly what should be avoided by the clinical observer.[21] An "interesting condition," for example, suggests the sensations called forth in the observer by contexts which emphasize a woman's physical and emotional vulnerability, so that childbirth is seen as an "interesting and painful function."[22]

The continuing presence of "interesting" cases illustrates how strongly subjective knowledge persists in clinical medicine. The discourse of the "interesting" points to a distanced, judicious observation while not quite concealing the emotion that motivates it. The term "interesting" in mid-nineteenth-century medical texts complicates their claim to a distanced objectivity even as this term is called upon to help execute the shift to that objectivity. "Interesting" substitutes for—and to some extent obscures—the tradition of "the curious" in the case history, but it does not eradicate it; in fact, like the sentiment that it evokes, the "interesting" enables the perpetuation of curious cases. An "interesting" sentimental rhetoric most often appears in difficult cases as a supplement, not a challenge, to clinical observation. This is perhaps why sentiment drops off sharply in the case history (although it does not disappear altogether) late in the century after the establishment of germ theory, which provided an alternate and powerful explanatory narrative for many fatal cases.

While "interesting" codes sentiment without directly referencing it, some medical texts display overt sentiment, more often in auxiliary texts such as prefaces or students' guides than in individual cases. For example, the preface to Alonzo T. Keyt's treatise on cardiac medicine offers a remarkable juxtaposition of clinical observation with an elegiac sentimentalism about the author, who died (ironically, of heart disease) before publication:

Alonzo Thrasher Keyt, M.D., died suddenly, without premonition, from paralysis of the heart, on the 9th of November, 1885, in the fifty-ninth year of his age. The post-mortem examination revealed calcareous granules in the segments, with incompetency of, [sic] the mitral valve, atheromatous degeneration in the heart and aorta, fatty and friable condition of the cardiac muscles, and dilatation of the left cavities.[23]

As the preface continues, more personal details emerge: "Dr. Keyt was aged prematurely from overwork"; "in this labor of his love and life he was insensible alike to the suggestions of hunger or fatigue"; and finally, after an extended encomium, "His life-work is ended, but its fruits remain" (iii). The preface goes on to discuss the organization of the book, in an odd return to functional knowledge after the heartfelt tribute. Such a passage combines the postmortem report on the corpse with a eulogy for the man, and suggests something of Keyt's grieving colleagues' difficult task in rendering appropriate homage while remaining professional.

Medical treatises do occasionally indulge in a sentimental or even melodramatic scene. In another example from cardiac medicine, Arthur Sansom warns that the pain of angina pectoris is "of terrible significance." He explains,

[I]f you have once seen a pronounced example of it, you will never forget it. The patient suddenly sits up in his bed, and with a cry of horror indicates his sense of pain at the praecordium.... The face wears a look of horror, the hue is pale or slightly leaden, and a cold sweat breaks out upon the forehead. Worse than the pain is the feeling of fearful sinking and depression; the poor patient gasps, "I shall die!" and, sometimes, as in a case which it was once my lot to witness, his short, but concentrated sufferings in a few minutes end in death.[24]

The practice of recording the last words of a patient like this nearly always results in a poignant scene. Sansom's description of dyspnoea in cardiac disease is affecting because the patient is reduced to gestures and moans. Dyspnoea begins when

the patient gasps restlessly, there is an instinctive craving for more air to oxygenate the sluggish blood in the lung; there is *air-hunger* as the Germans expressively term it.... [I]n the later stages ... the patient cannot lie down; perhaps can scarcely recline from the perfectly upright position: the whole mental energies seem bent upon the one task of getting air into the chest. (33)

The patient's extremity becomes here so pronounced that Sansom turns to a fellow-physician to convey the awful gravity of the situation. "I will quote the graphic words of Hope," he says.

> With eyes widely expanding and starting, eyebrows raised, nostrils dilated, a ghastly and haggard countenance, and the head thrown back at every inspiration, [the patient] casts around a hurried distracted look of horror, of anguish, and of supplication; now imploring in plaintive moans or quick, broken accents and half-stifled voice, the assistance already often lavished in vain; now upbraiding the impotency of medicine, and now, in an agony of despair, dropping his head on his chest, and muttering a fervent invocation for death to put a period to his sufferings. (33–34)

James Hope, a former president of the Royal Medical Society of Edinburgh, does not end there in the original but describes the patient's "interval of delicious respite," his "hope that the worst is over," the turn for the worse, when "hope vanishes," with "slumber fraught with the horrors of a hideous dream," and the final curtain: "The patient gasps, sinks, and expires."[25] No melodrama could be as exciting, as horrifying, or as pitiful as the "paroxysm described" in this medical treatise by a respected clinical physician.

When sentiment appears in individual cases, the cases tend to be unusual; to indicate the limits of medical knowledge and practice; to examine consumption (tuberculosis), the heart, fatally ill children, or the process of generation; or to end badly. Such cases can shake the professional stance nominally conveyed by clinical discourse. Cases that combine any of these triggers are most likely to challenge professional competency and to employ sentimental language.[26] Puerperal fever is a potent site for divisiveness over medical knowledge and standards of care. It also courts sentimental rhetoric due to its pathetic combination of mother and child, sometimes both condemned by this agonizing infection, which could not be effectively treated before the antibiotic era and often ended in death. Worse, it was suggested (accurately, as it turns out) that the fever was transmitted by the practitioners themselves, compounding medical ignorance with actual culpability. It is not surprising, then, that many case histories of puerperal fever retreat into a sentimental mode at some point, no matter where they stand in the debate over its etiology.

Sentimental language is also surprisingly prevalent in cardiac cases. John Ferriar in 1810 offers a wrenching portrait of William Cavanagh, a nine-year-old boy who suffered from "Dilatation of the Heart." Ferriar's description is pathetic in the details he chooses to tell, rather than in extraordinary rhetorical flourishes. "Every pulsation shook him strongly," Ferriar explains,

> and he was so much distressed, as to be unable to lie down, or to rest above a few minutes, in any other posture than leaning on a table breast-high, upon his forehead and elbows.... He never complained of any pain in the chest. Under these complaints he struggled upward of three weeks, growing worse from day to day, and at last expired without any agony.[27]

In another of Ferriar's cases,

> E.H. aged eleven, belonged to an unfortunate family, which was reduced to pass the winter of 1789 in a cold damp cellar, without beds, and very thinly clothed. They slept on tattered pieces of carpet, covered with a little straw. A fever soon arose among them, but it was this girl's lot to be seized with a violent palpitation of the heart. Every stroke of the pulsation raised up her clothes, so as to be visible at some distance, but the apex of the heart was felt nearly in the usual place. (205–6)

In Ferriar's cases, the juxtaposition of medical observation ("the apex of the heart") with hints of sentiment ("he never complained," "it was this girl's lot") demonstrates how the demands of clinical narrative conflict with those of human sensibility. He does acknowledge, however, in discussing "the sufferings of the patients," "[s]ometimes, as was Cavanagh's case, it is dreadful to witness them" (209). Tellingly, Ferriar does not admit his subjective involvement in Cavanagh's case while describing the case itself. Rather, he acknowledges his sympathy in a later passage. While sympathy is thought to enlarge the heart, Ferriar thus suggests that his own, figurative "dilatation of the heart," while an admissible element of a physician's sensibility, must wait until his clinical observation is done.

Indeed, sentimentalism also appears in cases that are not "interesting"— that are not obviously pitiable. Charles J. B. Williams, for example, turns to an evocative, emotional discourse in 1870 to demonstrate his insight when his patient, the late Earl St. Maur, dies amid accusations about the efficacy of Williams's treatment. The earl died of suffocation due to aneurysm; the earl's mother accused Williams of malpractice, and he sued her for libel. Although Williams generally relies on clinical observation and discourse, at critical moments he allows his rhetoric to flower to express the extremity of the situation, as when he considers "the painful duty of fully communicating my fears to the Duchess," specifically "the formidable nature of the suspected malady, and of the fearful results to which it would probably lead."[28] Williams's narration of the deathbed scene is especially sentimental. When Lord St. Maur suffers "the most severe laryngeal spasm that I ever witnessed," Williams describes him as "throwing his arms about in great distress" and adds, "In a hoarse whisper, he said, 'Do something for me, or I shall die.' These were his last words." Even a slight stirring some time later is "but the flickering of the lamp before its final extinction" (24, 27–28). To excuse his inability to prevent "the death of the sufferer," Williams offers a double-barreled description of "this strangling spasm—this awful death-blow" drawing equally on clinical and sentimental discourses. "[I]n the course of two or three minutes of frightful struggle for breath through a tight hissing glottis," he explains,

> the voice was reduced to a hoarse whisper, then silenced for ever; the eyes fixed in a ghastly stare, with widely dilated pupils; the face overspread with the pallid hue and clamminess of death; the features set in rigidity; the jaws firmly closed; and consciousness so suspended that even the surgeon's knife elicited neither movement nor sound. (29)

To cap the case, he offers a dramatic analogy to the unwise exertions of his friend and colleague, Liston, who, "[a]lthough strongly and repeatedly warned ... would not abandon his favorite exercises, and in six months the strong man was a corpse" (30). Remarkably, Williams follows "this melancholy history" with a statistical analysis detailing "34 cases of aneurysm of the arch of the aorta, attended with fits of difficult breathing," a conjunction that attests to the contested imperatives this particular case strives to fulfill (28, 36ff).

Williams's use of sentiment here likely defends against the perceived threat to his professional authority. In another source, discussing the "intellectual and moral greatness of [the medical] art," he similarly draws on sentimental rhetoric to finesse a challenging situation: "[I]f you would see the moral influence of medicine depicted in its liveliest hues, I would ask you to contemplate a domestic scene—a family whose hearts are wrung with a dreadful anxiety for one vibrating between life and death." He exclaims, "What a ministering angel does the physician seem! How they watch his every look! With what breathless eagerness do they hang on his words! and those words, how they wing themselves, to the souls of the hearers for sorrow or for joy!"[29] Williams uses affect-laden phrases—"hearts are wrung," "ministering angel"—to paint the family's relief from "dreadful anxiety" as a type of the spiritual and moral healing that the physician can also accomplish. By dwelling so insistently on the family's pathetic sorrow and anxiety, Williams can elicit in his readers a similar pathos and relief, replicating in his prose the work of the imagined ministering physician. Such rhetoric prompts sympathy for the patient's family but also, more importantly, empathy for the physician. No matter how this particular case turns out ("for sorrow or for joy"), the physician cannot be at fault, in any sense of the term.

While sentiment has clear utility in fatal or disputed cases, it also moderates successful cases, as in a factory worker's injury reported in the *Dublin Medical Press* in 1846. The case history reports that "an accident of a very serious description took place at [a] chocolate and mustard manufactory" when

> William Paine, a youth of 18 years of age, engaged in what is called the mustard cellar, got into the chocolate department, and into the cutting-room. While there, he took up a cake of the prepared chocolate, and was about to place it under the 'cutters,' when a part of the machinery, with which he was surrounded, caught hold of his smock frock on the left side, and instantly whirled him into the most dangerous part of the works. The poor fellow's cries brought several of the workmen to his assistance, and the engine was promptly stopped; but ... his right arm was shattered in a very shocking manner.[30]

The surgeon amputated the arm cleanly and quickly, an operation which "the unfortunate youth bore with amazing fortitude," and he was reported as "going on favorably." Why, then, the sentimental evocations of "the poor fellow's cries," the "shocking manner," "the unfortunate youth," and his "amazing fortitude"? These could indicate the extreme trauma common to such factory accidents (a phenomenon virtually unknown just decades earlier), when human meets machine, combined with youth and inexperience. The boy was perhaps fresh from the country, still wearing the rural "smock frock" that many urban workers changed for safer clothing; and while not the youngest of factory workers in 1846, Paine is described as a "youth" and had apparently just started work in the cutting-room. Such cases may also trigger more-than-usual narrativizing (as in the relatively complex description of the events leading up to the accident) and express the narrator's sense of human commonality and vulnerability in an alien environment "surrounded" by deadly machines.

Sentiment also marks cases of disability, even when they report successes, as recent critical work on disability and melodrama also suggests.[31]

William Carpenter offhandedly refers to "[t]hose unfortunate beings, in whom the cerebrum is but little developed" and "those lamentable cases" of the deaf and dumb.³² Such comments imply the physician's identification with, even as they definitively mark his difference from, the patient. Similarly, in the Jacksonian Prize Essay of 1866, William Paul Swain comments, "It is every one's experience with what facility the unfortunate possessors of the most deformed knee-joints move about with the help of some simple apparatus."³³ His reference to "every one's experience" draws an imagined community of able-bodied physicians sympathetic to, but distinct from the "unfortunate" disabled.³⁴ Such cases attempt to recuperate the sensibility of the eighteenth-century physician, supplementing the limitations of clinical medicine with insight, here instantiated as sentiment.

Sentimental Medicine in Dickens

If the sentimental gaze is permitted in certain medical contexts, as an oblique gesture toward the tradition of physician insight or a means of drawing close a community of observers, it is welcomed in a particular current of the Victorian novel, marked by a spectacular, almost aggressive sentimentality. Such novels assert a complex causative link between curious sights, sentimental fiction, affective power, moral insight, and the social value of the genre. That current reaches a groundswell in Dickens, as his competitor Thackeray knew to his chagrin. An early biographer explains,

> [I]t was Thackeray's delight to read each number [of *Dombey and Son*] with eagerness as it issued from the press.... When it had reached its fifth number, wherein Mr. Charles Dickens described the end of little Paul with a depth of pathos which produced a vibratory emotion in the hearts of all who read it, Mr. Thackeray seemed electrified at the thought that there was one man living who could exercise so complete a control over him. Putting No. 5 of "Dombey and Son" in his pocket, [Thackeray] hastened down to Mr. Punch's printing-office ... dashed it on the table with startling vehemence, and exclaimed, "There's no writing against such power as this—one has no chance! Read that chapter describing young Paul's death: it is unsurpassed—it is stupendous!"³⁵

If the aim of sentimental fiction is to collapse the distance between page and reader in an act of identification, the death of Paul fails for at least one reader: for Thackeray, Dickens's writing apparently brought him not the "vibratory emotion" of the nerves associated with sympathy, but the "electrified" force of professional envy.[36] It pushed him to a more acute awareness of the narration as fiction and craft instead of pulling him into the scene itself.

Despite my caveat, this anecdote, if only in its retrospective insistence on the "vibratory emotion" in "all who read it," testifies to the cultural staying power of Dickens's particular brand of sentimental medicine. Other readers were similarly moved by Paul's death.[37] But death from what? Consumption? The novel is frustratingly unclear. Dickens describes only vague symptoms: Paul is "fragile"; his head "had long been ailing more or less, and was sometimes very heavy and painful" before he collapses at school, with the room reeling around him; the Apothecary proclaims his "want of vital power" and "great constitutional weakness"; he has a "palpitating heart" when anxious and is "very thin, and light, and easily tired," feeling "unwell and drowsy" the night of the party.[38] These are enough to suggest consumption, but not quite enough to realize, rather than spiritualize, the disease. His illness is rendered less real by its context in a chapter insisting on Paul's moral and emotional connection to all around him, as he drifts farther from the world of action. Instead of describing a harsh cough, sharp chest pain, hemorrhage, or night sweats, Dickens insists that Paul is "old-fashioned," that he wishes to be well remembered by his schoolmates, that he feels borne away by "the rushing river" and listens to "what the waves were always saying."[39] Such ambiguity is common in the deathbeds of sentimental fiction; when illness is specified it is usually one, like consumption or a weak heart, that is readily spiritualized.[40]

Little Nell's death is also renowned for its pathos.[41] After a protracted buildup, in which readers see the pathetic figure of the grandfather deluding himself into thinking that "she sleeps," Dickens permits his audience to view the death, albeit in retrospect:

> She had been dead two days. They were all about her at the time, knowing that the end was drawing on. She died soon after daybreak. They had read and talked to her in the earlier portion of the night, but as the hours crept on, she sunk to sleep.... Waking, she never wandered in her mind but once, and that was of beautiful music which she said was in the air. God knows. It may have been.
>
> Opening her eyes at last, from a very quiet sleep, she begged that they would kiss her once again. That done, she turned to the old man with a lovely smile upon her face ... and clung with both her arms about his neck. They did not know that she was dead, at first.

... [S]he had never murmured or complained; but with a quiet mind, and manner quite unaltered—save that she every day became more earnest and more grateful to them—faded like the light upon a summer's evening.[42]

The dearth of clinical detail in this depiction, its utter romanticization of loss, is precisely what Aldous Huxley critiqued when he famously contrasted Little Nell's death with that of the child Ilusha in Dostoevsky's *The Brothers Karamazov*. Huxley notes that Nell's "same sweet face ... [has] the same mild lovely look" and is "unaltered." In contrast, little Ilusha's death is conveyed through "the thin, pale, wasted hand ... the wasted, yellow face ... the enormous, feverishly glowing eyes," the "broken voice," "the rapid, hard breathing," and "dry lips."[43] Huxley is typical of later responses to Dickens in condemning his sentimental deathbeds as false.[44]

The most sentimental deathbeds in fiction, like Paul's and little Nell's, tend to involve vague, slowly progressing disease and invite the reader's eye to linger upon the family scene.[45] This is a "good death" in the Victorian context: not very painful, permitting reconciliation and spiritual readiness, and within the bosom of family and friends.[46] These deaths should result in the least trauma for survivors, yet these qualities amplify pathos in a fictional death. The lack of pain or anguish in a melancholy death like Paul's allows the narrator's and readers' visual consumption of the scene to be marked by the pleasurable sadness we know as sentiment rather than grief.

Huxley's criticisms are not entirely fair, however; Dickens does portray some deaths with both pathos and some clinical detail. The death of little Harry, a boy Nell encounters in her travels, foreshadows Nell's death with its clear overtones of spirituality, but also details his feverish, "very bright" eyes and "wasted arms," his "faint" voice, and his "small cold hand" at the end (25.196–97). Dickens was not unaware of the physical details of death, and not unwilling to communicate them. Indeed, as his letters make clear, he modeled the death scene of Little Nell upon the death of his sister-in-law Mary Hogarth, who had died unexpectedly at age seventeen, four years earlier.

The most specific and powerful aspect of Paul's disease narrative is not the description of his external symptoms, but its free rendering of his internal experience of illness. For example, during his first illness at school, "there seemed to be something the matter with the floor, for he couldn't stand upon it steadily; and with the walls, too, for they were inclined to turn round and round" (14.159); or when, upon leaving the party at Dr.

Blimber's, the faces of Paul's schoolmates "swam before him, as he looked, like faces in an agitated glass" (14.169). These passages are among Dickens's most evocative and most realistic, portraying illness from within, in a precursor of modernist attention to the experience of consciousness. By producing an identification with Paul, they help drive the powerful affective surge Thackeray admires. Similar envoys from within a mind in extremity mark the deaths of both Carker and Quilp (in *Old Curiosity Shop*), shifting these narratives' tenor from judgment of evil to a kind of sympathy for a fellow subject at the moment of its dissolution. These passages selectively blend realism and impressionism in their description of bodily extremity, as these narrators embrace an identification with the sufferer.

We find an even more realist portrait in Mrs. Skewton's illness and death in *Dombey and Son*. Dickens's depiction of Mrs. Skewton's illness is fanciful but powerfully conveys the symptoms of a "paralytic stroke" complicated by neurological disease or injury: the palsy, which "played among the artificial roses ... like an alms-house-full of superannuated zephyrs"; the "Paralysis" itself, which left her lying motionless and "speechless ... sometimes making inarticulate sounds" and with "unwinking eyes" (37.443–45). Even Dickens's jibes about her "leering and mincing at Death" accompany more accurate and oddly more pathetic descriptions: the old woman's fear of her daughter, "fit of trembling," and "wandering in her wits" (37.446). Just as in medicine, such symptoms point forward to her inevitable decline; in her next appearance, Mrs. Skewton "was more lean and shrunken, more uncertain in her imbecility, and made stranger confusions in her mind and memory," such as "confounding the names of her two sons-in-law" (40.477). If Dickens does select the symptoms that will allow him to sketch Mrs. Skewton most deftly and memorably, he is both accurate and effective. She complains of "numbness," which usefully ironizes her constant palsied motion. Similarly, in speaking, she "cut some of her words short, and cut out others altogether," a symptom of neurological damage that allows Dickens multiple bits of dramatic business depicting her as a pitiable tottering wreck (40.478). Dickens cannot resist satire, noting that "it was not easy to ... keep the bonnet in its place on the back of her poor nodding head, when it was got on," requiring that it be "perpetually tapped on the crown by Flowers the Maid" (40.477); but satire of course accords well with the deflationary, reformist aims of realism.

These symptoms retain the essential qualities of this character and the tone (satiric), Dickens's predominant tone, in discussing her; but they also ground this portrayal in reality, so that when he approaches the topic of her death, the waste of her life is allowed to resonate beyond itself. His last portrait of her focuses on her wild delusions, her "cries," her "restless head" on the pillow, her "incoherence," and her second stroke, that leaves her "crooked and shrunk up, and half ... dead," "making mouths" as she is wheeled about. Dickens uses poetic language to describe "the thickening of the veil before the eyes into a pall that shuts out the dim world" as death approaches, but his depiction of the failing vision and "wandering hands upon the coverlet" strictly replicates the clinical symptoms of the deathbed noted by Victorian physicians (61.488–89). Frederick Taylor, for instance, notes that the symptoms of "graver cases" of brain disease include "plucking at the bed-clothes," and he warns, "death may occur at any time"[47] Once Dickens approaches Mrs. Skewton's actual deathbed, he no longer mocks her symptoms, as he consistently does with Major Joe Bagshott, who "took his lobster-eyes and his apoplexy to the club, and choked there all day" (40.480). Rather, she has now become not a caricature of a foolish crone, but a real body, with all its human waste and suffering.

Dickens's references to the uncomfortable physical reality of disease increase up to the unuttered moment of Mrs. Skewton's death itself: "[H]er mother, with her girlish laugh, and the skeleton of the Cleopatra manner, rises in her bed. Draw the rose-colored curtains. There is something else upon its flight besides the wind and clouds" (41.490). This is so effectively Gothic in part because it has been prepared for by the drumbeat of symptom after symptom, accurately establishing a body and its failures. The major's timeworn compliment that "he'll die in despair" without her had been met by Mrs. Skewton's horrified revulsion from "such dreadful words" (40.479); she read his romantic remark literally, as a realist invocation of death. Just this occurs in her death itself, which transforms the fluttering conventional artifice of her girlish ways; they are made horribly real by her descent into a shaking, skeletal infant.

Something similar happens after Carker's death. The dazzling, impressionistic reports from his pressured thinking resolve into a somber, static scene anchored in dispassionate observation and realist detail. Carker, so lately alive to the reader primarily as a consciousness, is transfigured by death into sheer materiality, and unpleasant matter at that: "something covered ... lay heavy and still, upon a board," and "dogs ... sniffed upon the road [where he had lain], and [men] soaked his blood up, with a train of ashes" (55.653). Sentimental fiction offers no place for soaking up a puddle of blood; the novel has crossed over into another realm of knowledge altogether. These phrases close the curtain on sentiment and melodrama by pointing to the all-too-physical reality of illness and death, in which lively, live characters devolve into mere bodies, bags of bone and blood.

True, Dickens grants his protagonists Paul and Nell a death bathed in the soft focus of Victorian sentiment, but unlike his descriptions of Paul, he makes capable use of clinical observation in the depiction of Nell's illness before her death. He records the progression of the illness, which A. E. Dyson identifies as consumption, in precisely the kind of terms that Huxley desires.[48] Nell's spiritual and virtuous strength mingles with earthly, physical weakness: we see her "too bright eye," her figure "so very weak"; her confusion of mind and of memories; her "aching head" and "shivering with the cold and damp"; her "weak voice" and "bruised and swollen feet"; we hear of the "pains that wracked her joints"; her sense of being "weak and spent" and utterly passive; the lack of food that turns ominously to lack of hunger and then "loathing of food"; finally her "diminished powers even of sight and hearing," difficulty breathing, and dulled sensibilities even to the prospect of death.[49] While some of these symptoms, like Paul's, are vague ("so very weak"), others evoke a specific materiality of the suffering body: her "bruised and swollen feet," or the flu-like pains and shortness of breath that mark the consumptive.

Far from eliding these symptoms, Dickens masterfully stages them, coordinating them with Nell's journey through the devastated industrial landscape of the Black Country. He allows the symptoms to build in frequency and severity, rendering them not only through the eyes of others, like the narrator and the grandfather, but through Nell's experience as well. At the climax of her illness, Nell feels "a dull conviction that she was very ill, perhaps dying; but no fear or anxiety.... Objects appeared more dim, the noise less, the path more rugged and uneven, for sometimes she stumbled, and became roused, as it were, in the effort to prevent herself from falling" (45.341). The unremitting cascade of Nell's symptoms as she and her grandfather traverse the Black Country both grounds and contrasts to Dickens's figurative (but social-realist) depiction of the "ills" of that landscape, even as the morbid atmosphere of these chapters amplifies the gravity of her symptoms.

Any author who could provide this litany of Nell's symptoms, and imaginatively identify with the symptomatic experience of illness and death, is not evading unpleasant truths. Dickens does not fail to acknowledge physiological reality but rather strategically deploys clinical discourse in the service of a nonclinical aim.[50] Both Paul's and Nell's most detailed symptoms appear much earlier in the novel than their actual deaths, which are indeed elided. Dickens's strategic use of a realist clinical discourse in depicting their worsening illnesses effectively frames the set-piece of the deathbed, paradoxically enabling and enhancing its sentimental force.

Amanda Anderson has argued that, in nineteenth-century realist fiction, "the fallen woman appears as both hyperdetermined and disturbingly 'false' (painted, melodramatic, histrionic); this portrayal in turn creates an effect of greater verisimilitude around the nonfallen."[51] In just this way, the contrast between the more-realist illnesses and the more-sentimental deathbeds in Dickens generates a charge by which the children's symptoms are, in retrospect, made more real; their deaths, in contrast, more spiritual and melancholy; and the whole, a more forceful and memorable presentation of his social-realist vision.

Dickens's sentimental sights reference, and relish, eighteenth-century fiction. However, the field of eighteenth-century knowledge most relevant here is its medicine: curious, individualized, saturated with sensibility, in which a patient's pathological body provides an index to character. This is most evident in Dickens's grotesque characters—Quilp, Miss Mowcher, Uriah Heep, even Wemmick. Nell's progressive illness, set alternately in the bleak landscape of nineteenth-century industrialism or among historical curios and memento mori, readily points up an imagined contrast between an earlier, spiritualized ideal and the all-too-real disease of a sinful Victorian world in need of reform. Similarly, Paul's illness, referenced again and again by the phrase "old-fashioned," signals not only Dickens's rejection of the ambitions of clinical medicine, but also a necessary contrast to the spiritual barrenness of Mr. Dombey's insistently forward-pressing, philistine mercantilism.[52] In the medical context, the sentimental narrative usefully compensates for and supplements the inevitable failures of medical practice; but medicine's failure here powerfully supports Dickens's sentimental narrative and its message of social reform.

The framing of *The Old Curiosity Shop* clearly evokes this engagement with an earlier, eighteenth-century aesthetic. The novel was first conceived of as part of a miscellany. After the effort of writing *The Pickwick Papers*, *Oliver Twist*, and *Nicholas Nickleby* over four years, and out of a concern that his public would tire of his lengthy tales, Dickens started a serial miscellany. *Master Humphrey's Clock* was modeled on eighteenth-century periodicals like the *Spectator*, although Little Nell's story took over and became a full-length novel.[53] Like the antiquarians Thomas Warton or Thomas Percy, Master Humphrey publishes from a hoard of old documents. *The Old Curiosity Shop* was originally figured as one component of a project like Horace Walpole's *Miscellany*, or the "cabinets of curiosities" collated by eighteenth-century natural philosophers.[54] The novel is of course itself a "curiosity shop" in which the reader can browse among the oddities for some appealing reminder of Britain's distant, honorable past. But the story is also itself a curiosity, an old tale which derives its interest in the medieval from its figuration as part of an eighteenth-century antiquarian project. It is not surprising, then, that the novel reveals an eighteenth-century understanding of medical "curiosities."

As in the narrative of sensibility in the eighteenth-century novel, Dickens's sentimental narrative engages readers' hearts through a visual circulation of affect. His use of sentiment also recalls eighteenth-century medical narrative norms that sought to certify the physician's insight by demonstrating his sensibility and sentiment as healing and diagnostic tools.[55] In his letters, Dickens discussed his own sufferings over the death scene of Little Nell. He forced himself onward, convinced that by writing Nell's death he could heal British ills, bringing readers closer to a simple faith and a simple comfort.[56] Dickens expressed his desire to "try and do something which might be read by people about whom Death had been,—with a softened feeling, and with consolation."[57] He presented it as a work of moral hygiene: "I could substitute a garland of fresh flowers for the sculptured horrors which disgrace the tomb."[58] But in Dickens, sensibility spills over into sentiment. He thus betrays his affinity for the eighteenth-century tradition of curious sights, with its interest in the affective participation of the viewer. With the imagined ability of the sentimental aesthetic to solicit and direct the gaze and affect of the viewer, Dickens hopes to enlist viewers' hearts in his social reformist projects, marrying idealism to a goal often associated with realism.

Fever and Gaskell's *Ruth:*
The Limits of Clinical Realism

If Dickens seems to blend clinical and sentimental medicine in the interests of investing social realism with transformative affective force, Elizabeth Gaskell hews closer to the clinical details of illness but ultimately puts these in the service of an even more transcendent ideal. In her 1853 novel *Ruth*, as in her other novels, Gaskell combines various narrative techniques to construct a social realism blended with sentiment, faith, and moral clarity. Her handling of medical crises in *Ruth* illustrates her contingent, even strategic use of clinical realism in the service of a larger moral aesthetic, demonstrating how novelists could use medical discourse in ways distinctly opposed to the goals of clinical medicine and of realism in general.

In so arguing, I hope to extend and to nuance some influential critical claims about how sickness functions in the Victorian novel. First, Miriam

Bailin points out that "scenes of illness" in Victorian fiction "are employed as registers of emotional tumult, and crucial stages of self-development, and as rather high-handed plot contrivances to bring events to their desired issue" (1). Gaskell does often use medical crisis as a plot device, so that Dickens famously grumbled, "I wish to Heaven her people would keep a little firmer on their legs!"[59] But Bailin goes on to assert that the sickroom scene has a necessary relation to realism; that "the sickroom scene ... is staged to call forth (in the breach) the conditions under which both the intelligibility of realist aesthetics and the viability of realism's social ethics of cohesion could be affirmed" as a kind of "cure for self and narrative incoherence" (1).

While Bailin's claims have proven productive, I am more interested in how, in Gaskell, realism functions not just as end but also as means; not so much in the sickroom as a prompt for the "cure" of realism but in the realist sickroom as a step toward transcendence. The narrative figures clinical observation as a necessary grappling with the world, yet uses the very strength of these realist representations to drive home a sentimental moral aesthetic that eschews sight for insight and, ironically, transcends the world altogether in its efforts to spiritualize Gaskell's realist social vision. Furthermore, in *Ruth*, fever provides more than an opportunity to, as Athena Vrettos says, "answer questions about the material, social, and spiritual nature of human relations."[60] The fever discourse paradoxically permits the narrative and its concerns to rise above material and social relations, to that spiritual realm. Finally, Vrettos and Peter Logan have extensively shown that "to respond to a narrative ... may produce illness; [and that] conversely, to be ill is to produce narrative" (Vrettos 2). Remarkably, Gaskell's novel strives to both produce and to overcome the narrative of illness. Although Ruth's fever provides the impetus for narrative and its closure, Gaskell uses clinical observation in her fever narrative to affirm another narrative altogether, that of sympathy and moral virtue.

The medical narrative in *Ruth* is indubitably realist, steeped in the details of the medical and public health culture of her time. By choosing typhus as the climactic epidemic of *Ruth*, Gaskell reflects public health fears of her time even as she goes against the grain of sentimental cases. One index of Gaskell's aspiration to realism is Ruth's death from typhus rather than consumption, childbirth, or heart problems. Furthermore, Gaskell clearly references contemporary theories of contagion. In framing the typhus epidemic that sweeps through the novel, she describes the climatological change immediately preceding the fever: "The summer had been unusually gorgeous. Some had complained of the steaming heat, but others had pointed to the lush vegetation, which was profuse and luxuriant. The early autumn was wet and cold, but people did not regard it."[61] To an acute Victorian, a sudden succession from hot, steamy weather to cold, damp weather should raise alarms; indeed, the narrator faults the townspeople for not "regard[ing]" the change in weather. A clear-sighted observation is not only prudent but necessary; the novel clearly refers to the association of fever with an unhealthy environment. This was a commonplace of medicine, expressed in warnings against damp, and against sudden changes in temperature or climate. William Buchan offers such warnings repeatedly in his household guide, *Domestic Medicine,* which was reprinted frequently throughout the century under various titles. He devotes section after section to the dangers of wet clothes, wet feet, damp air, damp beds, damp houses, cooling off suddenly after hard work, drinking cold liquids on a hot day, and other variations on the themes of damp and the sudden transition from hot to cold. This concern with climate underlies terms like "autumnal fever" for typhus. While climatology may now seem a quaint aspect of popular medicine, it was a central element in nineteenth-century theories regarding consumption and fever.

Gaskell also demonstrates her familiarity with typhus epidemics or medical descriptions of them. The etiology of typhus—the fact that it is spread by lice—was not yet known; but Gaskell accurately characterizes its usual territory as "hidden, slimy courses," and "sad haunts of vice and misery," and she pinpoints its origin, again accurately, in "the low Irish lodging-houses" (347). Typhus was indeed endemic in Ireland throughout the early part of the nineteenth century, and physicians associated it with the Irish, who spread "Irish fever" when they migrated around Britain in desperate need of work. Crowded, filthy lodging and bedding helped spread the disease, which accordingly was also called hospital fever, spotted fever, jail fever, camp fever, and ship fever. As William Osler later explained, "The special elements in the etiology of typhus are overcrowding and poverty.... Overcrowding, lack of cleanliness, intemperance and bad food are predisposing causes."[62]

Gaskell's realism also cannily uses the fact that typhus, unlike typhoid, posed a particular risk to caregivers. Osler warns that "[t]yphus is one of the most highly contagious of febrile affections," and comments, "[I]n epidemics nurses and doctors in attendance upon the sick are almost invariably attacked" (40). Ferriar calls the "narrow and crouded streets" of poor districts "nurseries of the disease," and comments, "The hardiest vagrant would shudder at the idea of entering a fever-ward."[63] And indeed, in *Ruth,* "one of the physicians had died, in consequence of his attendance [and] the customary staff of matrons and nurses had been swept off in two days" (347). This accuracy about typhus epidemiology grounds the realism of this novel, propelling and amplifying Gaskell's moral narrative of selfless devotion, by raising the stakes when Ruth offers to work in the fever hospital.

Gaskell's portrayal of Ruth's nursing experience also rings true, probably drawn from her role as minister's wife during cholera outbreaks in Manchester. The novel does not shrink from the grisly physical realities of Ruth's work. These become a tribute to her skill as a nurse and, by analogy, to her ability to triumph over her own bodily narrative. "At first ... ," comments the narrator,

> there was a recoil from many circumstances, which impressed upon her the most fully the physical sufferings of those whom she tended. But she tried to lose the sense of these—or rather to lessen them, and make them take their appointed places—in thinking of the individuals themselves, as separate from their decaying frames; and all along she had enough self-command to control herself from expressing any sign of repugnance. She allowed herself no nervous haste of movement or of touch that should hurt the feelings of the poorest, most friendless creature, who ever lay a victim to disease. There was no rough getting over of all the disagreeable and painful work of her employment. (320)

Gaskell retains some delicacy here, but female readers, with likely some experience of household nursing, would recognize the ugly materiality of disease here. Britain had recently suffered epidemics of typhus, typhoid, and cholera, the third wave of disease over the previous two decades. The virulent typhus in Ireland from 1846–1849 coincided with a severe influenza epidemic that killed 13,000 people.[64] Households across Britain would have struggled with these diseases and their unpleasant symptoms, which included nosebleeds, vomiting, petechial eruptions, and copious diarrhea. *MacKenzie's Ten Thousand Receipts,* a domestic handbook, offers an explicit description of a fatal case of typhus:

> [s]evere chills, astonishing and sudden loss of strength, countenance livid and expressive of stupor, the skin sometimes burning to the touch, at others the heat is moderate, the pulse is quick, small and rarely hard, violent pain in the head, redness of the eyes, low, muttering delirium, the tongue is covered with a dark brown or black looking crust, blackish sores form about the gums, the breath is very offensive, and, in the latter stage, the urine also, which deposits a dark sediment; in extremely bad cases blood is

poured out under the skin, forming purple spots, and breaks out from the nose and different parts of the body, the pulse flutters and sinks, hiccup comes on, and death closes the horrid scene. (124)

It is no wonder that typhus was also known as "putrid fever." While Gaskell doesn't list these symptoms, she clearly acknowledges them, in the "repugnance" and "recoil" that Ruth must initially overcome in handling the loathsome bodies of the diseased. *Ruth* may be a novel about a fallen woman's redemption from the body, but first it writes the body back into the text.

The body does not appear in the novel to be considered in and of itself. Rather, by noting the "decaying frames" of Ruth's patients, the narrator recenters the novel on Ruth and her moral progress, her increasing ability to overcome the realities of her own body and others, not through ignorance, as with her sexual initiation and pregnancy, but by seeing through the body, beyond it, to the spirit. Gaskell insists on Ruth's sympathy for her patients here, but her identification with them miscarries rhetorically. The novel's interest in Ruth's ability to surmount the messy realities of her work ironically displaces the suffering of her patients with her own, because she must register her discomfort before overcoming it. Another moment later in the novel similarly outlines Ruth's courage and alienation from her own physical safety, more than the patient's suffering, even as it underlines her essential difference from the unruly bodies she nurses. Davis, the surgeon, reminds Ruth of "that night when Hector O'Brien was so furiously delirious" that he broke a piece of glass from the window "for the sole purpose of cutting his throat, or the throat of any one else." This anecdote provides a memorable image of the strength and cruelty of the fever; yet the purpose of the vignette is to highlight Ruth's courage—she calmly takes the glass from the murderous man—in the face of a threat that makes her "[go] very white" even in retrospect (359). Again, the narrative draws on Gaskell's knowledge of the ghastly realities of fever, but shifts attention away from the patient's suffering body to Ruth's mental and moral composure, and—at the very moment of physical detail—pulls away from a realist narrative toward the idealist moral trajectory of the novel.

However accurate the novel may be in referencing medical fact, *Ruth* suggests a gulf of experience separating clinical observation from human insight. In the case of Richard Bradshaw's stroke, "the medical man . . . was not so much impressed with the serious character of the seizure as the family, who knew all the hidden mystery behind," that is, Bradshaw's shock at his son's crime and sudden injury. The "medical man" is correct in that Bradshaw is soon on his feet again; but "the family" is more right to identify this medical crisis as the most significant "turn" in their patriarch's career. The physiological and emotional shock causes Bradshaw to lose not only his voice, temporarily, but also his customarily peremptory, authoritarian tone: "For a moment, it seemed as if he had not the right command of his voice," after the stroke; and his first words are an inquiry after the son he had disowned, implicitly rejecting his previous rigid moralism and adopting a "tone of wistful entreaty" (340).

Gaskell's writing was praised for its "fastidiousness [and] delicacy"; Deirdre d'Albertis, for example, asserts that Gaskell "rules out the expressive resources of medical ... discourse."[65] It is true that Gaskell uses mostly lay or even folk terms to describe the body and its ills. However, the novel's medical scenes often rely on detailed physical description like that produced by clinical observation. In the description of Bradshaw's "seizure," for example, the narrator offers a medically exact depiction of the physiology and symptoms of stroke. We hear that "Mr. Bradshaw had opened his eyes and partially rallied, although he either did not, or could not speak. He looked struck down into old age. His eyes were sensible in their expression, but had the dim glaze of many years of life upon them. His lower jaw fell from his upper one, giving a look of melancholy depression to the face, although the lips hid the unclosed teeth" (339). Gaskell's description here not only echoes medical textbooks but also takes up the clinical tone of medical authority: the man "Mr. Bradshaw" fragments into various symptomatic parts, and the references to "[h]is eyes" and "[h]is lower jaw" give way to more detached phrases, "the lips" and "the teeth."

Clinical observation and clinical realism originate in the masculine world of physiology and the clinic, and critics have argued that Gaskell "disavow[ed] a conventionally masculine knowledge of fact, [while she] claimed the conventionally feminine knowledge of feeling."[66] However, much medical knowledge was equally disseminated in a feminine tradition. Because women, and women servants, were traditionally tasked with nursing the sick of their family, medical knowledge circulates in women's genres, including domestic advice manuals like Elizabeth Hammond's *Modern Domestic Cookery ... with a Complete Family Physician* (1817). Buchan's text is another good example of this genre, written by a man but for a domestic audience. He cannily argues,

> The cure of diseases does not depend so much upon scientific principles as many imagine. It is chiefly the result of experience and observation. By attending the sick, and carefully observing the various occurrences in diseases, a great degree of accuracy may be acquired, both in distin-

guishing their symptoms, and in the application of medicines. Hence sensible nurses, and other persons who wait upon the sick, often foresee the patients [*sic*] fate sooner than those who have been bred to physic.... [A] medical education ... is doubtless of the greatest importance; but it never can supply the place of observation and experience.[67]

Indeed, Gaskell draws on her own medical knowledge—such as expectations about the course of disease—gathered from observations as the mother of four daughters and the wife of a busy minister in an industrial city marked by great poverty. But she draws on this knowledge to create an effect at odds with a medical perspective. This becomes clearest in Ruth's fatal illness, which makes some well-known medical facts ground the force of both its realism and its sentimental moral.

Both Gaskell's characters and nineteenth-century medical authors, in books for professional or lay audiences, argue that the body becomes more susceptible to infection from a fever like typhus when run down and when suffering under emotional strain. For example, when Ruth trembles to consider the cost to her son, Leonard, should she fall ill, Mr. Benson cautions, "[I]f you cannot still this agony of fear as to what will become of him, you ought not to go. Such tremulous passion will predispose you to take the fever" (349). A midcentury physician would offer the same counsel. John Elliotson thoroughly examines the predisposing factors for typhus. He acknowledges the malign influence of overexertion, excess in venery, want of food or of good food, and want of fresh air, and he makes special note of the danger of depressed spirits. "I have frequently seen persons die of fever, because the mind has been depressed and uneasy," he explains. "The first predisposing cause of the disease, is mental depression.... Intense mental suffering, or great anxiety relative to anticipated misfortune, corporeal depression, or over-exertion of the intellectual faculties, will have the same injurious effect."[68] This would have been common knowledge among Gaskell's readers. Buchan similarly warns, "Fear and anxiety, by depressing the spirits, not only dispose us to diseases, but often render those diseases fatal which an undaunted mind would overcome," and "Fear, anxiety, and a fretful temper, both occasion and aggravate diseases."[69]

Ruth knows and understands this relation between emotional strain and a vulnerable body. She promises Jemima at one point that "if you are ill or sorrowful, and want me, I will come—" which Jemima mistakes as another reference to Ruth's new identity as sick nurse. "So you would and must to any one, if you take up that calling." But Ruth distinguishes between nursing as a calling, and nursing someone whom you love. "But I should come to you, love, in quite a different way," Ruth insists. "I should go to you with my heart full of love—so full that I am afraid I should be too anxious" (319). Gaskell here sets up the climax of her novel with a reminder that a nurse who is too "full of love" or any other emotion endangers her own health.

Indeed, Ruth's serene demeanor protects her in the fever hospital, even as the other nurses fall sick. Buchan comments that "[n]othing tends so much to the health of the body as a constant tranquility of mind," and Ruth is no exception (112). Mr. Benson reports back to his household that "[t]he fever, it is true, raged; but no plague came nigh her. He said her face was ever calm and bright" (351). Ruth acknowledges both her danger and the protective virtue of serenity. She comforts Mr. Benson's anxieties over her work with typhus patients by asserting, "I believe I have no fear. That is a great preservative, they say" (348). Even in considering the cost to Leonard, Ruth asserts, "I will not be afraid" (349). Ruth's initial ability to resist the disease correlates well with Elliotson's caveat that "[m]any persons are exposed with impunity to the emanations from patients labouring under typhus, till their mind desponds."[70]

As Jaffe has noted, feelings themselves are infectious in this novel (83). Indeed, the narrator conflates fear of the fever with the fever itself, in places. When "the virulence of the fever abated" in the town, "the general panic subsided" and "the overwrought fear of the town was subdued" (352). If Mr. Benson's cautions are correct, the panic itself must have encouraged and hastened the spread of the epidemic. Ruth, a model of strength and selflessness, is credited with subduing the fear of the town, and with it the fever itself. In fact, Ruth receives a letter of approbation from the Board of the town, praising her self-possession for calming the townspeople when the epidemic was peaking: when "there was hardly time to remove the dead bodies before others were brought in to occupy the beds," and "the alarm of course aggravated the disorder" (354). Mr. Donne—previously known as Mr. Bellingham, Ruth's seducer—displays his lack of self-control in falling prey to fear and the fever that inevitably follows it. Victorian readers would recognize the physical and moral debility implied of him when he was "too much alarmed by what he heard of the fever to set to work" canvassing for votes (359).

But if faith and goodness can seal Ruth away from all fear, they do not protect her from the effects of love and regret, nor, ultimately, the realities of disease transmission. Bellingham's illness shakes her composure; when she volunteers to nurse him, the surgeon warns her, "You are not fit for it. You are looking as white as ashes" (360). The narrator underscores Ruth's emotional involvement in the case, both verbally—she admits to Davis that Bellingham is Leonard's father—and in reporting the physiological changes in her as she tries to persuade Davis to let her help—the "sharp pain in her voice," her flush to "deepest scarlet," her "dull persistency," her "quick hot tears." These register the strength of feeling Bellingham rouses in her, and her physical vulnerability. They broadcast the truth Ruth finally admits, that, if Bellingham is "ill—and alone—how can I help caring for him?" In a medical context, Ruth's offer to nurse Bellingham is reckless; Davis calls her a "tenderhearted fool" even as he accepts her offer (360–61).

Gaskell returns to the language of clinical observation to index the symptomatology of Ruth's fall into fever, just as she had with Bradshaw's stroke, and as Dickens does with Nell. The narrator registers the nuances of Ruth's bodily and emotional strain: after three nights of watching, she "had never left the room. Every sense had been strained in watching—every power of thought or judgment had been kept on the full stretch." As in Dickens, the novel records Ruth's perspective of the physical and mental effects of fever (a "whirling stupor of sense and feeling," a "heavy languor," "an oppressive headache"), although Gaskell juxtaposes this with Davis's trained eye, and its detached observation of Ruth's body: "the hurrying breath," "the fever-flush brilliant on her cheeks," wide eyes, and "distended" pupils (364).

However, the portrayal of Ruth's death itself, again as in Dickens, shrinks from recording the realities of the faltering body. Ruth's physical symptoms register only as a temporary nod to mortality, tragic and pitiful, before the narrator evokes the beatific vision that calls her forward into death, turning its back on medicine and its epistemology, and sealing her character as an icon of goodness and self-sacrifice. Unlike the earlier reference to the unpleasant physical symptoms that Ruth's patients suffer and that Ruth, too, must endure, the description of her death blinks the messy realities of death by typhus. The narrator does remind readers of the provenance of Ruth's illness—"utterly exhausted by watching and nursing, first in the hospital, and then by the bedside of her former lover, the power of her constitution was worn out"—but only to explain the gentleness and propriety even of Ruth's delirium, which "displayed no outrage or discord" (366). Other than this "sweet, child-like insanity," the only symptoms Gaskell acknowledges are that Ruth's "strength faded" and "the breath and the power to [sing] had left her" (366), until the moment when she raised herself up, reached out her arms toward "the Light," and died. In an inversion of Mrs. Skewton's death, the real becomes ideal, and this moment of her death literalizes, not the "decay" of her body but the resurgence of sweet faith.

Ruth's deathbed scene, like Paul's and Nell's, is more sentiment than realism, so that her decision, foolhardy in medical terms, registers as beatific self-sacrifice in the novel's moral index. Ruth deliberately puts herself into danger, sacrificing her health and life, to nurse Bellingham, her former lover, and return him good for evil. She enacts an utter disregard of the calculus of risk that the novel has so carefully laid out. Something similar occurs in Charlotte Yonge's popular novel *The Heir of Redclyffe,* where the saintly Guy selflessly nurses his heir and would-be enemy, Philip, through a bad case of malaria despite having "no constitution" and "a tendency to low fever" (429).[71] Sure enough, Philip survives the fever but Guy sinks under it; and as Gaskell does, Yonge shifts from realist to sentimental descriptions of Guy's symptoms as the end approaches, in a pointed transcendence of the material realm and its forms of representation.

Indeed, the logic of the mid-Victorian novel makes it necessary that Ruth's nursing endangers her; the medical fact of her vulnerability allows her to expiate her sin. In Yonge's *The Clever Woman of the Family* (1865), Rachel similarly contracts diphtheria after she insists on nursing a poor girl she had impulsively consigned to an abusive school, proving Rachel's bullheadedness but also her contrition and selflessness. The degree of these women's deviations from convention can be gauged by the severity with which the novels discipline them: Rachel merely falls ill, but Ruth, whose transgression was sexual, must die.

Gaskell deftly deploys the medical "plot" of fever epidemic and emotional strain, calling upon a clinical observation of the realist body, but she does so not to register Ruth's foolishness but to complete Ruth's rehabilitation, to index her utter moral transcendence from the body and from its cares and history, into a realm of pure insight. Here the closely observed disease becomes a window onto the spirit even as Gaskell works to shift social reality in the all-too-material world.

Sentiment, the Deathbed, and the End of Narrative

It is no accident that this chapter on sentimental medicine has focused on scenes of death. Evangelical Victorians considered the deathbed an unparalleled opportunity for reconciliation and spiritual rebirth, which also makes it an ideal site to convert skeptical readers to sentimental ones.⁷² Jaffe argues that "[w]ith its ostensible effacement of differences and asserted dissolution of individuals into a common humanity, sympathy [in the Victorian novel] . . . seeks to efface the social and political problems for which it is offered as a resolution" (15). The sentimental physician and the sentimental narrator also overtly demonstrate the process of sympathy, to spark sympathy for and with him and his project. The deathbed scene, it is clear, should heighten these sympathetic effects. How else can we explain the deathbed scene's ability to evoke a sympathetic portrayal of the most hardened or evil characters? How else understand the narrative's near-identification with Quilp (Quilp!) at the moment of his drowning?

Moreover, the deathbed is a haven of sentiment because it marks where clinical medicine *must* fail. It thus offers a reminder that the material facts of clinical knowledge must be subordinated to the unsounded truths of the spirit. Thus Dickens and Gaskell turn clinical realism to sentiment just as physicians do: sentiment usefully corrals the reader and insists on human connection at moments that strain the explanatory narrative.

Finally, like the deathbed, sentiment performs a kind of violence, even apart from its insistent demand for affective mirroring. If a scene is "moving," enacting a "dilatation of the heart," it also arrests life and forward motion. It forcibly reorients the text's values from a fact-based clinical knowledge, with its task of pursuing and representing and its open-ended, ongoing, and outward-looking interpenetrative movement between observer and observed, to a heart-based "truth," a truth of insight that refuses plot and seeks only to realize an identification between self and other in a relation that is closed and set.⁷³ Strictly speaking, despite the central trope of "the Great Change" that occurs in any deathbed scene, it portrays not a narrative but a tableau.

It is perhaps for this reason that, at these novels' deathbeds, when the text is most suffused in sentiment, the body often disappears. The clinical, material body becomes visible as only instrumental, a vehicle whose narration puts viewers in position to be moved. If Catherine Gallagher argues that fictionality enables sympathy ("nobody's story"), Jaffe modifies this by arguing that "it is not so much the absence of actual bodies in novels that produces sympathy as it is sympathy . . . that produces an effect of fictionality. . . . The cultural narratives that constitute sympathy themselves do away with the body" (13). In the novels I've examined, sympathy most frequently does "do away with the body" at the moment of death, but it is most effective when the illness narrative immediately preceding death has included a decidedly clinical observation of the body. The successful prosecution of a sentimental narrative in these novels relies largely upon its framing by the brisk force of an intermittent, situational realism.

In contrast, in physicians' sentimental case histories, the body can remain fully contemporaneous with feeling. Earl St. Maur's struggling body does not fade away in his deathbed scene, despite Williams's often-voiced pangs of regret. Medicine, then, precedes the novel in learning how to write a realist sympathy that does not require the end of narrative. As the next chapter will show, George Eliot took up this challenge and revised both clinical observation and sympathetic insight still further.

Chapter Four

George Eliot's Realist Vision

Mechanical Observation and the Production of Sympathy

> It is astonishing what a different result one gets by changing the metaphor! Once call the brain an intellectual stomach, and one's ingenious conception of the classics and geometry as ploughs and harrows seems to settle nothing. But then it is open to some one else to follow great authorities, and call the mind a sheet of white paper or a mirror, in which case one's knowledge of the digestive process becomes quite irrelevant.
> George Eliot, *The Mill on the Floss* (1860)

> Hunter in one of his lectures ... speaks playfully, but most truthfully of the various *theories* of digestion, which have arisen from exclusive views of different sets of facts. "Some physiologists will have it that the stomach is a mill;—others, that it is a fermenting vat;—others again, that it is a stew-pan; but in my view of the matter, it is neither a mill, a fermenting vat, nor a stew-pan—but a *Stomach*, gentleman [sic], a *stomach*."
> Worthington Hooker, *Physician and Patient* (1849)

George Eliot's rueful consideration of Tom's recalcitrant mind in *The Mill on the Floss* offers, and discards, a number of images—a field ripe for ploughing, a stomach plied with indigestibles, blank paper, a mirror—to illustrate the power and the pitfalls of metaphor as an analytical tool. It is instructive, however, that she does not eschew figurative language altogether. In contrast, the second quotation, by a midcentury American physician, Worthington Hooker, cites the great John Hunter in order to mock the use of any figure whatsoever. However, Hooker's slippage from "theory" to metaphor, in which metaphors for the stomach also represent various medical theories, bespeaks the difficulty of hewing exclusively to literal reference. Indeed, George Eliot also often turns to memorable metaphors as a mode of argumentation. Her very caution about the philosophical and logical validity of this strategy argues for her conviction of its power, and suggests that she carefully attends to the nuances of those figures she does choose to employ, especially those, like the web, that recur throughout her novels.[1] In this chapter, I will examine a particular chain of figures—mirrors and other visual or optical devices—in George Eliot's early fiction, to examine how she privileges sight over the other senses, and how she posits structures of vision as enabling or disabling realism and its (for her) necessary and desirable end, sympathy. In both her realist fiction and in midcentury medicine, these structures of vision stand in for a particular distanced, scrutinizing relation between the world and its representation, a relation that, despite external similarities, appears very different in the mechanical observation of scientific medicine and the deeply informed sympathy of the novel.

George Eliot's offhand reference to "the mind [as] . . . a mirror" wryly echoes a famous passage in her first novel *Adam Bede* (1859), where she argues that "observing" should be not so much "seeing" as "reflecting." As critics from Erich Auerbach to George Levine, M. H. Abrams to Jonathan Crary have shown, and as George Eliot suggests, authors theorizing about realist narrative have often turned to the metaphor of a mirror, whether the page or the mind act as a mirror of the world. In *Adam Bede*, she uses the mirror metaphor to revise the "great authorities" she mentions above.

Classic literary realism did not account for contemporary research on the imperfections of human vision. In *Adam Bede*, George Eliot incorporates an alternate realist tradition, drawn from clinical science, which also construes realist representation as a primarily visual process but emphasizes the inevitable flaws and distortions in human-mediated representations of the world. Clinical realism requires observers to compensate for these flaws through meticulous, laborious attention to reproducing detail exactly, attempting a mechanical observation, as chapter 2 discussed. This ideal shapes George Eliot's narrative technique in *Adam Bede*, where she describes a mirrored structure of observation in many ways like a camera obscura. Her use of this structure, and her explication of the flaws of the mirror at its heart, correct and focus the classic metaphor, as an optical device might compensate for and correct faulty vision. This allows her to insist on the problem of mediation at the heart of any observation, which had concerned scientists, and to distinguish between the mind's task in an *observing* process—when it acts like a mirror, in which the world is reflected—and its function in a *representing* process—when it acts like a sheet of white paper, on which the world is written. Either process may introduce the distortions of individual judgment. Crucially, George Eliot also rejects a central tenet of clinical realism by suggesting this skeptical, detailed, and mechanical perception of realist vision can and should evoke a "deep human sympathy" for others.

In 1799, when *Adam Bede* is set, British medicine was still in the midst of a strong empirical backlash against French theory, whereas in the 1850s–1860s, when the novel was published, medicine and science were gradually accepting the judicious use of speculation and imagination (in the form of hypothesis) as a revisionary element of a scientific process, as I will show in the next chapter. In the novel's revision of strict mechanical observation, it is of a piece with its time rather than its setting. However, what scientists provisionally endorsed at midcentury was a creative, even intuitive, but unemotional complement to the tedious labor of observation; whereas the novel urges readers (and novelists) to use that tedious labor to produce a specifically affective engagement with the world.

George Eliot engages with a tradition of verisimilitude in fiction stretching back to Defoe, a tradition explicated by Michael McKeon and others. But in the decade before *Adam Bede*, the debate about accurate observation and verbal representation was carried on as much in scientific communities as in literary ones. Hooker, for instance, reinvigorates a skepticism about fanciful representation, bringing up an old tale about the eighteenth-century physician John Hunter. Practitioners of science during the first half of the nineteenth century worked to codify a single "scientific method" that could be universalized across disciplines and would certify individual findings for use by a large and heterogeneous audience.[2] That method was grounded in skepticism about human observation and representation. Scientists like Hermann von Helmholtz concluded that "the eye has every possible defect that can be found in an optical instrument." Even physicians advised their students that "the senses. . . . require a special system of training and education before their evidence can be trusted."[3] Clinical medicine thus offered a realist methodology to guide perception and representation, outlined in physiologists' texts as early as the 1840s; that methodology could be of use to novelists with similar concerns.

In her repeated recourse to tropes of perception and optical devices in her early fiction, especially *Adam Bede*, George Eliot places herself in relation to her scientific colleagues, as fellow theorists of realist vision and representation. Her examination of the stages of moral observation in *Adam Bede* demonstrates how far she discards any notion of realism as simple mirroring. Her reconstruction of the mind-as-mirror metaphor disarticulates that metaphor into disjunct, potentially conflicting stages of observation and representation, and distinguishes them from their product, ideally a "deep human sympathy." She demonstrates a flexible, particularizing, and skeptical model of realism as anything but transparent or unifying, and she poses specularity as itself necessarily suspect, so that *Adam Bede* sets out to correct not only romance and the "silly novels" of her famous essay, but also classic realism itself. While critics disagree over whether her novels are classic realist texts, and over how to define classic realism itself, they agree that this category is central to understanding her work. Ironically, George Eliot's significance to classic realism may be clearest when her novels are unsettling its conventions.[4]

George Eliot's familiarity with science, especially physiology, is well known. If, as Sally Shuttleworth argues, "[s]cience permeated not only the social and psychological theory, but also the language, structure and fictional methodology of the Victorian novel,"[5] George Eliot's novels anchor much of the literary criticism on realism and scientific discourse. Her fascination with scientific methodology informs her narrative technique even when she is not explicitly addressing scientific issues. As Sidney Colvin said of her in 1873, "[T]here is something like a medical habit in the writer, of examining her own creations for their symptoms, which runs through her descriptive and narrative art and gives it some of its peculiar manner."[6]

Middlemarch foregrounds this interest, of course; both narrator and narrative are openly preoccupied with the questions of science, observation, and objectivity. Most critics turn to this novel as the site where George Eliot most pointedly interrogates science and society, optics and perception.[7] However, she had immersed herself in scientific culture long before. Much of her early fiction experiments with using clinical realism, with its pronounced and self-conscious interest in detail, fact, method, and visuality, as a literary methodology—that is, a textual strategy for establishing verisimilitude, producing authenticity, and gaining authority through narrative. She considers the benefits and pitfalls of a clinical realist vision as early as *Scenes of Clerical Life* and *Adam Bede,* where she engages with concerns about accuracy of perception and representation that derive from the early-nineteenth-century scientific community. Both texts build upon and critique contemporary debates over scientific objectivity, specifically the doctrine of "mechanical observation." My focus on *Adam Bede* in this chapter hopes to shift critical attention to the existence of this "medical habit" in George Eliot's early fiction as well as in her much-discussed later novels.[8]

The mid- to late 1850s, when George Eliot began to write fiction, overlapped with the period when her partner, the biologist and critic George Henry Lewes, began his physiological research (animal experiments) and writing.[9] With Lewes, she considered the major scientific debates of the mid-nineteenth century, including Darwinian evolution, the theory of positivism, and the development of physiology. George Eliot knew the controversial pathologist John Elliotson by 1853.[10] She had conversed with eminent researchers like Johannes Müller during her trip to Germany with Lewes in 1855. And she and Lewes, with T. H. Huxley, were instrumental in lobbying for a medical physiology laboratory at Cambridge and installing Michael Foster as its head in 1870.[11] Even after Lewes's death in 1878, she established a studentship in physiology in his name.[12] Although it is clear that she was familiar with other Victorian sciences, such as anthropology and economics,[13] clinical realism in medical specialties like physiology and pathology lends itself especially well to her project.

George Eliot's early discussions of the realist aesthetic resonate with the questions that were driving debates over the role of physiology in midcentury medicine. Both medicine and the realist novel struggled to balance accurate, objective vision with a humanist, intuitive understanding. Like Eliotian realism but unlike most other sciences, midcentury medicine struggled to fulfill the demands of its empiricist skepticism without renouncing its more idealist, humanist aims. Physicians and novelists both had to embrace simultaneously a stringent realist ideology and the idealist demands of their art.

Physicians disagreed about the complementarity of their humanist "art" and empiricist "science," an important concern in George Eliot's writing as well. She had doubtless read her friend Herbert Spencer's argument against the separation of science and art in 1854,[14] and her fiction often seeks to combine these pursuits. Many physicians gloomily forecast an incommensurability between the precise detail of clinical observation and the longer view of humanism. Charles Williams warns, "We have to consider, not merely *disease in the body*, but *the body in disease;* and it is by losing sight of this great practical axiom, that minute or microscopic inquirers ... signally fail in prognosis and in practice." Holland cautions that the unique conditions making it difficult to control and replicate research on living, thinking beings "must ever keep practical medicine in the rear of other physical sciences." Even staunch advocates of the sciences took care to acknowledge its relation to the *ars medica*. Bennett cautions his students, "[G]entlemen, I trust that, in studying [physiology and pathology], you will never lose sight of the important fact, that you are medical students, and that as such your ultimate object is to acquire an art."[15]

Williams's and Bennett's concern over "losing sight," above, registers the extent to which this debate over progress in medicine centered on questions of visuality, in particular the problem of reconciling different kinds of medical vision. As in literary realism, accurate observation was considered central to medical practice; Thomas Watson, for example, taught students that "[t]here is ... this peculiar to our art.... [I]t requires *skill in observing*." Edward Forbes argued that "[t]he two qualities most essential to the physician are *correct observation* and *accurate discrimination*.... The mind must be trained to reason justly, the instrument of the mind to observe correctly." And Holland considered that medicine owed its progress to "more cautious observation and more exact evidence."[16] Accordingly, medical progress was represented by mechanical aids to vision, like the microscope or otoscope, or by instruments which made the body visible in new ways—as the sphygmograph or kymograph recorded physiological forces and rhythms on the page. The trope of vision appears frequently in both paeans to and jeremiads against the new technologies and their effect on physicians' ability to "see" the body. Nineteenth-century physiology and pathology texts demonstrate, then, how such instruments symbolize scientific progress by extending and mechanizing human vision, even as they may co-opt that vision.[17] Just this kind of vexed investment in instruments of observation also grounds, and fractures, George Eliot's early aesthetic of realist vision and her view of realism as itself an instrument useful to a larger humanist project.

Adam Bede and Mechanical Observation

In *Adam Bede,* George Eliot demonstrates her commitment to a realism that she felt compelled to defend, famously, in chapter 17 of the novel. The passage combines classic literary realism with aesthetic and legal realism, which are explicit, and mechanical observation—a central trope of clinical realism—which is less explicit but equally important. The narrator rejects an imagined call for more idealized characters, like those who might populate the plot if the narrator were "a clever novelist, not obliged to creep servilely after nature and fact, but able to represent things as they never have been and never will be." This explains the choice of lowborn protagonists and the refusal to gloss over unpleasant facts. "But," the narrator continues,

> I have no such lofty vocation, and ... I aspire to give no more than a faithful account of men and things as they have mirrored themselves in my mind. The mirror is doubtless defective; the outlines will sometimes be disturbed; the reflection faint or confused; but I feel as much bound to tell you, as precisely as I can, what that reflection is, as if I were in the witness-box narrating my experience on oath.... It is for this rare, precious quality of truthfulness that I delight in many Dutch paintings, which lofty-minded people despise. I find a source of delicious sympathy in these faithful pictures of a monotonous homely existence.[18]

This passage defends the novel's realist content by espousing a realist technique of representation. The narrator conceives of the reality of the world primarily as a visual event: it enters one's experience visually and then is transposed as exactly as possible from the mirror of one's mind onto the page. Most critics focus on the question of realist subject matter here. Daniel Gunn, for example, argues that "Eliot's defense through the language of painting is ... primarily an argument about the subject matter of art."[19] It is significant, however, that George Eliot approaches the question of content through that of form and the problems of representation and mimesis. These are clearly serious issues for her, too.

George Eliot here references the tradition of discussing mimetic art through a metaphor of "mind as mirror," where the trope of the mirror imagines the ideal of an unmediated, exact replication of reality. This figures representation as a visual record, and as more a reflection than a creation. Her use of authenticating terms like "faithful account," "precisely," and "truthfulness" signals her interest in this kind of accurate rendering. Her repetition of terms like "outlines" and "faithful pictures," as well as her references to Dutch art and the legal figure of the "witness," the valued observer, marks how specifically visual constructions of knowledge lay the groundwork for her project of realist representation.

Besides referencing the mind-as-mirror tradition of visual mimesis and the visual evidence of the witness-box, George Eliot also adopts some basic tenets of John Ruskin's *Modern Painters*. She had reviewed it at length in 1856, praising its theory of *"realism*—the doctrine that all truth and beauty are to be attained by a humble and faithful study of nature, and not by substituting vague forms, bred by imagination on the mists of feeling, in place of definite, substantial reality." Like George Eliot, Ruskin had linked a realist interest in quotidian "facts" to the passive, mirroring imagination of the "great idealist." He explains,

> [H]e who seeks for frivolities and fallacies, will have frivolities and fallacies again presented to him in his dreams.... The whole of his power depends upon his losing sight and feeling of his own existence, and becoming a mere witness and mirror of truth, and a scribe of visions,—always passive in sight, passive in utterance,—lamenting continually that he cannot completely reflect nor clearly utter all he has seen....[20]

Here the artist's "imaginative power" and access to "truth" derive from his antiromantic observation, willingness to adopt a passive role as mirror, skepticism about his abilities, and sense of humility before his task.[21]

In *Adam Bede*, George Eliot's echo of Ruskin's "mirror of truth" seconds his endorsement of a realist aesthetic and his condemnation of the romantic "fallacies" that encourage artistic egoism. Narrative for the early George Eliot seems less about pleasure or charm than about rendering a truthful reflection of the world, resisting the active intervention of the romantic "touch." When her narrator scorns "picturesque sentimental wretchedness," and "picturesque lazzaroni or romantic criminals," the novel mocks not only the unlikely inhabitants of the romantic novel but also an overwrought or romantic discourse itself, contaminated by the desires and fantasies of the author and reader (178–79).[22] Her narrator admits, "The pencil is conscious of a delightful facility in drawing a griffin," but then firmly rejects the imagined plea of readers that "[t]he world is not just what we like, do touch it up with a tasteful pencil" (176–77). She suggests that realist narrative might introduce readers to another kind of pleasure: the pleasure of approaching the truth.[23]

George Eliot also tweaks Ruskin's mirror trope to suggest her greater skepticism about the artist's task. Her rejection of authorial "improvement" signals her concerns about the mediated structure of perception and representation. Like Ruskin, she emphasizes the artist's sense of inadequacy, challenging the mimetic tradition of a naïve classic realism by troubling the authority of the mirror. While Ruskin's artist "becom[es]" himself a mirror, George Eliot's narrator locates the mirror in his mind, emphasizing its subjective basis and its inaccessibility to others' inspection. Moreover, like many mirrors in George Eliot's work, it is unsatisfactory, even "defective."[24] *Adam Bede* describes at length the "queer old looking glass" that Hetty dislikes because it "had numerous dim blotches sprinkled over the mirror, which no rubbing would remove, and because, instead of swinging backwards and forwards, it was fixed in an upright position, so that she could only get one good view of her head and neck" (149). Pretty Hetty, like pretty Rosamond in *Middlemarch*, represents the blindness—the lack of foresight and perspective—of all human vanity, which, like the looking glass, provides only one angle of reflection. Hetty's blotched, stationary looking glass reminds the reader that human vision is not only incomplete, as Ruskin warns of imaginative vision, but also "queer," distorted, and fixed. George Eliot's interest in distortion demonstrates how, even as a novice fiction writer, she questioned the notions of transparency and control that critics associate with classic realism.[25]

Despite her emphasis on the need for a precise, mirrored rendering of the world, then, George Eliot insists that she cannot offer more than merely a distorted representation of "the real." Her narrator can "give a faithful account of men and things" only "as they have mirrored themselves in my mind."[26] This mediation between reality and its representation is implicit in the structure of perception, and it is necessarily ("doubtless") flawed. This structure of seeing requires not only a strict passivity in allowing "things" to "mirror themselves" on the mind, but also, paradoxically, a laborious, anxious attention. Her narrator's legal discourse conveys the responsibility of the observer, who is "on oath" to render that reflected image "precisely" by tracing or transcribing the reflected image with painstaking care to minimize additional distortion.

The opening to chapter 7 of *Adam Bede* performs just this kind of corrective acknowledgment of a distorted vision. The dairy offers

> a scene to sicken for with a sort of calenture in hot and dusty streets—such coolness, such purity, such fresh fragrance of new-pressed cheese, of firm butter, of wooden vessels perpetually bathed in pure water; such soft colouring of red earthenware and creamy surfaces, brown wood and polished tin, grey limestone and rich orange-red rust on the iron weights and hooks and hinges. But one gets only a confused notion of these details when they surround a distractingly pretty girl of seventeen, standing on little pattens and rounding her dimpled arm to lift a pound of butter out of the scale. (83)

This detailed, rich clarity of homely objects and surfaces mimics the tenor of the Dutch realist paintings that George Eliot later discusses. But the mind-mirror of the narrator warps at that "distractingly pretty girl" Hetty, bringing her into sharp focus and allowing the rest of the room to slide into a blur of colors and textures. The close observation shifts toward a more curious sight, in a move like what Amy King describes as the problem of "how to faithfully represent, or make real, the commonplace thing without succumbing to the lure of the individual and rare thing" (181).

The close attention of realist observation always runs the risk of making its object spectacular. George Eliot's narrator warns that interest may impede a "faithful account" of the room. The careful description of the dairy, above, somewhat counters the self-deprecating admission of "only a confused notion of these details," but the narrator notes only those pastoral elements most flatteringly framing her figure.

In these caveats over the accuracy of the mind-as-mirror, George Eliot adapts and revises the ideal of mechanical objectivity, grounded in skepticism about human perception, that had emerged in the new scientific culture around 1830. In the eighteenth-century notion of accurate representation, which the historians Lorraine Daston and Peter Galison term "truth-to-nature," the observer's judgment was needed to screen out misleading details. "Truth-to-nature" required the observer to shape his text or image toward nature in its ideal form: astronomical charts portrayed the heavens unobscured by clouds, anatomical atlases showed bodies unmarked by scars. The nineteenth-century ideal that Daston and Galison call "mechanical objectivity" (and I term "mechanical observation" given its interest in visuality) became standard training for medical students, as I established in chapter 2, and would have been familiar to George Eliot with its influence in physiology. Mechanical observation frowns upon human mediation, including judgment or selection. Daston and Galison define it as "the insistent drive to repress the willful intervention of the artist-author," noting that although its aim was to produce "a right depiction of nature," in fact "its primary allegiance was to a morality of self-restraint."[27] In order to suppress the observer's "temptation to impose systems, aesthetic norms, hypotheses, language, even anthropomorphic elements" on the observed image he must practice not just "self-surveillance" but also "self-mastery" to the extent of "self-elimination" or even "self-annihilation."[28]

George Levine has usefully examined how this "dying-to-know narrative" functioned in Victorian culture. However, the paradox of the observer's continuous, constrained agency—expressed through his labor and his attention—is at least as important in this narrative as his suppression or "death" as a subjective individual. To satisfy its extreme skepticism, mechanical observation "requires," as Daston and Galison explain, "painstaking care and exactitude, infinite patience, unflagging perseverance, preternatural sensory acuity, and an insatiable appetite for work"—or, as George Eliot puts it, for "creep[ing] servilely after nature and fact."[29] The narrator here opposes the realist novelist's work to that of the "clever novelist" by contrasting the low, dirty work of "creeping"—one imagines a closely observing botanist or entomologist, literally "grounded" in "nature and fact"—to the "lofty goals" of theory or fancy.[30]

The narrative position of a Victorian physician may seem more active; he expects to intervene in the case before him, to affect its outcome. George Eliot's realist narrator, on the other hand, stands at a remove from the plot, "reflecting" only; the novel demands only the faithful rendering of this miniature reality. However, clinical and professional norms similarly limit the agency of the midcentury physician. The principles of mechanical observation restrain and discipline his gaze and judgment in the examination and report, and even in practice he is enjoined from any promiscuous action. The great reform movement of 1840s and 1850s medicine, in a backlash against "heroic" medicine, valorized less treatment rather than more. Hippocrates' ancient caveat, "first do no harm," reappeared as "watchful waiting" or "letting Nature take its course," during the long pause between the abandonment of heroic measures like bloodletting or mercury early in the century, and the advent of efficacious treatments such as antibiotics at its close. Primary among the physician's tasks, then, is to recognize that his well-meant actions may make matters worse.

Crucially, George Eliot's observer may be "passive in sight," like Ruskin's artist, but she cannot be entirely "passive in utterance." Uttering requires agency, shaped by the call for a truthful rendering. That agency, ironically, is to bind herself over to slavish description of the reflection she sees, not only despite but because of its inherent distortion; because she cannot risk any further distortion in representing the image. Such faithful self-restraint becomes a kind of self-assertion. As in mechanical observation, her narrator must work incessantly to account for his inherent distortions, in a continuous process of self-abnegation that, ironically, reinserts his figure in the trace of his efforts to erase himself.[31]

Two important elements differentiate the clinical realist theory of mechanical observation from a naïve realist theory of simple reflection: this anxiety over the contested place of the observer, necessitating a skeptical stance toward his work; and the mechanical arrangements (moral, technological, social) that seek to compensate for this problem of the observer, not by fixing his errors but by paralyzing any attempt to do so—immobilizing his principle of judgment or selection as he transcribes the image. Thus the narrator's caveat about the mirror's production of a "disturbed," "faint," or "confused" representation of reality—his concern about the observer's mediation—places the novel closer to mechanical observation than to naïve mimetic realism. It is precisely because the observer's perceptions are so flawed that he must so anxiously strive to replicate that mirrored view exactly, lest he introduce further distortions in trying to "touch it up with a careful pencil." George Eliot's realism is acutely aware that it is situated and embodied, and inescapably mediated.[32]

Both mechanical observation and George Eliot's theory of realism emphasize that a realist methodology may underwrite an ethical, as well as scientific or aesthetic, goal. Daston notes how scientists' "language of self-restraint sometimes echoes that of Christian asceticism.... of manful self-denial, of speculation crushed and beguiling illusions willfully destroyed." Indeed, "the self-restraining and self-effacing counsels of mechanical and aperspectival objectivity reverberate with the stern voice of moral duty: the self-command required in both cases to suppress the merely personal is indeed the very essence of the moral."[33] The conjunction of selflessness with the valorization of mere fact and incessant meticulous labor renders mechanical observation a moral as well as intellectual and aesthetic ideal; it is perhaps this combination that appealed to what Andrew Miller has termed George Eliot's "moral perfectionism." As Amanda Anderson demonstrates throughout her genealogy of Victorian detachment, ethical concerns were not infrequently conjoined with questions of disciplinary method and procedure.[34] It is not, then, surprising that the ideology of mechanical observation might prove useful to an author like George Eliot.

However, literary critics did not valorize "mechanical" production. The proliferation of detail in texts produced by mechanical observation corresponds to what Peter Logan calls the "fullness of details" in midcentury literary realism, but any notion of automatism sat ill with most writers, readers, and critics.[35] While in the *Fortnightly Review* and elsewhere Lewes enthusiastically promoted a realist aesthetic grounded in mechanical observation,[36] the *Saturday Review* from the 1860s repeatedly criticized such fiction. The *Review* used the term "mechanical" in a pejorative sense, attacking the prolific output of a novelist like Trollope by reading realism's reproductions of visual detail as cheap mass-produced images, like stereotypes or photographs.[37] While George Eliot escaped the charge of "mechanical" plot or character, readers balked at her sometimes clinical prose as early as the *Scenes from Clerical Life,* one declaring her "very possibly a *man of Science* but not a practised writer."[38] With the mirror figure in *Adam Bede,* George Eliot counters this standard literary opposition of "mechanical reproduction" to "imaginative art." She argues that the reflective, automatic quality of her mirrored image makes it better art: it represents the world better, because more comprehensively.

We can see the similarity between George Eliot's realism and mechanical observation when comparing her words to those of Alfred Stillé, the pathologist discussed in chapter 2. While Stillé does not use the term "mirror," his "practical genius," as noted, "creates nothing ... it only *sees things as they are.*"³⁹ Like George Eliot, he prefers to plod in the "mechanical labour" of a realist narrative methodology, rather than leap with the flourish of a romantic one. He also foregrounds the nature of his genre as narrative; for, like the novel, the case history requires not simply one accurate image of reality, but a string of them. When Stillé, like Eliot, valorizes "faithful and exact transcripts of the truth" or "a faithful narrative," he acknowledges the linearity of the genre, and he puts into question the process of transcribing image into prose, so crucial to an understanding of realism's vulnerability. When Stillé warns of the possibility of "an unfaithful representation," he betrays his suspicion of human observation, warning that only "[a] faithful narrative ... described minutely what had actually been seen and felt, and in terms admitting of no double construction." Finally, he emphasizes the difficulty of his task. George Eliot warns, "Falsehood is so easy, truth so difficult"; Stillé likewise exclaims, "[T]here is no royal road to truth!"⁴⁰ For Stillé and George Eliot alike, "truth" demanded that the observer eschew "the temptations of aesthetics, the lure of seductive theories, the desire to schematize, beautify, simplify."⁴¹

ADAM BEDE AND OPTICAL DEVICES

Just this temptation drives the conflict in a crucial scene of *Adam Bede*, and unites the two central chapters, 16 and 17. During Arthur Donnithorne's conversation with Mr. Irwine in chapter 16, subjective response colors his representation of his relationship with Hetty. Arthur had determined that "[t]here must be an end to the whole thing at once.... He would go and tell Irwine—tell him everything" (139). But when it comes to the point, Arthur asks Irwine only about "witchery from a woman" in the most general way. He thinks, "The conversation had taken a more serious tone than he had intended—it would quite mislead Irwine—he would imagine there was a deep passion for Hetty, while there was no such thing" (171, 173). Arthur's swerve from his original intent here dramatizes the human ability to overlook unpleasant aspects of our reality and to edit our narratives accordingly. The narrator establishes Arthur's desire to be admired (he "lived a great deal in other people's opinions and feelings concerning himself") and his desire for Hetty, which was an "unrecognised agent secretly busy in Arthur's mind at this moment" (171, 173). Readers, schooled by the novel, know that Arthur needs to examine his actions and communicate them in all their uncomfortable detail to Mr. Irwine. But Arthur's subjective desires for reputation and for Hetty distort his mental mirror, muddying his reflections and thus also his narrative. After this watershed moment, which demonstrates that only a meticulous accounting for every detail can compensate for our fallibility in self-perception, the rest of the plot follows inevitably.

The novel signals its central interest in issues of perception by framing this important conversation between extended depictions of optical instrumentation, specifically devices which transmit images using a glass surface coated in a medium that blurs, filters, or otherwise alters vision.[42] Significantly, the mind-as-mirror passage of chapter 17 immediately follows this conversation, just as a passage on tinted glass lenses precedes and follows it; together they constitute a critical node at the heart of the novel, foregrounding the vagaries of perception and its necessary correctives.

Early in the conversation, Mr. Irwine warns Arthur of the need to construct a mental defense against temptation, one which, paradoxically, ensures clear vision by obscuring sight. He advises that "keeping unpleasant consequences before [a man's] mind … gives you a sort of smoked glass through which you may look at the resplendent fair one and discern her true outline" (172). This metaphor of a lens of smoked glass references astronomy, another clinical science, and suggests that one's attitude—if it is skeptical—may protect vision by excluding or blurring anything that could prompt a dangerously distorting subjective response. An observer can thus see a more "true outline" with a filtered than with an unfiltered gaze. The danger here is of an overwhelming world whose reality—like "that roar which lies on the other side of silence," postulated in *Middlemarch* or "The Lifted Veil"—overloads and distorts our perceptive apparatus, requiring an ingenious device for sensory correction.

Mr. Irwine's irony here, in calling a woman a romantically "resplendent fair one," is undercut by his optimism about his own ability to see past the glare of beauty. George Eliot's own skepticism prevails, as she shows through dramatic irony, grouping Mr. Irwine's advice with the fateful conversation in which Arthur misapplies his advice. Indeed, Arthur demonstrates the potential danger of any filter, keeping pleasant rather than unpleasant consequences more "before his mind." Mr. Irwine's well-meant comment only encourages Arthur's ill-placed faith in his own selective vision. Reporting only certain details from his scenes with Hetty, recording their relationship through his own, mistaken, defensive filter, ironically misleads Arthur into a fatal inattention to the "true outline" of his own case.

As though to confirm readers' awakened suspicions, the novel returns to and revises the figure of smoked glass after the conversation, this time clearly marking it as a dangerously misleading indulgence. This figure reminds readers, unambiguously, that optical instruments may not produce a reliable image, and that they do not always serve a scientific or even a truthful vision. After Arthur deceives himself and Mr. Irwine by denying any sexual entanglements, Mr. Irwine alludes to another form of tinted-glass filter, the transparency. He remarks,

> By the way, Arthur, at your colonel's birthday fête there were some transparencies that made a great effect in honour of Britannia, and Pitt, and the Loamshire Militia, and, above all, the "generous youth," the hero of the day. Don't you think you should get up something of the same sort to astonish our weak minds?

And the narrator comments, "The opportunity [for Arthur's confession] was gone" (174). Because they project vision without substance, these transparencies suggest Arthur's and Mr. Irwine's failure to see and to communicate the reality of Arthur's involvement with Hetty; they demonstrate the false or distorted perception that hinders Arthur's self-knowledge.

By referencing a different kind of translucent glass, then, the transparencies replace the metaphor of truth-telling smoked glass with one where the subjective, distorting medium of vision—glass or mirror—produces illusion rather than truth, a false image of Arthur as another "hero of the day" rather than the shamed paramour he will prove to be. A transparency projects the image of reality, but it produces a vision born of illusion and spectacle, closer to the romantic tales that "astonish" readers than to an earnestly accurate realist vision.

Furthermore, this figure of the transparency ironically literalizes George Eliot's suspicion of pleasurable fantasy. The "delightful facility" of imagining a griffin will be recognized as not just unproductive but immoral, when read in the context of Arthur's pleasant illusions about himself and his furtherance of others' pleasant illusions as well. The courage to face unpleasant facts, the persistence and determination to attend steadily to a reality not clearly perceived—these would be the strengths of the Eliotian, antiromantic hero.

These framing tropes in chapter 16, at the heart of the novel—focusing readers' attention on how optical devices aid and deceive perception—inflect the mind-as-mirror passage that immediately follows: there her emphasis on "faithful" and skeptical representation seems a corrective reminder of the illusions and distortions of vision. In fact, by reading chapter 17 as a response to the concerns of chapter 16, a new metaphor becomes apparent, one that enables George Eliot to dissect the structure of human vision more precisely.

In the light of the smoked glass and transparencies of chapter 16, the mind-mirror that opens chapter 17 becomes visible not simply as a mirror but as part of a structure that links an optical device—a mirrored mechanism—to its operator. It becomes evident that the mind-mirror functions very much like the mirror in a camera obscura, an optical instrument associated not only with parlor entertainment, like smoked glass and transparencies, but with scientific optics and pathology as well. Based on a principle known for centuries, the camera obscura "surged" in popularity after 1815 and commonly appeared in nineteenth-century media.[43] Many walk-in camera obscuras were open to the public at midcentury, in London (at the time of the Great Exhibition), Bristol, Edinburgh, and travel destinations such as Brighton and Margate. The camera obscura relies on the fact that light, streaming through a small opening into a darkened chamber, will project an image of the outdoors on the far wall of the chamber (Fig. 3). The camera obscura projects the image, in inverted form, on the far wall of the chamber. Many camera obscuras include a mirror angled to project the reflection onto a screen, so the operator may trace and preserve the image on the page, presenting to his audience the most accurate reproduction possible.

The mirror in a camera obscura thus points simultaneously back outward to the real world and upward to the site of representation distanced from the world; reality is at the same time reflected *in* and reflected *by* the mirror. This double function seemingly insures the accuracy of the image the operator will trace on the page.[44] However, the artist's rendering is hardly unmediated: it is a representation of a projection of a reflection of a projection of an image of the source. While the number, quality, and relation of objects will appear precisely as they are, angle or size may be distorted through projection, and direction will be reversed.

The human eye draws upon the same properties of physics, and the notion of the eye as a camera obscura was common at midcentury, especially among those interested in scientific topics. Helmholtz, in his 1868 lecture on "The Recent Progress of the Theory of Vision," centers his discussion around this analogy, the "natural camera obscura of the eye" (131), and his *The Description of an Ophthalmoscope* opens by directing the reader to "take any kind of small camera obscura well blackened within" and consider it "a *fac simile* of the eye."[45] The *Athenaeum*, for which Lewes reviewed regularly and which reviewed his books, published in 1856 a brief review

GEORGE ELIOT'S REALIST VISION

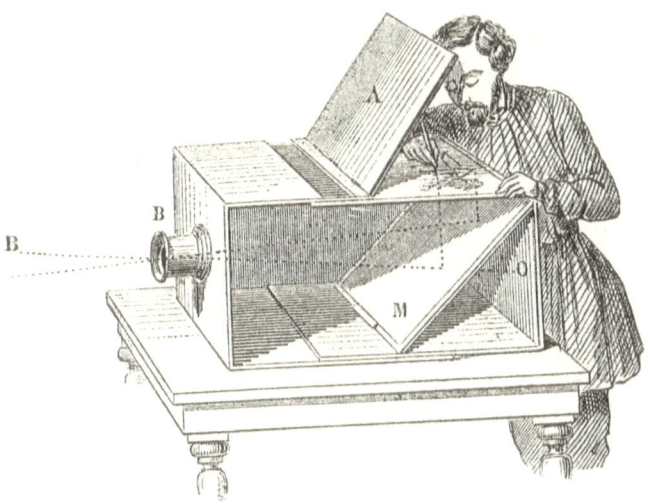

FIGURE 3. Illustration of camera obscura. From *The Museum of Science and Art*, ed. Dionysius Lardner (1855).

of a book by George Wilson, MD, titled *On the Extent to which the received Theory of Vision requires, as to regard the Eye as a Camera Obscura*.[46] In 1859 the surgeon John Spiller published a paper on his experiments in making a photograph in a camera obscura using the eye of a bullock as the lens.[47] It is likely, given George Eliot's and Lewes's involvement in the scientific community at that time, and her documented interest in vision and perception, that she may have known of these attempts. Such experiments were common enough that the Honorable Mrs. Mary Ward, in a manual for amateur microscopists, includes an extended discussion of a fish's eye—indeed, any eye—as "an exquisite miniature camera-obscura." She observed "all this mechanism [the camera obscura] shown with a cow's eye, cleverly arranged by a physician, who exhibited it to a large party."[48]

With this in mind, it becomes evident that, in the mind-as-mirror passage, George Eliot does not portray the mind as a simple mirror. While she does not make any direct reference to any particular optical device, she does emphasize those aspects of human vision that work like a camera obscura. In the optical structure described in *Adam Bede*, the image of reality enters the consciousness through the faculty of vision—the eye serving as the small aperture admitting light into a dark room—and the "mirror" of the mind registers a reflection which, projected outward, allows the narrator to painstakingly record this representation of the world for the readers.

What do we gain by recognizing the ways in which George Eliot's mirror trope works like a camera obscura, whether or not she brings that trope to the surface of her narrative? First, we can more easily perceive her interest in contested theories of vision and representation, since the camera obscura, like realism, suggests both ideal perception and its impossibility, which had become increasingly evident after the "epistemic break" of the 1830s and 1840s, when Victorians began to acknowledge the arbitrary nature of the visual stimulus.[49] George Eliot's specification of this structure highlights the mechanistic aspect of her theory of realism, linking it to mechanical observation by explaining vision as a structure, perhaps even implying an analogy that her readers might have expected in such discussions. The camera obscura was the conventional trope at midcentury for imagining, and questioning, the mechanics of vision. Crary points out that "for two centuries [the camera obscura] stood as model ... of how observation leads to truthful inferences about the world" but that "[b]y the beginning of the nineteenth century [it] is no longer synonymous with the production of truth and with an observer positioned to see truthfully." He argues that the camera obscura retained a kind of double valence in the field of vision: "For those who understood its optical underpinnings it offered the spectacle of representation operating completely transparently, and for those ignorant of its principles it afforded the pleasures of illusion."[50]

The camera obscura thus symbolized the questions of perception for midcentury thinkers; it stood, like nineteenth-century realist fiction, uneasily poised between the promise of transparency and the knowledge of illusion. The similarity between the camera obscura and realist narrative, in both their theoretical function and their cultural meaning, means that when George Eliot depicts this visual structure, which is like that of the camera obscura, she works out her relation to the tradition of realism, her interest in truthful perception, and her skepticism about the unreliability of both vision and representation.

Second, thinking about chapter 17 of *Adam Bede* in the light of a camera obscura allows us to see more clearly George Eliot's skeptical stance, another major link to theories of mechanical observation. We can more readily recognize the mind-mirror as a structure divided between an observer and the mechanism she operates, rather than a singular object. Although mechanical observation desires representation to be automatic, so that seeing and stating are collapsed, this particular mechanism explicitly distinguishes those tasks, suggesting that George Eliot theorizes perception and representation as separate challenges—an important distinction for a realist novelist, and one integral to clinical realism. The complexity of the structure she describes allows her to foreground her skeptical stance toward perception more readily than with a simple mirror trope. She complicates both realist vision and representation by drawing attention to the layers of mediation involved in what initially seems a simple act of exact mirroring. In fact, George Eliot is concerned not only with the role of the author and narrator, but also with the position of the reader and the possibility of a reading error. Her narrator comments, "Nature has her language, and she is not unveracious; but we don't know all the intricacies of her syntax just yet, and in a hasty reading we may happen to extract the very opposite of her real meaning" (155). In "reading" the observations imaged on our mind-mirror, we risk providing a transcription that distorts them further.

Thus, while the traditional "mind as mirror" trope proposes a simple mirror as the site of both observation and representation, George Eliot's narrative (like a camera obscura) separates its functions into the act of observation and the act of representation. The mirror of the mind is depersonalized and made instrumental; its function is not to "observe" or "notice" but merely to receive an image of the world, which the narrator then records on the page, much as the camera obscura was used to guide more accurate renderings of a scene. Thus, the optical structure she describes splits the narrator figure into a double function: the passively reflecting instrument and the narrative voice, with a limited agency guided by its structural role. In fact, one role can help police the other, as Bennett suggests in advising students always to record what they see through the microscope, "because drawing necessitates a more careful and accurate examination of the objects themselves." That is, the responsibility to record the image makes the observing more painstaking, although both observing and recording are inherently flawed.[51]

This distinction between "seeing" and "stating" allows George Eliot to revise the conventional mirror metaphor for realist narrative: she depicts narration more skeptically, because it is more complexly mediated, and insists that the multiple and conflicting aspects of human subjectivity inevitably inflect the structure at every point. As the narrator had earlier commented in "Janet's Repentance," "Do not philosophic doctors tell us that we are unable to discern so much as a tree, except by an unconscious cunning which combines many past and separate sensations . . . ?" (268). Even simple observation is both partial and multiple, and utterly reliant on its subjective origin.

George Eliot's interest in a distorting "mind-as-mirror" clearly constitutes part of a pattern of optical instrument tropes structuring *Adam Bede*, as well as her more famously scientific novel, *Middlemarch,* as a way of considering the abilities, and limits, of human perception. Reading chapters 16 and 17 in the light of these optical devices allows us to see that she and the proponents of mechanical observation share three central concerns: a skepticism about the distortions of human observation, an interest in a real or figurative "mechanism" of mirror-like vision, and an overall goal of a less biased representation. Clearly, George Eliot and clinical physicians draw from a common cultural reservoir of anxiety over truthful vision and representation. More interesting, both endorse a mirroring, slavish, mechanical observation as a means to accurate or "realist" representation. George Eliot's early use of the language of mechanical observation demonstrates her interest in adapting clinical realist vision, a model that—unlike naïve classic realism—could distinguish the disjunct steps of observation and representation, recognize the inherent distortions of the observing subject, prevent interpretive "improvements" to the record by enforcing a compensatory acknowledgment of the inherent situatedness and multiplicity of all human perception, and produce a moral imperative.

"The Secret of Deep Human Sympathy"

Adam Bede also represents an important departure from clinical realism. Crucially, George Eliot insists that a technique of mechanical observation can produce a sympathetic understanding of difference. In the novel, visual perception is transposed into subjective or even affective knowledge through a narrative of careful, clinical observation.

George Eliot does not echo scientists' optimism about the possibility and benefits of an objectivity supposedly enabling and enabled by mechanical observation. The French physiologist Claude Bernard, whose work helped shape George Eliot's later aesthetic,[52] demonstrates the extent to which an ideal of mechanical observation might require depersonalization. He refers to these principles in distinguishing between the crucial scientific processes of observation and experiment, in his *Introduction to Experimental Medicine* (1865). Bernard's experimental techniques introduced a number of changes to clinical medicine and its narratives, which chapter 5 will discuss, but he innovates by adding to the groundwork of mechanical observation, not departing from it.

As George Eliot had turned to a structure like that of the camera obscura to describe realist representation, Bernard calls upon the supposed objectivity of the camera, a later form of the camera obscura. While "the experimenter ... applies methods of investigation ... so as to make natural phenomena vary," in contrast

> [o]bservers ... purely and simply note the phenomena before their eyes.... To this end they use every instrument which may help make their observations more complete. Observers, then, must be photographers of phenomena; their observations must accurately represent nature. We must observe without any pre-conceived idea; the observer's mind must be passive, that is ... it listens to nature and writes at nature's dictation.[53]

Bernard's emphasis on the accuracy, lack of preconceptions, and passivity of the observer here, and his exhortation to "use every instrument," replicates the ideals of mechanical observation.[54] He values even greater automatism, however, in using not a camera obscura but its descendant, the camera, which seems to collapse observer and recorder, instrument and operator, in apparently recording images without mediation.[55] Furthermore, he warns, "the man of science wishing to find truth must keep his mind free and calm, and if it be possible, never have his eye bedewed ... by human passions" (39)—a recommendation George Eliot would hardly approve nor believe possible. By exaggerating the observer's physical and subjective distance from the object of study, Bernard distances clinical observation from the practice of medicine as an art. Similarly, by warning that physicians are better off "the less of ourselves we introduce" into observations, Stillé suggests that human subjectivity can be exiled from "mechanical observation" simply by refusing to "introduce" it.[56]

George Eliot, however, sees human mediation as inescapable and argues that a mechanical observation can and should actually produce subjectivity, in particular the desirable impulse of sympathy.[57] Although she posits that sympathy derives from the ideally impersonal, reflective stance of the detached observer, it is also clearly embodied (with the narrator's use of the "I"). Her truth of deep human sympathy is voiced as an expression of shared universal human community, but in the novels it emerges as also an intensely private response. If, as Daston says, the nineteenth-century "cult of objectivity" aimed to "suppress the self altogether," then George Eliot's sympathy offers a radical revision of objectivity; here it suppresses the self in order to bring forth the bridging of self to self. She uses the "mechanical" ideal to produce a humanist one, uses skepticism to produce trust, uses an intense disinterest in order to cultivate interest, and uses detachment and differentiation to produce an assertion of commonality.

Ironically, Ruskin (like Stillé and Bernard) also held that accuracy implies the evacuation of subjectivity, although he deplored this automatism and considered it antithetical to humanism. As he had warned in *Stones of Venice* in 1853, "Men were not intended to work with the accuracy of tools, to be precise and perfect in all their actions. If you will have that precision out of them ... you must unhumanize them." In fact, despite his injunction that the great artist must be "a mere ... mirror of truth," Ruskin scorned the Dutch realists "who do not feel at all, but who reproduce, though ever so accurately, yet coldly, like human mirrors, the scenes which pass before their eyes."[58] Ruskin's apposition of "coldly" with "human mirrors" condemns too-precise reproduction as dehumanizing: the artist's passivity as a "mirror" should signify his acceptance of the powerful imaginative faculty, not his rejection of subjectivity altogether.

In *Adam Bede* George Eliot champions the Dutch realism that Ruskin deplores, and she proposes that this mirror-like precision of observation need not require a frigid inhumanity. She argues that, paradoxically, the realist technique of mechanical observation actually produces a humanist sympathy, that it counters romanticism by teaching readers to "love that other beauty too, which lies in no secret of proportion, but in the secret of deep human sympathy" (181). The precise images produced by the camera obscura of realist vision are necessary but themselves inadequate; indeed, "[t]he keenest eye will not serve," she had earlier written, "unless you have the delicate fingers, with their subtle nerve filaments, which elude scientific lenses, and lose themselves in the invisible world of human sensations."[59] Thus the narrator of *Adam Bede* can substitute, for the "delightful facility" promised by a fantasy griffin, a "delicious sympathy" toward real people (177). This is her ultimate goal as a novelist, as she told John Blackwood—"the presentation of mixed human beings in such a way as to call forth tolerant judgment, pity, and sympathy"; this makes realism necessary but ultimately just instrumental.[60]

George Eliot argues here that lack of sympathy is actually a lack of knowledge. She implies that the accurate detail produced by a mechanical observation educates and enlarges the viewer, because it includes details that a selective eye might blink; and that this fuller knowledge promotes identification and elicits sympathy. Rather than empowering the viewer in a typically Foucauldian relation, then, George Eliot's version of mechanical observation disarms that viewer, rendering him subject to the unmanning effects of sympathy: these lead the "I" to assert the needs not of the self but of the other.

How would a precise, mirroring observation produce sympathy? Characters in the novel model the process by first providing, through dispassionate detail, a clear image of another character, and then soliciting an affective response by asserting sympathy with him. When Adam hears the details of his fiancée Hetty's crime, Mr. Irwine looks into Adam's face and is silenced, for

> the sight of Adam before him, with that look of sudden age which sometimes comes over a young face in moments of terrible emotion—the hard bloodless look of the skin, the deep lines about the quivering mouth, the furrows in the brow—the sight of this strong firm man shattered by the invisible stroke of sorrow, moved him so deeply that speech was not easy. (409)

Here George Eliot has Mr. Irwine show us exactly the kind of particularizing observation her narrator proposes in chapter 17, especially clinical in his initial, distanced description of the details of "the" skin, mouth, and brow. But after detailing how the body is marked and humbled by tribulation, the narrator (still speaking from Mr. Irwine's perspective) swerves away from clinical detachment and the systematic notation of symptoms, to an affirmation of interest in "this strong firm man shattered." The passage calls upon readers to match Mr. Irwine's emotions, when it emphasizes how "deeply" he is "moved" by Adam's grief.[61] Similarly, in chapter 21, the narrator allows us to watch Adam gazing around Bartle Massey's "night-school," the details of which he "knew by heart" and notes as his gaze touches each one. These deliberate observations yield sympathy: "a momentary stirring of the old fellow-feeling, as he looked at the rough men painfully holding pen or pencil with their cramped hands, or humbly labouring through their reading lesson" (232). What Mr. Irwine and Adam model, George Eliot asks her readers to share.

Paradoxically, then, *Adam Bede* argues for the mirroring realist technique Ruskin deplores, but offers it as an antidote to the effect—the cold, unfeeling art—he thought it would produce. George Eliot proposes this kind of realist vision as a cure for both the sentimental, self-absorbed fantasies of romantic narratives and the refusal of humanist subjectivity in clinical realism. Building on the eighteenth-century notion of sympathy as the visual circulation of affect, she expands upon Hume and Smith in arguing that the painstaking detail of a clinical representation may call forth a stronger sympathetic identification.

Furthermore, while Stillé articulates the goal of clinical narrative as differentiation—"penetrating into all things within our reach and knowledge, and ... distinguishing their essential differences" (46)—George Eliot wishes her sympathetic realism to transcend difference, to provide both diagnosis and cure. She vows, "[T]he only effect I ardently long to produce by my writings is that those who read them should be better able to *imagine* and to *feel* the pains and the joys of those who differ from themselves in everything but the broad fact of being struggling erring, human creatures."[62] She illustrates this difference between realist vision that produces difference, and one that produces sympathy, in the scene where Adam sees Hetty in court:

> In the corpse we love, it is the *likeness* we see—it is the likeness, which makes itself felt the more keenly because something else *was* and *is not*. There they were—the sweet face and neck, with the dark tendrils of hair, the long dark lashes, the rounded cheek and the pouting lips: pale and thin—yes—but like Hetty, and only Hetty. Others thought she looked as if some demon had cast a blighting glance upon her ... and left only a hard despairing obstinacy. But ... to Adam, this pale hard-looking culprit was the Hetty who had smiled at him in the garden under the apple-tree boughs—she was that Hetty's corpse. (431)

Here Adam articulates the elements of Hetty's appearance, using the impersonal article "the" to check off, one by one, her face, neck, hair, lashes, and so on. But his tabulation does not, as might be expected, dissect her into a mere litany of parts and symptoms. The passage avoids this effect largely due to George Eliot's insistence that Adam sees a continuity that embraces Hetty's life-shattering change, just as he recognizes the organic whole, "Hetty, and only Hetty" underlying these differentiated features. He knows her likeness beneath the terrible fact of her new and unalterable difference, rendered as likeness not to Hetty but to a cadaver. The narrator's assertion of human perspective ("to Adam"), of grief for the loss of pastoral innocence and "the Hetty who had smiled at him in the garden under the apple-tree boughs"—these crucially shift the tone of the passage. They insist that the catalogue of visual details should intensify, rather than deny, readers' sympathy for Hetty and for Adam. The "others" in the courtroom permit her to oppose the harsh "illusions" of the observer devoid of sympathy to what she sees as the redemptive power of Adam's truly humanist realist vision. Overall, the passage argues that mirroring (the recognition of likeness) is necessary but inadequate—a mere preliminary to the sympathy it enables in Adam.

The early George Eliot and clinical medicine thus both draw on a scientific ideal—realist vision as mechanical observation—but they use it to construct two very different cultures. With other clinical realists, Stillé valorizes an ethics of objectivity birthed through patient, painstaking labor. He considers that the skeptical, mediated quest for accuracy produces, and enforces, difference: that of one body from another, observation from subjective response, scientific from literary ("poetic") discourse, truth from falsehood. George Eliot, however, proposes this technique as a path to commonality. She argues that visual accuracy produces sympathy; that the laborious techniques of mechanical observation prompt us to build bridges over the chasms between us. She thus revises mechanical observation into a technique inextricably steeped in subjective relations. That is, George Eliot appropriates a mechanism, and a metaphor, associated with clinical realism; but she employs mechanical observation to produce a "deep human sympathy" in herself and her readers, while the physician uses it to suppress any emotional involvement with his subject.

George Eliot's analysis of sympathy here suggests some inherent resistance to it, a kind of antisensibility. The flow of sympathy is innately impeded, which is why the narrator must exhort the readers to open their eyes to all human experience, not just romantic experience. This innate resistance makes the self-discipline that produces sympathy a moral rather than just natural act: it overcomes our innate selfishness and self-absorption. Dickens, on the contrary, suggests that sympathy should naturally flow once he has gained us access to the sentimental scene. Neither he nor his readers need to work as hard as George Eliot does here. But both she and Dickens assume that to make us feel, they must make us see. For George Eliot, clinical realism offers an important and necessary antecedent to both seeing and making readers see.

Ironically, George Eliot fails to consider that the production of sympathy might actually hinder realist representation, just as Stillé and Bernard warn. When Mr. Irwine tells Adam of Hetty's crime, the sympathetic realist vision Eliot promotes does in fact endanger realist representation. Mr. Irwine's sympathy "moved him deeply," so "speech was not easy." Indeed, Mr. Irwine does not speak again, and we do not hear his thoughts, until Adam has worked himself into a rage and is almost out the door, on the way to accost Arthur. Furthermore, Mr. Irwine's silence affects the narrative itself. The technique of free indirect speech aligns him with the narrative voice here. The narrator breaks off Mr. Irwine's train of thought and begins again after clinically listing the changes in Adam's face, starting the sentence again, as if "that look" and "the sight" were too much to bear.

The courtroom passage suggests a similar breakdown of meaning in which deep human sympathy may be at odds with realist representation.

The narrator (speaking for Adam) repeats, "[She was] like Hetty, and only Hetty.... This was... Hetty... she was that Hetty," asserting Adam's recognition of and sympathy with the girl he loved. But the final word "corpse" ("she was that Hetty's corpse") interrupts, diverts, even reverses the redemptive process that George Eliot has worked so hard to establish. It points instead to the insistent doubleness of Hetty's identity, established never more clearly than in Adam's desperate desire to recognize, and assert the truth and identity of, the Hetty he knew, by discerning traces of her within that "pale hard-looking culprit." It permits the cadaver which grounds all clinical medicine to surface as her "corpse," and as a kind of refusal of Eliot's efforts to infuse it with Hetty's fled spirit. These examples suggest that the realist representation George Eliot recommends and the deep human sympathy that she valorizes may in fact not coordinate as readily as she suggests.

Sympathy and Narrative Perspective

George Eliot's complex engagement with observation and perspective in *Adam Bede* also positions her in relation to yet another important tradition. Daston reminds us that "the divergence, integration and transcendence of individual perspectives were the province of moral philosophy and aesthetics" in the eighteenth and early nineteenth centuries through the work of Hume and Shaftesbury. However, while the philosophical eighteenth-century and the scientific mid-nineteenth-century versions of perspectivity might "agree in both their means (de-individualization, emotional distance) and ends (universal knowledge of one sort or another)... they treat very different objects: moral and aesthetic claims on the one hand, and scientific claims on the other."[63] George Eliot's interest in moral and aesthetic claims clearly allies her with the philosophers, but she just as clearly uses elements of the later, scientific tradition of mechanical observation: her fetishization of detail and exactness, and her emphasis on the laboriousness and tediousness of the novelist's mirroring, passive labor. Furthermore, Daston notes that the philosophical tradition seeks a universal beauty, while the scientific one pursues the reality of nature. George Eliot combines these by arguing for a universal beauty grounded in the low, material reality of "nature and fact."

More important, Daston differentiates mechanical observation from the nineteenth-century scientific ideal of aperspectival objectivity, which seeks to escape any individualized angle of vision. She explains, "The difference between perspectival and mechanical objectivity is brought into sharp focus by their contrasting responses to photography. The photograph is the emblem of mechanical objectivity, because it appears to be a direct transcription of nature, free of meddlesome human interference. But perspectival objectivity rejects the photograph, because it preserves [the angle of vision]."[64] George Eliot's realism also explicitly rejects this scientific aperspectivalism, through an insistent privileging of the individual viewpoint. In *Adam Bede,* George Eliot argues that it is impossible to escape the individual angle of vision. Because the narrator's reflecting mirror is "in my mind," its view is inescapably an individual one.

Daston also distinguishes scientific aperspectivalism from Hume's early, aesthetic version of aperspectival objectivity. Humean sympathy reaches for a "perspectival suppleness, the ability to assume myriad other points of view, rather than the total escape from perspective implied by the 'view from nowhere'" cultivated by nineteenth-century scientists (604). This perspectival suppleness is just what the narrator models in a significant passage of "Janet's Repentance," roughly contemporaneous with the novel. In discussing the town's judgment of the evangelical preacher, Mr. Tryan, the narrator muses on the flaws and frailties of "real heroes."

> So it was with Mr. Tryan: and any one looking at him with the bird's-eye glance of a critic might perhaps say that he made the mistake of identifying Christianity with a too narrow doctrinal system; that he saw God's work too exclusively in antagonism to the world, the flesh, and the devil; that his intellectual culture was too limited—and so on; making Mr. Tryan the text for a wise discourse on the characteristics of the Evangelical school in his day. But I am not poised at that lofty height. I am on the level and in the press with him, as he struggles his way along the stony road, through the crowd of unloving fellow-men. (266)

Here the narrator explicitly refuses the "birds-eye" view of judgment associated with a de-individualized, distanced aperspectivalism. Rather, the narrator aggressively claims a local, individual perspective, down "on the level and in the press." The same movement of repudiation occurs in *Adam Bede* when the narrator scornfully refuses to be considered a "clever novelist," instead proudly embracing the "creeping," tedious labor of close observation, choosing the "low" view over the "lofty" one.

The similarities between these passages are instructive. The narrator's refusal to judge and prettify is thus associated not only with a clever novelist's inappropriate aesthetic evaluation but also with a critic's inappropriate moral judgment. The Tullivers' bourgeois taste in *The Mill on the Floss* is similarly associated with their poor moral judgment and lack of sympathy for Maggie. By asserting an individual perspective as well as assuming the labor of mechanical observation, the narrator also refuses the scientific ideal of aperspectival objectivity.

Significantly, George Eliot's refusal to enforce an emotional distance from her observed subject marks her difference from both mechanical observation and scientific aperspectivalism. Indeed, the narrator of "Janet's Repentance," after claiming that spot "in the press" with Mr. Tryan, continues by modulating into a more emotional key, moving yet closer to an identification with him:

> He is stumbling, perhaps; his heart now beats fast with dread, now heavily with anguish; his eyes are sometimes dim with tears, which he makes haste to dash away; he pushes manfully on, with fluctuating faith and courage, with a sensitive failing body; at last he falls, the struggle is ended, and the crowd closes over the space he has left. (266)

There is no hint of irony or undercutting here, as in other passages of free indirect discourse in the early fiction. The narrator here imaginatively and wholeheartedly inhabits not only Mr. Tryan's viewpoint but also his feelings, in a memorable display of the loss of the observing self in a deep human sympathy. This knowledge of Mr. Tryan's "struggles" overlays the narrator's local perspective with his, as it invests it with a powerful affective energy. In contrast to the scene in the courtroom, where the clinical gaze, alongside Adam's evident emotion, produces Hetty's "corpse" as much as Hetty, this scene does not borrow a dry, factual, clinical tone, and the emotional and rhetorical effect is not undercut.

If, as Daston argues, mechanical observation "battles the general, all-too-human tendencies to aestheticize, anthropomorphize, judge, interpret, or in any other way 'tamper' with the givens of nature,"[65] George Eliot's realism is similarly all about the self-restraint in renouncing preconceived notions of beauty or the little aesthetic "touches" that might nudge reality closer to them. It is true that the narrator is not entirely successful in either evading judgment (that "vilely assorted cravat and waistcoat"! that "high-shouldered, broad-faced bride"! [179, 177]) nor compelling sympathy (the repeated references to "poor Rosamond" in *Middlemarch* seem forced, and the references to "poor Hetty" tilt dangerously close to mere pity). But this aesthetic shudder, as a stutter in the narrative vow of communal sympathy, allies the narrator with other willing-but-flawed characters such as Mr. Irwine or Mr. Tryan. Like the distortion in the mirror, it suggests, our biases are inevitable but can be compensated for by acknowledging them. The narrator's determined embrace of even the bourgeois shopkeeper exemplifies just the kind of sympathy that the novel endorses, both real (flawed, human, and individual) and ideal (in its insistence on mastering the merely personal).

Certainly it seems strange to consider that a novelist, especially a novelist invested in ethical responsibility, might ask the reader to opt out of interpretation, if by interpretation we mean evaluation and judgment. But given George Eliot's skepticism about our perceptive abilities (physical, aesthetic, and moral), it is likely that she asks the reader to distrust the apparatus of interpretation, because—however impossible any true realist vision may be—it can only be achieved by refusing to "touch up" our perceptions with judgment. It is only by hewing to the principles of a mechanical observation of our fellow humans and of the novel that we may attain a true sympathy with them.

Both George Eliot's mechanical observation and her sympathy are grounded, then, in a refusal to judge, whether aesthetically (that cravat!) or morally (Hetty). Although the narrator does not always live up to the high standard she sets, Adam, Dinah, even Mr. Irwine are models for us because, while they do testify "on oath," they do not judge—they leave that to the trial and to God. George Eliot suggests that a full and complete record of Hetty's actions will call forth from the reader a more sympathetic understanding of her. The narrator's move from a discourse of mirroring to a legal discourse, "in the witness-box," thus reinforces the message of mechanical observation by reminding us of our proper place in the world—as witnesses to the world, not judges of it.

CHAPTER FIVE

Speculation and Insight

Experimental Medicine and the Expansion of Realism

> [P]oets should
> Exert a double vision; should have eyes
> To see near things as comprehensibly
> As if afar they took their point of sight,
> And distant things, as intimately deep,
> As if they touched them.
>
> Elizabeth Barrett Browning, *Aurora Leigh* (1857)

In *Middlemarch,* the novel in which she most intently examines figures of vision, George Eliot again suggests that the quest for a realist vision needs to both incorporate and exceed the methods of clinical realism. However, she refocuses her visual instrumentation away from the sympathy-producing mechanical observation of *Adam Bede.* Replacing the mind-mirror of *Adam Bede* with a pier-glass or a microscope's illuminating mirror, she sharpens her skepticism about human perception, shifting away from the need to produce sympathy and toward the obligation to correct for the distortions of egoism. The figure of the microscope replaces the purely passive observer-as-mirror with an active observer who must manipulate the apparatus of vision. Finally, she describes a subjective, idealized understanding that is not produced by but supplements mechanical observation with an imaginative insight that goes beyond sympathy in expanding the visual and affective depth of field.

Middlemarch reflects an important tenet of the new experimental medicine in its skepticism about clinical observation alone, but enthusiastic faith in its possibilities when combined with this intuitive, interpretive, even speculative inner vision. The novel registers how far George Eliot has come from a classic-realist text, in her acknowledgment of the provisional nature of vision, and in her insistence on both our egoistic complicity in deforming that vision, and the need to destabilize our standpoint and enlarge our visual range in order to remedy it. In this way *Middlemarch* accords with an important development in midcentury clinical medicine. In their valorization of empirical detail and method, early-nineteenth-century physicians had institutionalized a realist methodology—opposing a "mechanical" observation to speculation and "caprice"—that would become central to medical and literary writing. But, facing an unattainable ideal of perfect truth and complete knowledge, Victorian physicians are led to supplement their clinical vision with the more versatile and wide-ranging sight called speculation, in a creative tension that would trouble physician narratives throughout the century.

In *Middlemarch*, George Eliot interrogates marriage and vocation through the entwined lives of the townspeople, some gifted with extraordinary sympathy and ability, but nearly all marred by a myopia of "egoism" like the distorted romantic visions she had warned about in *Adam Bede*. To explain how egoism clouds vision, she offers not a mental but a physical mirror, in her famous parable of the pier-glass (a tall, narrow mirror). The narrator explains,

> An eminent philosopher among my friends, who can dignify even your ugly furniture by lifting it into the serene light of science, has shown me this pregnant little fact. Your pier-glass or extensive surface of polished steel made to be rubbed by a housemaid,[1] will be minutely and multitudinously scratched in all directions; but place now against it a lighted candle as a centre of illumination, and lo! the scratches will seem to arrange themselves in a fine series of concentric circles round that little sun. It is demonstrable that the scratches are going everywhere impartially, and it is only your candle which produces the flattering illusion of a concentric arrangement, its light falling with an exclusive optical selection. These things are a parable. The scratches are events, and the candle is the egoism of any person now absent—of Miss Vincy, for example.[2]

Here George Eliot revises the visual relation of observer and mirror, familiar from *Adam Bede*. Like her earlier trope, this "parable" poses an observer as both looking at a flawed mirror and looking at the world via this mirror, complicating the received notion of realist vision as a simple reflection of the world. The mirror, like most of those in these novels,³ represents our faulty perceptions—in this case scratched by the rub of events—but it is our egoistic reflection upon these traces of our experience that obscures our view of the world. The "little sun" of egoism, by highlighting the random abrasions "with an exclusive optical selection," disrupts the very function of the mirror, which should be to reflect the outside world beyond the candle, and the self. The distorted vision decried in *Adam Bede* is here altogether blinded by reflecting upon its own "flattering illusion[s]." The romance mocked earlier reappears in the explicit egoism of a Rosamond or a Casaubon, and the idealistic ambition of a Lydgate. In both novels, then, the narrators challenge our preference for self-flattering illusion and our failure to understand others' realities.

More important, George Eliot here subverts clinical realism more directly. She addresses her critique pointedly to science, turning the analytic instrument of mechanical observation on its source. She does privilege scientific terms as truth-terms—"concentric arrangement," "exclusive optical selection"—albeit with an ironic flair. And by framing this demonstration with the authority of the "eminent philosopher" of "science," the parable makes an experiment out of what was, in the source, merely an aperçu: Herbert Spencer and Ruskin had discussed a similar illusion: an observer of the moon over a body of water sees a reflective path of light leading to him.⁴ If "observation is investigation of a natural phenomenon, and experiment is investigation of a phenomenon altered by the investigator," then George Eliot here adopts the logic of experiment, in order to challenge it.⁵ By revising "moonlight on a lake" into "a candle held inquiringly to a mirror," she elaborates her mirror trope, strengthens her attack on egoism, and focuses her critique of science.

For the scientist is implicated in the very phenomenon he observes, by the narrator's wry gesture toward universality in saying, "[T]he candle is the egoism of any person now absent." The ironic exception of those present does not seriously excuse them from this structural distortion in human vision. Of course, the narrator implies that "the serene light of science" is a privileged order of illumination, one that would, like daylight, either illuminate all the scratches or permit the viewer to see through them to the larger reflection behind them. But in fact, the experiment depends upon candlelight, suggesting the "serene light of science" is absent; for if the experiment succeeds, the observer is dazzled. The narrator's experiment proves, paradoxically, the impossibility of an impartial clinical vision.

Most striking, the narrative evades two central questions: Under what circumstances may we view and record these scratches, the traces of our experience, without selection? And how may we compensate for the real-world events—like the humble housemaid's polishing—that left these traces? The experiment suggests that we are prevented from ever achieving a true and complete view of the world—a realist vision—by the mechanics of vision, which can only perceive the world by mediating it through a mind-mirror that is disabled by the effects of the light (the ego) we require, ironically, to see. Such a pessimistic assessment of human vision would accord with the conclusions of Johannes Müller, whose 1833 *Elements of Physiology* declared that, as Jonathan Crary puts it, "[O]ur physiological apparatus is again and again shown to be defective, inconsistent, prey to illusion and in a crucial manner, susceptible to external procedures of manipulation and stimulation that have the essential capacity *to produce experience for the subject.*"[6]

It is no accident that the "reality" effaced by this defective, "egoist" vision is precisely that apostrophized in *Adam Bede:* the world of "a monotonous homely existence"; we see the scratches on the elegant mirror but not the housemaid who made them. George Eliot's "parable" permits her sympathetic humanism to enlarge the landscape of clinical realism, embracing householder, scientist, and housemaid in one sweep of the narrator's eye. The pier-glass parable resonates throughout the novel as a trope of the romantic egoism that disables vision in many of George Eliot's characters. When the physician Lydgate succumbs to this blinding halo of light in his courtship of Rosamond Vincy, the narrator comments,

> Young love-making—that gossamer web! Even the points it clings to—the things whence its subtle interlacings are swung—are scarcely perceptible: momentary touches of finger-tips, meetings of rays from blue and dark orbs, unfinished phrases, lightest changes of cheek and lip, faintest tremors.... [A]nd subtle as it was, the light made it a sort of rainbow visible to many observers.... (IV.36.325)

As with the pier-glass, this optical illusion blinds Lydgate with light. Lydgate's almost clinical attention to Rosamond's body—eyes, blood flow to cheek, pulse or tremor—is distracted by the egoism of desire into registering only her lovely illuminated aura, woven of minute ("subtle") thread-like surface traces, and bright with the reflected light of her flattering interest in his person. His "personal pride and unreflecting egoism" and "that naïveté which belonged to preoccupation with favourite ideas" limit the depth and accuracy of his perceptions. His observations, honed in Paris, the mecca of clinical medicine, fracture under his self-flattering misperceptions, as he shatters his early idealist vow that "henceforth he would take a strictly scientific view of woman." This passage mocks not so much Lydgate's failure to live up to his scientific ideals, but the romantic naïveté of those ideals in promising that "illusions [could be] at an end for him" (144). Denying the subjective bias of his vision perversely renders Lydgate more vulnerable to its effects. These passages are more pessimistic than *Adam Bede* was on the possibility of realist vision, and they more pointedly critique the ideal of mechanical observation as unrealistic. No longer is it adequate to "tell you as precisely as I can what that reflection is" and assimilate that representation to a "rare, precious quality of truthfulness." Instead, the mirror's reflection of the world, its (even the narrator's) limited perspective on truth, is always-already obscured by the "little sun" of the self. In her trope of a microscopic vision, George Eliot works out an understanding of perception as necessarily provisional and contingent, and requiring both depth of field and a flexible, mobile standpoint.

The Microscope and Its Lenses: Clinical Vision and Speculative Insight

Mark Wormald notes that "we cannot separate [*Middlemarch*] from the discourse of microscopy."[7] If the pier-glass metaphor allows George Eliot to articulate a focused attack on egoism, the sustained conceit of the microscope suggests a skeptical, pragmatic response to the problem of realist vision. By portraying the narrator as overwhelmed by the visual material and the observing apparatus, the novel undermines a crucial feature of the classic realist text—its investment in "the positions of the subject in a relation of dominant specularity" to a given reality[8]—through reference to the preeminent instrument of nineteenth-century clinical realism.

What a mirror does well, one might conclude from the pier-glass experiment, is to reflect light; in a microscope this propensity to reflect and focus light may be harnessed and disciplined to augment, rather than hinder, vision.[9] A microscope's mirror provides a uniquely powerful trope for the mind-mirror, since, unlike a pier-glass or camera obscura, it does not frame and reflect but illuminates, by concentrating ambient light onto the world to be examined (Fig. 4). Thus the narrator of *Middlemarch* plaintively comments, "I at least have so much to do in unravelling certain human lots, and seeing how they were woven and interwoven, that all the light I can command must be concentrated on this particular web, and not dispersed over that tempting range of relevancies called the universe"

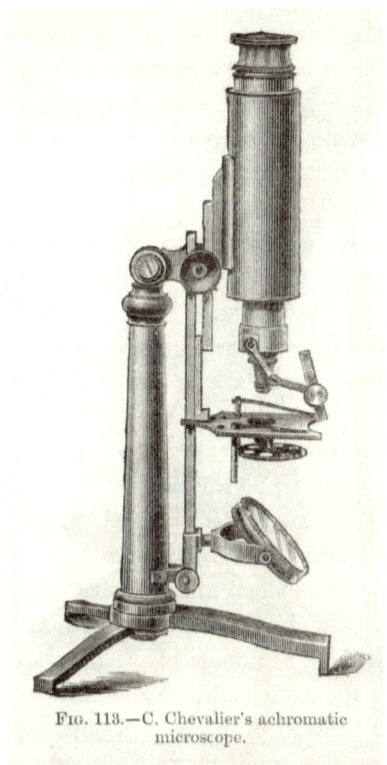

Fig. 113.—C. Chevalier's achromatic microscope.

FIGURE 4. Chevalier achromatic microscope, c. 1824. From William B. Carpenter, *The Microscope and Its Revelations*, 7th ed., edited by W. H. Dallinger (Philadelphia: P. Blakiston, Son, 1891), 148.

(II.15.132). However, the frazzled tone and suggestion of inadequacy in this passage suggest that "all the light I can command" may be insufficient and needs to be directed with care; the emphasis falls on adjusting and focusing the microscope rather than observing and narrating events.[10] This figural suspicion of light complicates the tropes of perception throughout the novel.

Indeed, *Middlemarch* draws attention to many problems of microscopic vision, both practically and figuratively. These were notorious. Bennett comments, "The art of observation is at all times difficult, but is especially so with a microscope," and Laycock remarks, "All experienced microscopists agree as to the fallacies to which the use of the microscope inevitably gives rise." The image could be distorted by something as trivial as the changing viscosity of the observer's corneal fluid. A pathologist described the blurry images as "something like the specters of an imaginative eye, or the refined delusions of a complex optical mechanism."[11] Light could be a liability in the microscope just as in a pier-glass, causing a glare or halo—a confirmation of George Eliot's figural suspicion of light and reflection.[12] Abundant light is "almost a defect" in the lens most useful to medical microscopists (¼"), where "the field of vision is often dazzling, and always presents a glare most detrimental to the eyes of the observer," enough even to "incapacitate" the researcher.[13] Both illumination and magnification—the strengths of the microscope—contribute to the many artifacts that can trip up the unwary observer.

Ironically, then, the microscope seems to offer greater specificity and greater objectivity when in fact, as George Eliot points out, its specificity is relative and the apparatus requires more intervention from the observer. The microscope thus displaces rather than dispels the problem of subjectivity, by providing a locus of observation that apparently distances the human observer but in reality requires significant manipulation and introduces the possibility of additional visual errors. In this context, self-abnegation is no longer possible. George Eliot moves away from Ruskin's purely passive observer toward an observer who needs to intervene, to "tune" the image, in a shift from Claude Bernard's conception of the "observer" to that of the "experimenter."[14] Theorists of science had begun to emphasize the need for human agency to direct experiments, a shift that Lewes registered in his work. By assessing realist vision through the figure of the microscope, George Eliot can begin to revise the meaning of human mediation: no longer perceived as "distortion" as in the theory of mechanical observation, the observer's engagement is now required to guide microscopic vision.

The novel leverages one other serious flaw in microscopic vision to suggest how crucially realist vision may require subjective involvement. The narrator first implicates the microscopic perspective by suggesting that the illumination and focus of a mirror and lens might be superseded at a higher resolution. That is,

> [e]ven with a microscope directed on a water-drop we find ourselves making interpretations which turn out to be rather coarse; for whereas under a weak lens you may seem to see a creature exhibiting an active voracity into which other smaller creatures actively play as if they were so many animated tax-pennies, a stronger lens reveals to you certain tiniest hairlets which make vortices for these victims while the swallower waits passively at his receipt of custom. (I.6.55)

Microscopic vision is relative, then, with gradations of "weaker" and "stronger" lenses; observations depend upon the observer's choice of perspective. The contrast between "you may seem to see" and "reveals to you" codes the stronger lens as the truthful one. It would seem to be the prototypically realist moment at which the novel "fixes the subject in a point of view from which everything becomes obvious" and "closes" the text by allowing us to "read the previous discourses in a 'final'—that is to say *once and for all*—manner [and] see the real identities which are mistaken."[15]

But by framing this remark with the narrative eye initially at fault, George Eliot considers that even the stronger lens might be superseded by another. There is no "once and for all" in this scene. Even the narrator's first interpretation cannot be dismissed as wrong; it is merely "coarse." Observers must sample the range of different visual truths or images at different levels of magnification or perspectives. And observers must judge only cautiously, since truth is never certain and possibly contradictory.[16] This passage gestures toward the unsettling midcentury visual theories of Helmholtz, which "made some forms of image resolution impossible." Microscopes frequently included multiple objectives with lenses of different strengths, requiring microscopists to navigate between different images of any single object viewed at different resolutions. Helmholtz's research threatened to render these correlations "unreliable" and unwise.[17] Furthermore, the various magnifications are irreconcilable. It was not possible to slide along a continuum from lesser to greater magnification; instead, one objective must be exchanged for another, and the observer must map the previous image onto the new one.[18] Indeed, the object often is invisible to the naked eye, and the observer can only imaginatively construe any perceived microscopic image as "seeing." Furthermore, what the eye perceives in a compound microscope is not the material object, simply magnified, but instead a virtual image created inside the tube of the instrument by the combination of lenses. The tempting suggestion of precision and minute examination in microscopy is complicated by the fact that the carefully rendered image may not even be veridical. Thus Carpenter's well-regarded treatise on the microscope argues, "[M]icroscopic vision is *sui generis*. There is and there can be *no* comparison between microscopic and macroscopic vision."[19]

The trope of microscopic vision thus leads the novel to consider the existence of simultaneous conflicting realities not all visible at once or in the same way. This phenomenon of the stronger and weaker lens insists on the situated, contingent vision of George Eliot's narrator, by making that narrator visible as a microscopist shifting between these "two contradictory articulations of the world."[20] George Eliot returns to the image of an oscillation between incommensurate lenses to mark Lydgate's fall from science. His friend Farebrother remarks on his sudden lack of "definite things to say or to show which give the way-marks of a patient uninterrupted pursuit, such as . . . 'there must be a systole and diastole in all inquiry,' and that 'a man's mind must be continually expanding and shrinking between the whole human horizon and the horizon of an object-glass'" (VII.43.602). It is just this need to switch scale, to view any scene both microscopically and from a universal perspective, that renders truth ultimately undeterminable; and it is the ability to do so, and to acknowledge the shifting ground of perception, that Lydgate loses and that George Eliot strives to display.[21]

This injunction to compare one perspective with another recalls a crucial flaw in vain Hetty's looking glass: that "instead of swinging backwards and forwards, it was fixed" and could offer only one limited view of her world. But it also marks a significant change in George Eliot's philosophy of realist vision. Rather than hoping that a clinical vision could *produce* the deep human sympathy she had sought since the days of *Adam Bede*, *Middlemarch* calls for *supplementing* clinical vision with a speculative insight borne of a subjective, imaginative sensibility, a mode of perception that can provide the needed depth in the visual field.[22]

The instances of this insight in the novel have become critical touchstones. Studying "Louis' new book on fever" early in the novel, Lydgate indulges

> that delightful labour of the imagination which is not mere arbitrariness, but the exercise of disciplined power—combining and constructing with the clearest eye for probabilities and the fullest obedience to knowledge; and then, in yet more energetic alliance with impartial Nature, standing aloof to invent tests by which to try its own work. (II.16.154)

This passage, as critics have noted,[23] serves as George Eliot's paean to imagination. Instead of the "involuntary" imagination of Ruskin's passive artist, the novel celebrates the agency of an intellect that delights in its "exercise" and "energetic" action.

The passage resonates with scientists' new insistence on the centrality of hypothesis in the scientific project. In France, Claude Bernard was promulgating new experimental methods based on observation and experiment, directed by hypothesis. In England, William Whewell, John Tyndall, and George Henry Lewes emphasized the importance of hypothesis—an imagined solution—in directing skeptical scientific experiment and analysis.[24] Bernard had famously argued that "we must give free rein to our imagination; the idea is the essence of all reasoning and all invention. All progress depends on that." Free rein within limits, of course; Lydgate's imagination carefully "stand[s] aloof" during the "tests" because, according to Bernard, "the results of an experiment must be noted by a mind stripped of hypotheses and preconceived ideas."²⁵ Nevertheless, Lydgate's imaginary vision powers, illuminates, and focuses his clinical realism. It is, in fact,

> the imagination that reveals subtle actions inaccessible by any sort of lens, but tracked in that outer darkness through long pathways of necessary sequence by the inward light which is the last refinement of Energy, capable of bathing even the ethereal atoms in its ideally illuminated space.... [Lydgate] was enamoured of that arduous invention which is the very eye of research, provisionally framing its object and correcting it to more and more exactness of relation. (II.16.154)

Lydgate's imagination, trained on the inaccessible object, is more powerful than "any sort of lens."²⁶ Yet George Eliot still employs the trope of the microscope to figure this sublime vision, which Lydgate must tune, "framing its object" and "correcting" his focus "to more and more exactness." Like the microscope, Lydgate's ideal vision allows for the change of scale and perspective, from minute details to unimaginable distances. Although the actual instrument must be supplemented by Lydgate's speculative insight, its mode of perception—its accommodation of varying magnifications and even perspectives—still governs George Eliot's figure here.

In all of these visual structures—camera obscura, pier glass, microscope—the observer is symbolically split into the mirror-of-nature and the observer or register of that image, although the camera obscura distinguishes further between observer and representer. In *Middlemarch*, George Eliot makes sense of the distinction between mind-mirror and observer, by positing that realist vision must be compounded of both clinical observation (the mirror, the would-be mechanical observation) and the interpretive insight—the observing subject—that humanizes it, thus comprehending both the clinical detail and the broader landscape of human lives.²⁷

Rethinking Imagination: Speculation and Insight in the Clinical Case History

Despite the emphasis in early Victorian medicine on empirical methods, later physicians argued that mechanical observation can be partnered with a more inventive vision. That vision ranged from intuition to speculation to hypothesis, all denounced by ardent empiricists. Authors dismissed attributes like insight, intuition, invention, ingenuity, and imagination most skeptically early in the century. They began to acknowledge the importance of "speculation" and "hypothesis" at midcentury, when clinical medicine began to be influenced by the tenets of experimental medicine, even before Bernard's influential 1865 treatise, *Introduction à l'étude de la médecine expérimentale* (*Introduction to the Study of Experimental Medicine*), and well before Tyndall's famous 1870 speech on "The Scientific Use of the Imagination." Physicians writing in the 1860s and 1870s are much more likely than earlier writers to encourage a judicious use of imagination, and to respect the intuition and interests of the individual physician-narrator. They reached a kind of compromise position in the 1890s, drawing back from the enthusiasm of the previous decades.[28] Of course subjective knowledge always persisted to some extent in even the most determined effort toward objectivity. More interesting is that Victorian physiologists came to recognize, to tolerate, and eventually to welcome it, in the form of speculation.

Most physicians writing through the 1840s renounced an imaginative or intuitive sensibility. Alfred Stillé asks the observer to exclude not just his correction, judgment, or illusion, but specifically his imagination and creative invention—his "natural and inherent power of seizing truth intuitively."[29] Even the reasoning of hypothesis was rejected. The *Dublin Medical Press* damns an 1845 treatise on gout because in its pages "[h]ypothesis is piled on hypothesis, conjecture on conjecture, speculation on speculation." Stillé argues that "the science of medicine is founded *alone* upon the observation of facts, to the *entire exclusion* of all hypothetical reasoning, and ... *as a science*, [medicine] has as little to do with the imagination or the conscience, as has the determination of a comet's orbit with the 'Music of the Spheres.'" This hostility to imagination sees it as not just incompatible with medical reasoning but a perversion of it. "[E]ach has its appropriate sphere," he explains. "[T]he poet should hold ... sway in his own realm, the scientific investigator ... in his. They cannot wield a common and united scepter." Not only is there "no necessary connexion between medical and intuitive truth, between the physical sciences and poetry or religion," but "[t]o assert such a connexion, is to pervert or degrade them all."[30] His choice of the terms "pervert or degrade" suggests the monstrous degeneration of a medicine that should be dedicated instead to healthy progress.

Many early-century medical writings then use the pejorative term "speculation" as shorthand for "inductive reasoning unfounded on facts." In 1818, for example, Dr. Crampton writes that he is not "inclined to speculate" on extra data, because "cases to illustrate this matter would have been liable to objection ... and I am unwilling to advance any thing but facts, or such reasoning as is evidently deducible from them." In 1828 Sir William Lawrence praises a colleague who observed "the nature of life" "not with the wavering outline and undefined forms of speculation, nor in the gaudy and delusive tints of hypothesis, but with the firm touch that real observation alone could give.... He seldom ventured into the regions of speculation." As late as 1844 Thomas Watson (whom George Eliot had read) warned his students against "ingenious refinements ... the speciousness of novelty, or the boldness of speculation" (15).[31] "Speculation" is of course a loaded term, suggesting unfounded fancy or risky investment, especially given its strongly negative financial associations with the failed 1840s "railway mania."

Remarkably, just a decade later, physicians begin to use the term approvingly in the sense of an informed, reasoned, yet imaginative projection into the unknown. "Speculation" provides yet another mode of seeing. To "speculate" is derived from the Latin *speculat-*, which implies scouting out, spying upon, exploring, or observing from a vantage point. Thus a text that "speculates"—unlike the aperspectival objectivity discussed in the previous chapter—expresses a particular angle of vision, the angle provisionally adopted by its particular observer and narrator, one susceptible of change and likely to range widely across the visual field. The term becomes associated with the new experimental medicine and Bernard's distinction between passive observation and active experiment, although physicians seem to use "speculation" for preliminary, exploratory reasoning, and reserve "hypothesis" for a more formal process.

In this sea change, individual experience, judgment, and even the supple, exploratory perspective of speculation could now be tolerated. Speculation helps develop a hypothesis and focus further inquiry. Edward Meryon, surveying the history of medicine, comments, "[T]he speculation, or even the bare analogy of one day, becomes the scientific induction of the next.... [H]ypotheses ... have been of high value as partial interpreters and provisional guides to higher truths." William Carpenter accordingly remarks, "[T]he speculation of M. Dugès can at present only be received as a stimulus to further inquiry." In a later edition he revises the sentence to read, "[A]nd the speculation of M. Dugès derives confirmation from the researches of Helmholtz...."[32] Speculation, then, works with observation so that investigation may be both far-reaching and still grounded in fact, with the physician casting his gaze out into obscurity, then bringing his minute, material observations up underneath that gaze to either support it and project it out further, or collapse it to go ranging elsewhere.

Despite its possibilities, speculation had to be used judiciously and it must supplement, not replace, mechanical observation. Laycock explains the necessary balance: "[Y]our researches must be ... philosophical in their nature and aim, while they are laborious and minute." William A. Guy argues that medicine requires not only precision and accuracy but also must allow "great scope for individual judgment, foresight, and decision. To the correctness of a good observer the medical witness must add the intelligence and invention of an acute experimenter." Henry Holland, a skeptic, warns more ominously that "strict attention to the laws of evidence" is "a matter of peculiar obligation" given that contemporary physiology was examining "the more abstruse questions connected with vitality, the nervous power, and the relations of mental and material phenomena—inquiries justifiable in themselves, but needing to be fenced round by more than common caution as to testimony, and ... conclusions." He laments, "[S]uch precautions have been disregarded," whether from "the real difficulty of the subject" or "the incompetency" of the researchers, including "many who wander merely on the confines of science, believing they are within its pale; and whose speculations on what they see are little checked by collateral knowledge, or by a due estimate of the laws and limits of scientific inquiry." Speculation is especially dangerous in curious researches: "The mystery of the subject is in itself a charm and seduction to the mind," Holland explains. "The feelings are thereby excited even more than the reason; and belief is hurried on, and results accredited, with little care for the sufficiency of proof."[33]

Many physicians demonstrated this anxiety about "wander[ing]" at the borders of medicine and this need to "fence round" their more speculative moments. William Brinton, writing on the alimentary canal, hedges admirably when he writes,

> It is a serious objection to any theory which would constitute irritation the first link in the chain of cause and effect, that ... we cannot name any morbid state or affection of the bowels in which irritation is not present.... Nor can we show, or even plausibly speculate upon, any differences in the degree or kind of irritation in the different diseases of the bowel.... On the other hand, since we find a physical fact ... to be the necessary condition of a peculiarly physical phenomenon ... there are considerable grounds for suspecting some immediate physical causation in this circumstance....[34]

Brinton's intricate, nuanced, and cautious syntax suggests that although "theory," "speculate upon," and "suspecting" are admissible rational activities, they require careful handling.

By midcentury, however, physicians began to consider speculation as even a necessary supplement to mechanical observation. Thomas Laycock explains, "Our observations are imperfect, our knowledge is imperfect—our conclusion, therefore . . . is never true, but always hypothetical or theoretical." John Rutherford Russell warns, "There can be no greater mistake than to suppose, that the avoidance of speculation secures a practitioner from error. Men of mind must speculate, because speculation is a name for thought."[35] Similarly, Laycock argues, "What is common to [all great thinkers] . . . is this—the combination of accurate, sedulous, minute observation with theories and hypotheses." Even Holland admits that "a certain amount of speculation, duly guided, enters into the purest form of inductive science." "Even could the mind be restrained from excursions beyond the strict bounds of evidence," he continues; "such restraint would be a wrong done to that genius, which has often through these speculations opened a path to new and more certain knowledge."[36] A more complete revision of Stillé's "practical genius" is hard to imagine.

Indeed, the age of hypothesis ushered in a new, romantic role for the physician, one that was unthinkable earlier: the role of intrepid explorer. American physicians especially embraced it, as is evident in the opening to the Medical Society of Pennsylvania at its 1872 meeting. Robert Crawford, a local physician, celebrates the adventurous spirit and laments the lack of recognition of his colleagues:

> When . . . a band of heroes . . . launch[es] forth on a voyage . . . to explore the dark and unknown regions of a far-off country . . . all the world are alive to the history and success of the enterprise. . . . And yet to every individual of our race . . . the discovery of islands, or even of continents, are of little value to him, compared with . . . the successful investigations and discoveries of that noble band of volunteers who constitute the medical profession, whose voyage of observation and exploration lasts from youth to old age, and whose life-long struggle has been against the enemies of human life and human happiness.[37]

Words like these enable Freud's romantic view of the scientific explorer, decades later.

By the end of the century, then, Thomas Huxley could describe speculation not as an unwelcome intruder disrupting the scientific process, but rather as a necessary and even pleasurable part of the scientific tradition. He explains,

> [F]rom the dawn of exact knowledge to the present day, observation, experiment, and speculation have gone hand in hand; and, whenever science has halted or strayed from the right path, it has been, either because its votaries have been content with mere unverified or unverifiable speculation (and this is the commonest case, because observation and experiment are hard work, while speculation is amusing); or it has been, because the accumulation of details of observation has for a time excluded speculation.[38]

Unlike the early George Eliot, whose distrust of pleasurable fancies led her to eschew griffins for carpenters, or Holland, who rejected the "charm and seduction" of speculative subjects, Huxley admits both duty and pleasure in the pursuit of knowledge. Balance is necessary between speculative and empirical stances. He echoes earlier writers' characterization of speculation as seductive, and agrees that it must be reined in (it is "amusing" but must not be "unverified or unverifiable"). Crucially, though, he warns that science will "halt" or "stray from the right path" without it.

In late-century medicine, although physicians could not deny the importance of hypothesis, they express more anxiety about speculative vision. Byrom Bramwell, lecturing in Edinburgh, cautions,

> No one is a truly great clinical observer who is not scrupulously truthful and exact. Let me beg of you, then, from the very first to strive above all things to elicit and record the facts *as they are in nature,* and to be on your guard against seeing the facts in a false light, colouring them, and making them fit in to the supposed nature of the case.[39]

He warns against deceptive vision here—"seeing the facts in a false light"—from an angle that might shade them into a false "colour." His repeated intensifying phrases—"from the very first," "above all things," "as they are in nature" focus urgency on the danger. He does not merely urge students to "elicit and record the facts"; he wants to impress upon them what they must struggle *not* to do, *not* to see, in the process. Bramwell's language often recalls Stillé's. Telling students to "cultivat[e] the habit of minute observation," he celebrates the "real and practical" knowledge of a medical treatise. A physician, he explains, must be scrupulously objective, must "conscientiously ... consider every doubtful and disputed point" and "weigh evidence correctly," with the "most persevering industry." In contrast, "mere cleverness, mere ability, mere literary skill, will never enable any man to write anything which is really worth reading ... on any subject connected with practical medicine." Most important, he argues, "is the training and disciplining of the mind, and the cultivating ... of the power, the habit, the method, and the love of work."⁴⁰

Despite these encomiums to a mechanical observation characterized by tedious labor rather than poetic or intuitive genius, Bramwell demonstrates an ambivalence characteristic of his time:

> [F]irst impressions and hasty conclusions, though they sometimes lead to very brilliant results and dazzle students, are apt to be erroneous. A sharp man of wide experience has no difficulty ... in drawing conclusions with so much rapidity and precision, that his knowledge seems intuitive, and his conclusions almost miraculous to the inexperienced.... The temptation to be brilliant in this way is a strong one—for after all there is no genius required—but it should not be encouraged; men who are in the habit of diagnosing cases off-hand, every now and again make huge mistakes.... It must not, however, be forgotten that "the experience of years ... gives to the physician ... a power akin to that of the artist, incommunicable by words; an instinct of divination, so to speak, by which the true character and the history of the organism may be read."⁴¹

This passage offers a remarkable oscillation between the censure of intuition and an acknowledgment of its seductive power; between "hasty conclusions" and "brilliant results"—"no genius required" and "almost miraculous"—"huge mistakes" and, as the last word, "a power akin to that of the artist." Bramwell is very much part of his time in suggesting that students should cultivate both "minute observation" and "very brilliant" first impressions, both "the habit, the method, and the love of work" and the "instinct of divination."

Speculative Insight and the Depth of Focus

Although George Eliot set *Middlemarch* in the early 1830s, when the doctrine of mechanical observation and the science/art debate were at a peak, she was writing in the 1870s, when the principle of hypothesis was securely established.⁴² As a result, she allows her physician protagonist to model an imaginative intellection unlikely to be shared by many of his 1830s peers. When Lydgate's "imagination reveals subtle actions inaccessible by any sort of lens," he anticipates his peers by a few decades at least. Although he will never discover "the primitive tissue" (I.12.102), he represents the future of scientific work. Lydgate may be permitted his anachronistic imagination because it provides a narrative model for the authorial gaze, probing and interpreting these "subtle actions" of motivation and character. Just as the microscope seemed miraculously to unfold a heretofore invisible world at the cellular level, George Eliot's aesthetic discerns unseen structures of thought. She models the supplementation of objectivity with speculative insight, for the narrator can only articulate the nature of Lydgate's "arduous invention" by moving beyond the kind of mirror-vision that described Hetty, to a speculative vision informed by a mobile standpoint and a variable interpretive lens.

Speculative insight carries unsettling implications for the realist author, however. As Lewes explained, "[T]he truth is that Science mounts on the wings of Imagination into regions of the Invisible and Impalpable, peopling these regions with Fictions more remote from fact than the phantasies of the Arabian Nights are from the daily occurrences in Oxford Street."[43] He figures the scientific imagination as even more fantastical than the classic romance that George Eliot so scathingly dismisses in *Adam Bede*. How far is Lydgate's "delightful labour of the imagination"—or George Eliot's—from the "delightful facility in drawing a griffin" she had resolutely rejected earlier? Clearly the relations of pleasure and knowledge have become complexly imbricated for her. While both *Middlemarch* and *Adam Bede* insist on the problems of human perception and representation, and both seek to make a place for the observer's subjective responses, *Middlemarch* proposes different terms, in different relations, from those in *Adam Bede*, where "a sympathetic realist vision" was clearly opposed to "an egoistical romantic gaze." Now the energy underpinning the bid for a "deep human sympathy," so central to the early fiction, has been redirected into an attack on its opposite, egoism; and sympathy itself has been revised into the broader sensibility of speculative insight. With the pier-glass scene's exposure of the romanticism of even scientific inquiry, and the narrator's endorsement of the scientific imagination, the realism/romance dyad has collapsed altogether.

What does the novel gain from adopting that farther range of perspective promised by speculative insight? George Eliot is not willing to give up the close focus associated with mechanical observation. However, the novel suggests that—as in Victorian medicine—these two modes of vision may complement one another. If it is possible to work with both a "stronger" and a "weaker" lens in microscopic vision, why cannot unassisted vision also vary from a close focus to an infinite one, just as physicians do in oscillating between the detail work of mechanical observation and the longer vision of speculation? The novel persistently imagines different levels of images, background and foreground, superimposed or combined to be simultaneously available.[44] Dorothea notices Featherstone's funeral procession in the distance, and the narrator muses, "Scenes which make vital changes in our neighbours' lot are but the background of our own, yet ... they become associated for us with the epochs of our own history" (IV.34.306). Later in this scene, Casaubon enters the room to sit "in the background," where his presence is acutely felt by Dorothea (IV.34.307). This expanded focus on near and far underlies Dorothea's most terrible moment, when she mourns her love for Ladislaw, whose "nearness" is also a "parting vision," who is "aloof, yet persistently with her" (VIII.80.739). While this vision is overpowering to her at first, her "vivid sympathetic experience returned to her now as a power: it asserted itself as acquired knowledge asserts itself and will not let us see as we saw in the day of our ignorance" (VIII.80.741). Dorothea's expanded, sympathetic vision is realized here through precisely this kind of expanded focus comprehending both near and far. At that moment,

> there was light piercing into the room. She opened her curtains, and looked out towards the bit of road that lay in view, with fields beyond, outside the entrance-gates. On the road there was a man with a bundle on his back and a woman carrying her baby; in the field she could see figures moving—perhaps the shepherd with his dog. Far off in the bending sky was the pearly light; and she felt the largeness of the world and the manifold wakings of men to labour and endurance. She was a part of that involuntary, palpitating life, and could neither look out on it from her luxurious shelter as a mere spectator, nor hide her eyes in selfish complaining. (VIII.80.741)

The narrative gaze here, like Dorothea's, starts with her immediate standpoint near the curtains and the window frame but rapidly moves out to the road and its figures, the field and its figures, and the "bending sky." That her gaze does not simply travel outward, adjust its focus to infinity ("the largeness of the world"), and stay there is evident in that the passage returns more than once to her spot at the window, to assert that "she was a part" of that larger world—that is, to assert the existence of a continuum of life that reaches from the window to the world and back again—and also to note her standpoint, in a "luxurious shelter." This expanded vision occurs at her apotheosis of sympathy and understanding, in which her largeness of spirit finds its greatest expression. In a reversal of mechanical observation,

Dorothea's affective response enhances her vision, making it clearer and more powerful. Her speculative insight is also clearly at work (wondering about that shepherd with his dog). In contrast, the egoist of the pier-glass has a much more constricted range of focus, bounded by the nearest surface and blinded to events "beyond" that mazy glow.

The expanded focus thus combines a close, realist look at one's own immediate surroundings and an imaginative reaching out to the bounds of vision. Other characters also demonstrate it at critical moments. When Bulstrode is on the verge of exposure, he "felt the scenes of his earlier life coming between him and everything else, as obstinately as when we look through the window from a lighted room, the objects we turn our backs on are still before us, instead of the grass and the trees. The successive events inward and outward were there in one view: though each might be dwelt on in turn, the rest still kept their hold in the consciousness" (VI.61.578). Although the past is distanced from the present, Bulstrode achieves an unusual clarity and depth of focus in this moment of extremity, in which the "background" of the past seems to come forward and claim equal attention with the "foreground" of the present.[45] Lydgate experiences a similar suddenly expanded focus at his "moment of vocation," when the minute details of the valves of the heart reveal to him the extent of knowledge promised by those tiny folding doors. With his mind's eye still fixed on the "finely-adjusted mechanism in the human frame," "the world was made new to him by a presentiment of endless processes filling the vast spaces planked out of sight by that wordy ignorance which he had supposed to be knowledge" (I.15.135).

What George Eliot strives for in these scenes, and implicitly urges her readers to strive for as well, is what photographers and microscopists call "depth of focus." A visual instrument—a camera or microscope—with good depth of focus can image objects both far and near with good resolution throughout the field. Jabez Hogg explains, a "*large angle of aperture* is necessarily incompatible with the far more generally useful quality of *penetration*. *Penetrating power* is synonymous with *depth of focus,* that is, [the] extreme distance of two planes, the points of which are *at the same time* sufficiently in focus for the purpose of distinct vision." Depth of focus combines a long field of vision with the selecting, intensified attention of focus. However, because "illumination . . . diminishes with [the] angle of aperture," a microscope adjusted for greatest depth of focus will need more light.[46] Thus George Eliot's narrator exclaims, "[A]ll the light I can command must be concentrated on this particular web, and not dispersed over that tempting range of relevancies called the universe" (II.15.132). "This particular web" is, then, not just a web but also a field of vision, one that requires constant adjustment to maintain both focus and illumination in a continuous striving toward the clearest, most comprehensive vision.

Depth of focus produces in the Victorian novel its characteristic diversity of discourses and standpoints, and its ability to accommodate seemingly incommensurate subjects, from the nettlesome details of bourgeois furniture and horse-trading to the most sweeping questions of human existence. Henry James may refer to the unmatched depth of focus in Victorian novels when he designates them "large loose baggy monsters, with their queer elements of the accidental and the arbitrary."[47] But a principle of selection in the best of these novels belies the descriptions of them as indiscriminate collections of clutter. George Eliot strives in *Middlemarch* to demonstrate how the combination of focus and range that characterizes depth of focus enables a powerful illumination of human lives, with their simultaneous experience of the trivial and the profound. It is something like depth of focus that allows her "literary language" to shift "with great flexibility from level to level, achieving much of its intensity by means of allusion and connotation across levels."[48] Increasingly skeptical but also increasingly ambitious, George Eliot produces in *Middlemarch* a clinical realism enlarged by and corrected with sympathy and imagination, combined with them in a depth of focus that ties the close examination of mechanical observation to the broad and deep vista of speculative insight. If her realism is founded on the apparent incommensurability of clinical vision and its necessary supplement, speculation, it is also fully aware of the contingency of all vision.

CHAPTER SIX

Mapping an Unnavigable River

Freud, Rider Haggard, and the Imperial Romance

Twentieth-century historians of medicine, developing a more analytic historiography, shifted the field away from the "great men of medicine" toward the examination of medical cultures and practices. However, any reading of the case history must grapple with one major figure: Sigmund Freud, whose struggle to establish a science of psychoanalysis also redefined medical narrative. His influence on the novel has hardly been less.

Freud reopens debates about the form and authority of the case history at a crucial point in its development. As Steven Marcus has argued, "[T]he case of Dora is first and foremost an extraordinary piece of writing.... [I]t is a case history, a kind or genre of writing—that is to say, a particular way of conceiving and constructing human experience in written language—that in Freud's hands became something that it never was before."[1] In this chapter, I discuss the literary nature of psychoanalytic work: its inherently metaphorical mechanism; its figuration of the psychoanalyst as reader, interpreter, and editor; its reliance on narrative and a figurative logic as cause, diagnosis, and treatment; and its structural similarity to romantic literary genres, despite Freud's frequent invocations of realist narrative technique. In particular, Freud uses the late-nineteenth-century imperial romance to authorize his search for truth as an incessantly textualized, labyrinthine descent into a primitive past.

Placing Freud within the historical arc I've laid out clarifies how elements of his case history endangered his bid for professional authority. Psychoanalytic work is not only literary work, as other critics have noted, but a discursively hybrid literary work: Graham Frankland points out that "[a]s well as a self-deconstructing postmodernist, Freud can equally be seen as a creator of mythopoeic narratives, an introspective Romantic, a nineteenth-century bourgeois realist, a modernist experimenting with stream-of-consciousness technique, and as many variations on the theme as there are critics."[2] This chapter will argue that Freud's early psychoanalytic case history juxtaposes the realism of the clinical report with antirealist genres like the sentimental novel, roman à clef, or imperial romance. He recuperates precisely those aspects of the eighteenth-century case history that were ostensibly repudiated by clinical medicine. Freud foregrounds his close observation but, by also valorizing judgment and interpretation, he departs from the principles of mechanical observation. In fact, he stages not only his speculative insights but also the curious sight presented by his patients, and his own spectacular heroism in tracking and mapping the unknown territory of the mind. Ultimately, Freud's case history revolutionizes the role of medical narrative by not only recording but also conducting the work of psychoanalysis; but it does so by drawing on visual and representational modes that were no longer collectively recognizable as clinical medicine.

Sigmund Freud strove to position himself as the founder of a new science, an accomplishment for which (he was convinced) he was unrelentingly and unfairly attacked. As he explained, "[P]sycho-analysis is my creation ... and all the dissatisfaction which the new phenomenon aroused in my contemporaries has been poured out in the form of criticisms on my head."[3] His provocative combination of clinical observation with a curious sight and an intuitive, speculative insight, and his insistent discursive hybridity, forced him into the role of an embattled prophet as he sought a secure site of narrative authority on which to found his science. The unconventional lineaments of Freud's psychoanalytic case history not only hindered his attempts to establish psychoanalysis as a science but also allowed clinical medicine to disavow these elements in itself. After Freud, clinical medicine could externalize its curious past by relegating these discourses to the marginalized practice of psychoanalysis.

This chapter focuses on Freud's earliest full-length case histories, written as he was still developing the basics of psychoanalysis and trying to ground it as a science. These early case histories focus on hysteria, in *Studies on Hysteria* (coauthored by Freud's early collaborator, Josef Breuer, and published in 1895) and *An Analysis of a Case of Hysteria* (the case history of "Dora," written in 1901 but not published until 1905). *Dora*, now a canonical text in studies of literature and medicine, hysteria, and feminist theory,[4] displays his growing sense of opposition. Both these texts persistently romanticize psychoanalysis, its procedures, its practitioners, its detractors, and its texts, to establish a Freudian "empire" in the scientific realm.

FREUD AND THE HISTORY OF THE CASE HISTORY

Freud's unique experiment in genre can only fully be understood within the historical trajectory of the case history. He claimed that psychoanalysis was an entirely new medical science. Early in his career, he explains, "I regard [my initial views] as valuable first approximations to knowledge. . . . [A]ny one interested in the development of catharsis into psycho-analysis [should] begin [here] and thus follow the path which I myself have trodden."[5] If his theories are new, however, his case histories mine the history of the genre. This genre demonstrates capaciousness and generosity in its relation to the past of medical narrative. He references not only ideals of clinical medicine such as mechanical observation and speculative insight, but also norms of eighteenth-century medicine such as a curious sight and an expansive prose style. In fact, Freud elevates his literary style—characterized by anecdotal argument, discursive hybridity, a nonlinear structure, and figurative language—to the status of a new methodology. Finally, he offers a new model of vision, which goes beyond even the surveying impulse of speculation in its active intervention, its imaginative projection, and its conflation of diagnosis and treatment: Freud unravels, traces, and maps the knotty puzzle of the troubled mind, using the romantic rubric of the labyrinth and its heroic explorer.

This chapter aims to complicate the critical convention that "[i]t was not until towards the end of the century and the advent of psychoanalysis that medical discourse adopted, in the case study, a form that approximated literary narrative."[6] Setting aside for the moment the covert persistence of literary norms such as sentimentalism in nineteenth-century case histories, the relation of the psychoanalytic case history to literary narrative is vexed, to say the least. In some ways, Freud's discursive hybridity expands the range and power of his narratives. The clinical case history strove for a realist narrative based on clinical observation, but privileging clinical norms hampered its ability to narrate some kinds of cases. Freud's case histories, which examine difficult diagnoses like hysteria, call upon multiple genres, many of them associated with literary work: theory, observation, interpretation, confession, manifesto, jeremiad, biography, autobiography, memoir, and outright fiction. This discursive hybridity creates one of the most flexible and extraordinary explanatory narratives of the fin-de-siècle. But Freud contested and denied his investment in literary forms, doubtless because his failure to maintain discursive purity troubled clinical norms and undermined his ability to establish psychoanalysis as a science.

Thus Freud's innovations change the relation of clinical medicine to the medical case history. His case history shows up the narrow visual and representational choices available to the clinical case history. It encumbers him with material associated with the nominally prescientific period of medicine, while he strives to found a new medical science; and it allows clinical medicine to marginalize these unwanted practices while not eschewing them altogether. It is no wonder, then, that Freud portrays himself as embattled. In his "History of the Psycho-Analytic Movement," he remarks, "I have long recognized that to stir up contradiction and arouse bitterness is the inevitable fate of psycho-analysis" (8). Although psychoanalytic theory eventually became influential, Sander Gilman comments that for a long time it "was seen as a Jewish pseudoscience and as [itself] a form of mass hysteria."[7] What does it mean for the psychoanalytic case history, and for Freud himself, that he constructs his new science as continually under attack?

Freud as a "Man of Science" and Clinical Physician

Despite figuring his work as new, Freud does not abandon the goals of clinical medicine; in fact, he embraces them to authorize his own project. As Sarah Winter shows, he did present psychoanalysis as a departure from psychiatry and neurology, and he worked to distinguish the psychoanalyst from the physician.[8] But his narratives required extraordinary authorization, given their methodological and discursive hybridity.

Freud attempts to gain authority for psychoanalysis by attempting to secure it as "science," despite his ambivalence toward and uneven reception in that community. Winter argues that his "masterful mobilization of scientific professionalism worked to legitimize psychoanalytic expertise."[9] He says, for instance, "You will realize, I am sure, that one cannot properly deny the findings which follow from this modification of Breuer's procedure so long as one puts it aside and uses only the customary method of questioning patients. To do so would be like trying to refute the findings of histological technique by relying on macroscopic examination."[10] Here Freud aligns his own strange technique with the seemingly unarguable evidence of the microscope—the foremost advance of late-nineteenth-century science, already an icon of immense cultural authority.[11] By posing an analogy between cathartic theory and the microscope, he makes his critics seem not only illogical in their reluctance to test his system, but also backward in their ignorance of modern scientific technique.

In *Dora*, Freud overtly aligns himself with scientific progress, and his critics with its enemies. He reassures us that "[w]hat is new has always aroused bewilderment and resistance."[12] It is true that medical advances often met controversy. The physician Henry Holland comments, in a separate debate, "The frequent revival of controversy on these points among modern writers shows at once their importance, and the incompleteness of the knowledge yet obtained on the subject."[13] The structure of Freud's psychoanalytic case history does carefully identify him as a researcher in the tradition of nineteenth-century clinical science.[14] In *Studies on Hysteria*, he ostensibly separates the historical from the more theoretical sections of the case history; he divides each patient's case history into the history proper and his "discussion" of the case. Dora's case is further divided into "Prefatory Remarks," "The Clinical Picture," analysis of her dreams, and a "Postscript." Freud prominently uses specialized terminology and links his discussion to other sciences, such as mathematics, when he explains, "If we ... try to represent the ideational mechanism in a kind of algebraical picture, we may attribute a certain quota of affect to the ideational complex of these erotic feelings which remained unconscious, and say that this quantity (the quota of affect) is what was converted."[15] His reference to a "quantification" of affect also suggests clinical representation, by promising to objectify the patient's emotions.

However, Freud proves to be less consistent than strategic in his use of scientific methodologies. Clinical observation certainly grounds some of his work; in the case history of "Fräulein Elisabeth von R.," he devotes one long paragraph to clinical observation of the type and location of the pain in his patient's legs ("a fairly large, ill-defined area of the anterior surface of the right thigh").[16] He is likely to draw attention to the clinical rigor of his methods. In "The Aetiology of Hysteria," he claims the virtue of a mechanical observation. He warns his critics, "Whatever you may think about the conclusions I have come to, I must ask you not to regard them as the fruit of idle speculation." Instead, "[t]hey are based on a laborious individual examination of patients which has in most cases taken up a hundred or more hours of work."[17] By formally substituting "laborious" for "idle," and "examination" for "speculation," Freud (like Byrom Bramwell in chapter 5) anchors his theories in the rhetoric of early mechanical observation. He strikes a similar empiricist stance when he boasts, in *Dora*, that he "approached the study of the phenomena ... without being pledged to any particular psychological system" and that "the material for [his] hypotheses was collected by the most extensive and laborious series of observations" (103). Sarah Kofman notes his ambition to "transform the initial untreated material of the text into a laboratory-controlled scientific fact."

But Freud's critics, then and now, attack his claim to empiricism. His research relies almost entirely on his patients' self-presentations and draws from a narrow demographic; and his agile and ingenious interpretations of his data look more like a leap of faith than a step of logic. Freud mentions that another physician considered his *Studies on Hysteria* "an unjustifiable generalization of conclusions."[18] His biographer Ernest Jones characterizes the reviews of *The Interpretation of Dreams* (1899) as "annihilating" in their critique of Freud's science: one psychologist jibed that "uncritical minds would be delighted to join in this play with ideas and would end up in complete mysticism and chaotic arbitrariness," while another more soberly considered that "the imaginative thoughts of an artist had triumphed over the scientific investigator."[19] Such criticisms persist; the twentieth-century literary critic Richard Webster (who is openly hostile to Freud's project) chastises him for theorizing beyond his evidence, arguing, "By far the most extraordinary feature of Freud's own theories is their almost complete disregard for any ... empirical factors."[20] Even Vern L. Bullough, a historian of sexology who is largely complimentary to Freud, remarks, "What he did was to seize on selected and historically transient evidence and generalize it into universal law."[21]

Freud's allegiance to clinical representation is also mixed. While some critics have found Freud to use a type of plain speech, a closer investigation of their examples does not support this claim. Steven Marcus waxes poetic about Freud's "splendid extended declaration about plain speech," part, he says, of "a tradition coming directly down from Luther."[22] But the passage he quotes from *Dora*, in which Freud proudly declares, "I call bodily organs and processes by their technical names.... *J'appelle un chat un chat*" (41), not only "disappear[s] into French" (as Marcus himself acknowledges) and into a metaphorical idiom, but, more importantly, refers more to a refusal to euphemize physiological organs and processes—that is, refers to a plain *vocabulary*—than to the plain *syntactical structure* that is part of the tradition of plain speech. Likewise, when Ursula Reidel-Schrewe praises Freud for "his skill in articulating observations of extremely complicated systems in a clear and inventive language," she refers primarily to his "similar, strikingly simple but perfect comparisons"—that is, his use of perfectly apt metaphors, his commitment to literary figuration rather than syntactical simplicity.[23]

Freud's ambivalent relation to clinical methodology is evident even when he signals a commitment to objectivity:

> If we ... enter into a girl's feelings, we cannot refrain from deep human sympathy with Fräulein Elisabeth. But what shall we say of the purely medical interest of this tale of suffering, of its relations to her painful locomotor weakness, and of the chances of an explanation and cure afforded by our knowledge of these psychical traumas?[24]

Here he claims both a sympathetic stance and its replacement, the more pragmatic—and, indeed, professionally necessary—detachment of the physician, signaled in part by the replacement of a sentimental rhetoric that demonstrates his sensibility ("enter into a girl's feelings," "deep human sympathy," "tale of suffering") with a clinical discourse that obscures it ("locomotor weakness," "psychical traumas"). Indeed, he continues,

> As far as the physician was concerned, the patient's confession was at first sight a great disappointment. It was a case history made up of commonplace emotional upheavals, and there was nothing about it to explain why it was particularly from hysteria that she fell ill or why her hysteria took the particular form of a painful abasia. (144)

This remarkable statement erases any trace of his earlier sympathetic eye, demoting her "tale of suffering" to "commonplace emotional upheavals." This passage nudges the distanced, skeptical relation of the clinical physician toward his patient to a frankly oppositional one. The "commonplace" nature of Fräulein Elisabeth's problems render her both more difficult to treat and of less medical interest to Freud, who evaluates the patient with an eye to the development of his theories. Freud's identification of himself in the third person ("the physician") re-places him as a distanced, generic observer.

Although Freud codes this juxtaposition of the sympathetic eye with clinical observation as a rejection of sentiment, it allows him to reintroduce a sentimental narrative, but with himself in the role of sufferer. By syntactically replacing Fräulein Elisabeth's "tale of suffering" and "confession" with a more clinical "case history," Freud also displaces her "suffering" with his own "great disappointment," a setback that he suggests is weightier than his patient's "commonplace emotional upheavals." After having dismissed his initial emotional response as a person, he introduces his subjective response as a physician, which indicates his objective interest in the case. Such a mixture of clinical and sentimental vision, like the conjunction of clinical and figurative language, indicates Freud's contested relation to the traditions of medicine upon which he draws.

Despite Freud's claim to inaugurate a "new" science and his careful references to clinical norms, his cases look back to eighteenth-century medicine in several ways. Indeed, his rhetorical strategies perform what he might consider a return of the repressed. Freud recuperated many norms of eighteenth-century medical practice: his interest in the "singular" case and in theoretical systems; his literary prose style; his revival of "curious sights" in his own overtly interested, sexualizing gaze; and the curious and controversial disorder he studied (hysteria). Freud values the singular, individual case; he privileges the anecdote rather than the quantification associated with clinical medicine. His texts compulsively theorize despite their declared allegiance to empiricism. He reintroduces the first-person narrative more common to the curious than the clinical case history, now in the form of the dream; and he otherwise returns the patient's voice to the page in his frequent textual use of dialogue.

Freud's representational practice recalls the "man of letters" as much as the "man of science." He retrieves the eighteenth-century practice of using illustrative quotations from and allusions to literature. He presents psychoanalytic evaluations of literary texts and characters, in the tradition of John Connolly's treatise on insanity, which examined Macbeth and other literary figures alongside actual patients.[25] And Freud establishes the importance of the physician's sympathy as a prerequisite for treatment of some disorders: "I cannot imagine bringing myself to delve into the psychical mechanism of a hysteria in anyone who struck me as low-minded and repellent, and who, on closer acquaintance, would not be capable of arousing human [read: his own] sympathy," he says; "whereas I can keep the treatment of a tabetic [syphilitic] or rheumatic patient apart from personal approval of this kind."[26] His emotional investment in his cases is evident. Despite his pose of dispassionate analysis, his narrative voice frequently throbs with passion, whether sympathy for his patient, anger at his critics, curiosity about the case, or the disappointment chronicled above.

Freud also returns to the overtly subjective, "curious" modes of vision disclaimed by nineteenth-century physicians. He seemingly replaces the visual relations of eighteenth- and nineteenth-century medicine with aural investigation, for the psychoanalyst must above all be a good listener. But his case histories nonetheless indulge a specular economy. They encourage the voyeuristic curiosity of eighteenth-century medicine and construct his patient as a spectacular, curious sight. Freud restores the "secret history" to center stage; one medical review even chided him for "usurp[ing] the confessional."[27] The peculiar symptoms of hysterical patients provide the kind of fantastical spectacularity common to the curious sight of the eighteenth-century case history. Frau Emmy von N., for example, "every two or three minutes . . . broke off [her narrative], contorted her face into an expression of horror and disgust, stretched out her hand . . . spreading and crooking her fingers, and exclaimed, in a changed voice, charged with anxiety: 'Keep still!—Don't say anything!—Don't touch me!'"[28] Another patient, a young singer, found herself first unable to close her mouth, and then, once it had been forced closed, unable to open it again.[29] Perhaps most famously, Breuer's patient Fräulein Anna O. "lost her command of grammar and syntax . . . [and] became almost completely deprived of words. She put them together laboriously out of four or five languages and became almost unintelligible." After becoming "completely dumb" for a fortnight, she began to speak again, but—without realizing it—in English instead of German. She lost her ability even to understand German, and, if forced to read a text written in French or Italian, "produced, with extraordinary fluency . . . an admirable extempore English translation."[30] The unusual manifestations of the disease here produce phenomena formerly associated with sideshows and religious revivals, and it is difficult for the narrator to maintain his stance as a distanced scientific observer—rather than a fascinated spectator—in the face of such theatrical extremities.

Freud's interest in these subterranean peculiarities of the spirit revives a "curious sight" as a specifically sexualized and sexualizing scrutiny. In this way his case history retrieves the old definition of "curious" as a euphemism for "sexual," as "curious books" refer to what the *OED* calls "erotic or pornographic works."[31] Freud insisted that sexuality was central to hysteria and defense neuroses. "Whatever case and whatever symptom we take as our point of departure," he trumpets," "in the end we infallibly come to the field of sexual experience."[32] While the medical consensus was for centuries that hysteria was rooted in an unruly uterus, most late-nineteenth-century physicians focused on biological and social causes for the disorder. Freud, however, notoriously focused on the sexual history of his patients. As he famously pronounced in *Dora*, "[S]exuality is the key to the problem of... the neuroses in general. No one who disdains the key will ever be able to unlock the door" (105).

This focus on sexuality provoked skepticism, even suspicion, in Freud's colleagues. The *British Medical Journal*, reviewing psychoanalysis in 1908, attacks the "most important point of his whole later teaching," the sexual root of neurosis. The article offers two quotations from Freud: "With a normal *vita sexualis* a neurosis is impossible" and "Without repressed sexual events of early childhood, no hysteria." While the reviewer remarks on the length of psychoanalytic treatment, he comments,

> We do not believe, however, that physicians will be deterred from adopting Professor Freud's method on account of the time involved, but for other, more obvious and certainly graver reasons. Although the patients are directed by Professor Freud to relate the incidents which come into their mind "without selection," the whole trend of the interrogation is... in one direction [e.g., sexual], and that a very undesirable one.... [T]his method of psychoanalysis is in most cases incorrect, in many hazardous, and in all dispensable.[33]

Such a response from the medical establishment is not surprising, but it was unwelcome.

Due to these incursions upon the unstable border between nineteenth-century science and its others, Freud must continually reimpose a clinical discipline on his text and its readers. Freud's anxieties about his tenuous position in the medical community strained his prose with the attempt to fulfill his vision of psychoanalysis despite its conflict with the precepts of clinical medicine. Frederic Jameson notes, "No small part of the art of writing, indeed, is absorbed by this (impossible) attempt to devise a foolproof mechanism for the automatic exclusion of undesirable responses to a given literary utterance."[34] Freud might argue that this originary trauma—the rejection of his peers—motivates his own continuous, impossible, and ultimately pathological compensatory task of proving psychoanalysis to be scientific even as he indulges in proscribed modes of seeing and stating.

Freud's Literary Vision: Reading as Seeing

Freud's eccentric and figurative methodology draws heavily on narrative and metaphor and owes as much to literary traditions as it does to nineteenth-century notions of what constituted scientific proof. Critics have amply praised Freud's agility and skill in writing and his acute sense of an aesthetic, especially a literary one.[35] Peter Mahony remarks that "the only prize Freud received from Germany in his life was the Goethe Prize for literature" (1). Marcus notes of *Dora* that "the actual case itself was full of such literary and novelistic devices or conventions as thematic analogies, double plots, reversals, inversions, variations, and betrayals" (79). And Graham Frankland devotes half a book to the proposition that Freud is not only a psychoanalyst but also a literary critic and even a would-be poet (*Dichter*). Critics have focused on Freud's literary style more than his theory of narrative. Mahony offers a brief survey of continental critics' debate over whether Freud was "above all a scientific writer" or an aesthetic one; these debates try to define Freud's writing in the face of "the supposed antithesis between science and art."[36] I am, however, less interested in judging Freud's case history as either "science" or "literature" than in how this "supposed antithesis" shapes disciplinary aspirations in Freud's prose and elsewhere. As Sarah Winter examined Freud's professional aspirations and how they inflected his construction of psychoanalysis, I would like to explore how his reliance on particular modes of vision and representation obstructs his disciplinary ambitions and drives his overdetermined insistence upon (and anxiety over) his professional status. In other words, when Freud refused to deny his texts, his readers, or himself the pleasures of a curious sight and romantic literary representation—or fully acknowledge these pleasures—he precipitated in his case histories a battle over disciplinarity that shaped not only psychoanalysis but also medical discourse as a whole.

In psychoanalysis, narrative and metaphor become more than merely representation; they help cause disease and cure it. Freud's texts evince a trust in narrative and a delight in metaphor that the clinical case history cannot at this point acknowledge. Clinical physicians did of course write on "case-taking" and its form, as my previous chapters have shown. But Freud made narrative and figuration newly central to the work of medicine.[37] Freud's model of vision requires not only seeing but reading or interpreting. Reading replaces the passive record of mechanical observation; reading is his X-ray for diagnosis and his scalpel for dissection.

Freud's early use of the "cathartic method" (which he and Breuer owed to Breuer's patient Anna O.) turns upon the construction of narrative. If hysteria derives from traumatic past experiences that haunt the patient, the physician helps her exorcise them by bringing them to consciousness and talking them out. As he puts it, "The patient is, as it were, getting rid of [her memory of a trauma] by turning it into words."[38] Freud cures the patient by working with her to construct a narrative of her history, or rather several narratives: the disjointed story of her past emerging from her randomly recalled memories; the more linear story of her past that the physician reconstructs from her statements; and the narrative he produces in the case history, framing the story of her past with the story of her treatment. While clinical physicians collected histories in order to reach their diagnoses in order to make a cure, Freud made the history become the process of both diagnosis and cure.[39] Unlike his colleagues in clinical medicine, he works with rather than against the truth that narrative grounds the practice of medicine, framing and mediating the physician's understanding of the patient. But his recognition of the narrative underpinnings of psychoanalysis is complicated by his cautious awareness of the precepts of science.

Freud seems to betray the ideals of empirically based science by relying so much on a narrative—the case history—rather than a "matter of fact." His use of the case history underscores an epistemological instability foundational to psychoanalysis that alienates it from both clinical and curious medicine: psychoanalysis works from the fundamental truth that the facts from which the physician proceeds are necessarily uncertain. "No one could distinguish between truth and fantasy in narratives elicited from the unconscious," says Freud in a letter to the surgeon Wilhelm Fliess.[40] Freud's emphasis on the case history as a tool of diagnosis and cure founds his science on the shifting sands of what the eighteenth-century experimentalist Thomas Sprat scorned as "Fancies" and "Fables."

If Freud makes narrative central to psychoanalytic treatment, he makes metaphor central to his theory of mind. Critics have noted the elegant, persuasive similes he uses to explain his theories.[41] *Studies on Hysteria* bristles with these. For example, Freud uses a simile to explain the patient's resistance to treatment: "A most important piece of information is often announced as being a redundant accessory, like an opera prince disguised as a beggar" (279). Once the patient has discussed a troubling memory with the physician, "the picture [representing that memory] vanishes, like a ghost that has been laid" (281). The psychoanalytic treatment itself "works like the removal of a foreign body from the living tissue"—or it "is exactly like putting together a child's picture-puzzle."[42] Freud clearly enjoys explaining himself through figurative language and draws his similes from a wide variety of contexts. Analogy had been common in eighteenth-century nosologies, but only to link similar diseases. Freud reanimates analogy in inventive similes, connecting medical findings to unexpected, nonmedical contexts; this suggests he finds metaphor precise and effective as a means of description. While precise and effective description was indeed an aim of the clinical ideal of mechanical observation, Freud's metaphors require an imaginative interpretation—a leap of re-vision; this goes beyond even the judicious use of speculative insight by scientists.

More important, hysteria becomes for Freud a figurative language the physician must learn to read. He cannot map the patient's narrative onto the body as simply and directly as he could within clinical medicine. In a clinical-realist case history, symptoms translate reliably into signs through a metonymic logic based on identity and contiguity. A pain in the chest implies heart trouble; a cough, lung disease. But hysteria works through another logic, one of figuration and symbolization, where slippage becomes possible. When the mind fails to abreact (or adequately digest) undesired events, Freud explains, mental snags become symbolized by physical ones—tics, coughs, limps, and the like. As in nineteenth-century clinical medicine, to discover the cause of illness, the physician must closely observe and record the clues offered by the patient's visible (legible) signs of ill health. But Freud can only cure the patient's physical problems by inducing her to uncover, or remember, their hidden cause, one step removed, in the mind. Symptoms no longer point to a localized illness; stomach pain, for example, does not indicate a stomach disorder, whether cancer, ulcer, or mere indigestion, but acts as a synecdoche in referencing a problem of another order altogether, in the mind. The proximate cause of illness is thus not just hidden (as in an internal tumor) but invisible, untraceable by any but the mind's eye, just as the ultimate cause is lost in the past. So Freud's work differs from the judicious speculations of midcentury clinical physicians; their imaginative insights were at least grounded in the physical body. While Freud, too, must begin with clinical observation, the difficult, deceptive nature of hysterical symptoms taught Freud to distrust a literal, realist reading of the body. He offers instead a figurative reading based in his imaginative reconstruction of the disease process.

This is not to say that hysteria, for Freud, is entirely divorced from physical causes. The hysteric's symptoms and their meaning are determined partly by the nature of the troubling event, and partly by the history of the body. For example, in explaining Dora's hysterical cough, Freud argues, "[W]e must assume the presence of a real and organically determined irritation of the throat—which acted like the grain of sand around which an oyster forms its pearl" (74). The hysteric body's "somatic compliance" with the mind means that "every hysterical symptom involves the participation of both sides [i.e., both body and mind]": the body's injury grounds the hysterical complaint.[43] As Freud explains Dora's leucorrhoea (vaginal discharge), "[W]e are here concerned with unconscious processes of thought which are twined around a pre-existing structure of organic connections, much as festoons of flowers are twined around a wire."[44] Freud's memorable similes here—the oyster's pearl, the flowers twined on a wire—make the point that hysteria, and psychoanalytic theory generally, rely on both a literal and a figurative reading of the body. In other words, Dora's hysterical cough or leucorrhoea grows over a "real" irritant, or twines itself around a "real" bodily injury[45]—much as Freud's similes furl themselves delicately over, around, and through the more direct, literal clinical prose that precedes and grounds them.

By shifting attention from simply physical symptoms to mental symptoms read through the lens of the body, Freud makes figuration the fundamental structure of hysteria and of psychoanalysis as a whole. And by requiring that these symptoms be translated yet again, this time into a narrative, in order to reach a cure, the Freudian case history insures that the word—the language of the mind, as opposed to the physical language of the body—becomes central as well. In fact, it is in many ways more important; more interesting, at least. In Freud's metaphor about the flowers on the wire, for example, the body becomes inorganic (the wire), whereas the "unconscious processes" which "festoon" and "twine" the wire provide the more aesthetically pleasing, intellectually intricate and living structure.

However, the work of untangling that structure is challenging and may seem arbitrary to the uninitiated. Since "a single symptom corresponds quite regularly to several meanings simultaneously," both physical and mental, the physician's work can require multiple layers of translation.[46] Dora's cough is "a real and organically determined irritation of the throat" in a complex "psychological wrapping" made up of several layers: "her sympathetic imitation of her father" and "her subsequent self-reproaches"; "her regret at [the] absence" of Herr K., her father's friend; and her sexual identification with Frau K, her father's mistress (74). Moreover, since the jumps and glitches of the mind are hidden, the body translates them into bumps and itches based on its own frailties; but the translation is a poor one, carried out in a dialect of bad puns and dramatic clichés. Frau Elisabeth von R.'s painful legs and difficulty in walking, he concludes, stem from her conviction that a "whole series of episodes ... had made the fact of her 'standing alone' painful to her," and that "her feeling of helplessness" meant "that she could not 'take a single step forward'" (152). Here the patient's body acts out a metaphorical phrase describing her state of mind, in an overblown game of charades. This "symbolization" in the case history of Frau Cäcilie M. provides a plethora of unsubtle symptoms. He traces her "extremely violent facial neuralgia" to an insult flung at her by her husband, which was, she said, "'like a slap in the face'" (176, 178). A "violent pain in her right heel" resulted from a fear that "she might not 'find herself on a right footing'" in a strange situation (179). A "penetrating pain in her forehead between her eyes" came about when the patient's grandmother "had given her a look so 'piercing' that it had gone right into her brain" (180). Other traumatic experiences caused pain in her chest "(meaning 'it stabbed me to the heart')" (180). A hysterical choking feeling, "when that feeling appeared after an insult, was [due to] the thought 'I shall have to swallow this'" (180). Language itself triggers symptoms through suggestive idiomatic phrases. The process of treatment—and the case history that is its record—becomes another process of translation, decoding Frau Cäcilie's clumsy references back into language from the physical clues she provides.[47] Because the hysteric's original message can be glimpsed only in its garbled, translated form, it demands (Freud tells us) patience, skill, and wisdom to read.

In such a situation, reading—teasing out the language behind the puzzling and often contradictory signs that the patient reluctantly offers—becomes a physician's paramount skill. Observation is central to clinical medicine because it works, despite the occasional cases in which pain in one organ is deceptively referred elsewhere. But within psychoanalysis, while observation is still necessary, it is not sufficient and must be supplemented by interpretation. This goes beyond the traditional rational work of the physician, beyond even the informed speculation of hypothesis, and requires instead art or intuition explicitly based in language. The physician is made necessary as the skilled reader, who can tease meaning from the symptoms and stories offered to him. The more difficult the text—that is, the constellation of mysterious hysterical symptoms and random reminiscences offered by the patient—the more important the physician's role. While Freud's theory of the figurative nature of hysterical illness conflicts with the realist logic of reading on which the clinical case history is founded, it usefully guarantees the physician both a job and a measure of authority.

But the more Freud becomes necessary for his particular vision in reading the patient, the more he relies upon an essentially subjective and singular—rather than professionally objective and reliably reproducible—aspect of the analyst's skill. While individual skill and experience had always differentiated physicians by ability, the convention of clinical medical knowledge, like that of any science, was that it was reproducible and generalizable—thus Byrom Bramwell's ambivalence about spectacular intuitive diagnoses, in chapter 5. Freud's theory, however, simply valorizes the individual practitioner as an artist, with a peculiar genius for interpretation that may well not be either communicable or teachable.

By 1893, when Freud published *Studies on Hysteria*, literary work attracted a sure disapprobation in scientific circles, the traces of which are also visible in marginalized scientific discourses like sexology. When the poet John Addington Symonds wrote to Havelock Ellis about their collaboration on *Sexual Inversion*, for example, he directed, "[A]nything you think fit to use ... shall be worked over so as to erase it's [*sic*] bias and to eliminate its literary quality."[48] The literary suggested an interested look and ornamental, fanciful style at odds with the dispassionate gaze and direct, precise style of scientific discourse. Freud's willingness to center his methodology on figurative representation and interpretation verged on literary work, rejecting the constraints of nineteenth-century clinical discourse.

Perhaps due to this contested status of literary work in science, when the hysterical symptom becomes most clearly metaphorical, Freud begins to display some ambivalence about his analyses, by vocally refusing to doubt his interpretations. He says, in one particularly unconvincing example, that "[t]he pain that occurs in hysteria of nails being driven into the head was without any doubt to be explained in her case as a pain related to thinking. ('Something's come into my head.')"[49] But the slips, reversals, inversions, displacements, and other "faults" (gaps, holes) in this translation call attention to the ambiguities—the near misses of meaning—inherent in any translation that transmits the thoughts of one language in the guise of another. Thus, as he continues, Freud warily avoids a wholehearted embrace of the figurative. He warns:

> [T]he hysteric is not taking liberties with words, but is simply reviving once more the sensations to which the verbal expression owes its justification.... [T]he expression of [these feelings] in words seems to us only to be a figurative picture of them, whereas in all probability the description was once meant literally; and hysteria is right in restoring the original meaning of the words. (181)

Here, like the seventeenth-century experimentalist John Wilkins and his project of a "Real Character," Freud imagines a golden age of language, when the slippage of meaning inherent in signification has not yet sundered the word from the thing itself. He displays his discomfort with his theoretical reliance on metaphor by proposing an originary moment in which sensation and expression coincide, and the "figurative picture" is literally the truth.

CHAPTER SIX

Freud's Problem with Genre: The Roman à Clef

If Freud's model of vision is a kind of reading, he forces the question of what genre, exactly, he is reading and asking us to read. He returns again and again to an opposition between scientific and literary work, without acknowledging that, in psychoanalysis, this is a failed and unsustainable binary. In "The Aetiology of Hysteria," after discussing two cases of hysteria, Freud sheepishly admits they are fictional:

> I have to confess that [these examples] are not derived from any case in experience but are inventions of mine.... But I was obliged to make up fictitious examples for several reasons, one of which I can state at once. The real examples are all incomparably more complicated; to relate a single one of them in detail would occupy the whole period of this lecture.... [T]he traumatic scenes do not form a simple row, like a string of pearls, but ramify and are interconnected like genealogical trees.... (196)

The falsification or fabrication of evidence is of course a mortal sin in scientific ideology, since it undercuts the reliability and truth of the entire empirical project. It is remarkable, then, not that Freud attempts to excuse his transgression with the shield of scientific necessity (for he "was obliged" by the canons of clinical medicine to present evidence for his claims), but that he then turns so readily from his guilty fictionalization to fanciful similes ("not ... like a string of pearls, but ... like genealogical trees"), continuing his reliance on literary work to defend what is neither true nor accurate.

Likewise, Freud's defense of his literary work as scientifically necessary often collapses back into the literary. In discussing Dora's suppressed homosexuality, he says:

> I should certainly give no space [to it] if I were a man of letters engaged upon the creation of a mental state like this for a short story, instead of being a medical man engaged upon its dissection. The element to which I must now allude can only serve to obscure and efface the outlines of the fine poetic conflict which we have been able to ascribe to Dora. This element would rightly fall a sacrifice to the censorship of a writer, for he, after all, simplifies and abstracts when he appears in the character of a psychologist. But in the world of reality, which I am trying to depict here, a complication of motives, an accumulation and conjunction of mental activities—in a word, overdetermination—is the rule. (52)

Freud here ostensibly argues that aesthetic goals like beauty of form are incompatible with his scientific goal of truth. But this championing of science against literature is undermined by his provisional adoption of a fictional role ("if I were a man of letters"). In fact, he doubles up the masquerade so that the fictional "man of letters" himself appears in disguise or on stage, "in the character of a psychologist." Ironically, Freud claims that the writer, unlike the psychologist, "simplifies and abstracts" the multiple layers and complicated relations of the real world; whereas this passage demonstrates how easily the literary accommodates and even celebrates such an "accumulation and conjunction" of roles. Everywhere Freud asserts "science" in this passage, the literary intrudes; and in the moment of his claiming the title of "medical man," his role collapses back into that of the "man of letters."

Most significant, even the opposition between science and literature that Freud attempts to set up here resolves itself into a division of genre, between a poetic romanticism he rejects ("the fine poetic conflict") and a realist representational methodology he admires ("trying to depict" the "world of reality"). It is ironic, then, that Freud's impulses tend so decidedly toward the romanticism of the poet rather than the realism of "the medical man."

Freud's problem with genre emerges especially clearly in his case history of Dora, which betrays an uneasy slippage between medical text and roman à clef, exacerbated by his efforts to fix it as clinical science. Freud sighs that, even with his audience limited to medical men, he must guard against the

> many physicians who (revolting though it may seem) choose to read a case history of this kind not as a contribution to the psychopathology of neuroses, but as a *roman à clef* [*Schlüsselroman*] designed for their private delectation [*Belustigung*]. I assure readers of this species that every case history [I will publish] will be secured against their perspicacity [*Scharfsinn*] by similar guarantees of secrecy. (3)

The roman à clef is the "book with a secret" originating with seventeenth-century French historical romances, which hides its characters' true identity, often because of lurid details about their lives. Here Freud performs his usual narrative gesture. He ostentatiously registers his scorn for the "bad reader," opposing the scientific audience to one hungry for literary curiosities. Yet he instructs us in the precise reading he wishes to avoid even as he rejects it; and he lavishes his most memorable and interesting prose—"revolting" yet "perspicacious," "private delectation"—on the forbidden, novelistic reading which he opposes to the perhaps duller but morally stainless "contribution" to science.[50]

In *Studies on Hysteria*, Freud and Breuer warn the reader that "the subject matter with which we deal often touches upon our patients' most intimate lives and histories. It would be a grave breach of confidence to publish material of this kind ... [and it] has therefore been impossible" to include it (xxix). In *Dora*, Freud adopts another tactic. He laments, "[W]hereas before I was accused of giving no information about my patients, now I shall be accused of giving information about my patients which ought not to be given" (1). Ironically, this opening disclaimer serves to advertise the "most intimate" material to follow. The rest of Freud's "Prefatory Remarks" to *Dora* display a similarly ambiguous attempt to forestall or, if necessary, rebut such accusations through (paradoxically) a systematic foregrounding of the private, sexual secrets revealed in the text. He acknowledges that the intimate quality of these stories means "[t]he presentation of my case histories remains a problem which is hard for me to solve" (2). He speaks of the hysteric's "most secret and repressed wishes" and warns that "the complete exposition of a case of hysteria is bound to involve the revelation of those intimacies and the betrayal of those secrets [*so kann die Klarlegung eines Falles von Hysterie nicht anders, als diese Intimitäten aufdecken und diese Geheimnisse verraten*]" (2). Freud's suggestive terms shift the clinical physician's concern for his patient's privacy toward a promise to satisfy the reader's voyeuristic curiosity. The moral ambiguity of his position emerges in his "revelation" and even "betrayal" of Dora's "intimacies"—terms that present her secrets as spectacle and implicate him in a voyeuristic economy.[51] Freud must strenuously assert his narrative to be an experimental report rather than a roman à clef in order to avoid attracting, or appearing himself to enjoy, a prurient view of the case. But his introduction of the term "roman à clef," followed by a coy refusal to provide all the details or condone his readers' desire to (like Freud himself) "penetrate" Dora's mysterious history, implicitly replicates the structure of the very genre he claims to despise.

Freud works so hard in *Dora* to define his readers and his text as "scientific," partly to displace a persistent alternate reading of this case history as a particularly juicy novel. Ironically, it is just this kind of limiting of readership that Gillian Beer identifies as an important rhetorical marker of the scientific text, in an attempt "to exclude, or suppress, feasible meanings" of his words.[52] *Dora* is shaped by Freud's insistence that his interest in sex is intellectual rather than physical or emotional; objective rather than prurient; scientific rather than literary. But his answer to his challengers is more rhetorical than scientific, and his anxiety is not only of discipline but also of genre.

Freud's Romantic Quest: The Psychologist as Archaeologist

If Freud works hard to deflect the charge that he has written a roman à clef, he invites speculation about another literary genre; for his early writings resonate with the quest or adventure narrative associated with romance. He knew and enjoyed much of the corpus of classical and European literature, which accounts for his familiarity with romance tropes.[53] His case history shows remarkable similarities with the late-century incarnation of the genre, the imperial romance. Nina Auerbach notes that "his clinical work with women was intensely affected by an essentially literary mythology," the late-century romance.[54] Indeed, Freud's identification with the romantic hero runs deeper than his tendency to loom over and figuratively master his women patients; it extends to an identification of his entire intellectual project with the probing expeditions and visual mapping of the explorer.

Freud courts the role of the hero as archaeologist and explorer, who surveys, brings to light, and ultimately maps the hidden secrets of a dark, feminized land, extending the speculations of experimental medicine into an active, interventional quest. It is perhaps not surprising that both Freud and a British author like H. Rider Haggard, both living in powerful empires at the close of the nineteenth century, and both interested in promoting and defending what they saw as a moral, necessary, and bold venture, should turn to some of the same romantic conventions to realize their vision in prose. Frederic Jameson argues that "a genre is essentially a socio-symbolic message ... [and] form is immanently and intrinsically an ideology in its own right" (141). Freud's romance of psychoanalysis, then, like Haggard's imperial romance, is an ideological document with its own interests. Indeed, by adopting the structure and discourse of romance, Freud's narratives permit psychoanalysis to be staged as an imperial project.[55]

That imperialism begins in Freud's insistence that the psychoanalyst secure visual as well as linguistic mastery of the case. Although the work of psychoanalysis is carried out through narrative, he imagines it as a primarily visual task: as the mapping of a disordered psyche, bringing its traumas to light and to order. His visual emphasis extends to the figures that track his progress through the hysterical psyche. Freud's theoretical chapter on "The Psychotherapy of Hysteria" in *Studies on Hysteria* abounds in visual metaphors explaining the structure of the disease. Memories, he explains, are grouped into "collections arranged in linear sequences (like a file of documents, a packet, etc.) ... [and] stratified concentrically round the pathogenic nucleus" (289). Memories obey yet another "arrangement ... the linkage made by a logical thread which reaches as far as the nucleus and tends to take an irregular and twisting path" (289).

Freud acknowledges the need to diagram these complicated images:[56]

> While these [first two arrangements] would be represented in a spatial diagram by a continuous line, curved or straight, the course of the logical chain would have to be indicated by a broken line which would pass along the most roundabout paths from the surface to the deepest layers and back, and yet would in general advance from the periphery to the central nucleus, touching at every intermediate halting-place—a line resembling the zigzag line in the solution of a Knight's Move problem, which cuts across the squares in the diagram of the chess-board. (289)

However, he never offers this diagram, preferring metaphorical to geometric figures. Although such a diagram would certainly be difficult to render, Freud admits that his preference—the simile of the Knight's Move—falls short of accuracy:

> The logical chain corresponds not only to a zigzag, twisted line, but rather to a ramifying system of lines and more particularly to a converging one. It contains nodal points at which two or more threads meet and thereafter proceed as one; and as a rule several threads which run independently, or which are connected at various points by side-paths, debouch into the nucleus. (290)

Freud turns to scientific terms here ("nucleus," "nodal points") but derives them from other sciences, rendering their use essentially metaphorical. He complicates his analogy by mixing metaphors: the "chain" is not only a "line" but also a "system" made up of "threads" which "debouch" into a "nucleus." The confusing combination of differing geometries and analogies (a chain, a thread, a river, a cell) here renders a diagram, invoked but not realized, even more necessary. Given his need to prove himself and psychoanalysis adequately scientific, and his insistence that the physicians' task is to map the patterns of the patient's memory, Freud's failure to produce even a rudimentary diagram of his theory seems inexplicable except as one more instance of his preference for verbal representation, even of the visualizing work central to analysis.

It is possible, however, to identify a general pattern to these diverse paths; to trace the logic of psychoanalysis, which directs the narrative structure of Freud's case histories, as a centripetal motion inward to a "nucleus" of secret memories, from which the hysteric's symptoms originate. Each memory coheres in "an unmistakable linear [reverse] chronological order," like the strata of an archaeological dig, and the physician's journey is organized as a penetration through the memories "stratified concentrically round the pathogenic nucleus" like an onion (289). This task cannot be rendered as a straightforward path to the core and origin; it must be achieved by "an irregular and twisting path ... along the most roundabout paths from the surface to the deepest layers and back, and yet would in general advance from the periphery to the central nucleus" (289). While with his medical training in neurology, Freud may have been influenced by the convoluted structures of the brain, this model of narrative also looks back to the late seventeenth and eighteenth centuries, whether in novelists' "secret histories" or in experimentalists' pursuit of the winding ways to nature's secrets. More immediately, the similarities between this plot and the labyrinthine paths of romance make explicit what Freud's narratives share with other late-nineteenth-century romances of exploration and empire, in particular how they mystify visual discovery as a way of naturalizing the process of mastery.

Structurally, Freud's case history accords with many of the characteristics of romance that Northrop Frye notes in his classic analysis of the genre. Freud typically presents a male narrator analyzing a female character, in order to understand or solve a problem in the present. He travels deep within her psyche, along a knotted and winding path, to track down a secret, the origin of which lies in her past, which is sexual or otherwise taboo (and which at this time Freud still believed to originate in sexual abuse by a father figure). The process of discovery is thwarted by obstacles including her own resistance to treatment but concluded by the triumphant disclosure of her secret, which resolves her troublesome symptoms.

This narrative of psychoanalytic treatment matches the quest/adventure plot Frye sketches as typical of romance, including the hero's difficult journey, crucial struggle, and exaltation. The dialectic structure between good and evil that Frye comments on emerges in Freud as a version of the dragon-killing theme, which involves perilous descent through a dark labyrinthine underworld "inhabited by a prophetic sibyl and ... a place of oracles and secrets" as part of a quest for buried treasure or to retrieve a bride from a "perilous, forbidden, or tabooed place" where she is "rescued from the unwelcome embraces of another and generally older male." The tangle of memory is the labyrinth where Freud accomplishes both aims: the origin of disease serves as the treasure he uncovers, and the hysteric represents the damsel in distress, whom he must rescue from the snares of her illness. Freud plays both the hero and another familiar character type from romance, the "old wise man."⁵⁷ The case history thus works both as autobiography and biography, for Freud plays the hero of his own story by intervening in somebody else's story. Although he registers his most imaginative flights as "work" and science, again and again he indulges in a romantic narrative of heroic discovery.⁵⁸ In this context his complicated imaginary diagrams of the mind become recognizable as maps of an unknown territory, one that he is staking out and claiming for psychoanalysis.

This romance of the psychoanalytic case history takes on an imperialist hue when its hero is an intrepid archaeological explorer of dark lands and ancient cultures. Freud's interest in archaeology is well known. He amassed an impressive collection of antiquities, having "often fantasized about emulating Heinrich Schliemann, the archaeologist who realized his childhood ambition of discovering the city of Troy." He also cultivated a friendship with Emanuel Löwy, an archaeologist and scholar of Greek art. In 1906 he wrote "Delusions and Dreams in Jensen's *Gradiva*," on William Jensen's lowbrow archaeological romance.⁵⁹ And Freud commented, in *The Interpretation of Dreams,* on the significance and promise of Rider Haggard's quintessential imperial romance, *She* (1887). He had offered it to an acquaintance to read, calling it "a *strange* book, but full of hidden meaning ... the eternal feminine, the immortality of our emotions...."⁶⁰

Thus it is not surprising that Freud figures his investigation of the hysteric's mind as an expedition into either the past or "the interior" of some wild land. In an early lecture on "The Aetiology of Hysteria," he explains the work of the psychoanalyst by comparing it to "another field of work" (e.g., archaeology, Egyptology) but, typically, romanticizes that work:

> Imagine [he says] that an explorer [*Forscher*] arrives in a little-known region where his interest is aroused by an expanse of ruins, with remains of walls, fragments of columns, and tablets with half-effaced and unreadable inscriptions.... [H]e may start upon the ruins, clear away the rubbish, and, beginning from the visible remains, uncover what is buried. If his work is crowned with success, the discoveries are self-explanatory: the ruined walls are part of the ramparts of a palace or a treasure-house; the fragments of columns can be filled out into a temple; the numerous inscriptions ... reveal an alphabet and a language, and, when they have been deciphered and translated, yield undreamed-of information about the events of the remote past, to commemorate which the monuments were built. *Saxa loquuntur!*⁶¹

In this lecture, Freud makes his characteristic move: even as he allies himself with "another field of [scientific] work," he begins with "Imagine." This passage is suffused with curious discourse reminiscent of the eighteenth-century case history. It solicits and admits to an affective response, from the explorer's "interest" being "aroused" or "awoken" (*Interesse erweckte*) to his "undreamed-of" (*ungeahnte*) access to the past, culminating in his excited, figurative cry, "Stones talk!"

More strategically, the figure of the Egyptologist or archaeologist serves Freud's needs beautifully. He probably models this "explorer" on German Egyptologists Adolf Erman, Hermann Grapow, or Heinrich Karl Brugsch. Their philology, translating and deriving a vocabulary of hieroglyphics, parallels his interest in "numerous inscriptions," "an alphabet and a language," and the work of "decipher[ing] and translat[ing]." Heinrich Brugsch combined the explorer and the scholar, respected for his role in establishing Egyptology as a science. The nineteenth-century archaeologist compacts the excitement and rigor of scientific discovery with a recuperation of past cultures and traditions that lends authority and implies mastery of the "field." He combines the most exciting new scientific methodologies with a respected tradition of inquiry, recalling the travel narratives that filled the Royal Society's *Philosophical Transactions*. Freud can thus imply not only the utter originality of his work but also its links to the distant past, its connection both to a romantic historicism and to a respectable, familiar tradition of scientific inquiry. The role of scientist as misunderstood hero is even in Freud's time a cliché.[62] With it, however, he can cast himself as both a pathbreaking explorer and one in a venerable lineage of similar explorers, keeping alive the ancient flame of knowledge. The cool reception of this lecture only prompted him, later, to reassert his role as a "lonely discoverer."[63] Indeed, Freud makes this analogy frequently in the early years. He comments that he and Breuer "had often compared the symptomatology of hysteria with a pictographic script which has become intelligible after the discovery of a few bilingual inscriptions. In that alphabet being sick means disgust." Here Freud uses a simile—the hieroglyphic alphabet—to express the metaphoric nature of hysteria itself. Likewise, he presents his work as archaeology: "This procedure [the cathartic method] was one of clearing away the pathogenic psychical material layer by layer, and we liked to compare it with the technique of excavating a buried city."[64]

Freud romantically figures the archaeologist's "discoveries" as revelatory. But he must first "clear away the rubbish," must assert ownership and establish mastery over the site by regularizing it and reordering it to Western standards, and discarding as "rubbish" whatever does not belong to a mystified, originary past. This labor transforms the "half-effaced and unreadable inscriptions" into a rich archive: "an alphabet and a language" with "undreamed-of information" that his reading, of course, will provide. Unlike mechanical observation, which would require the scientist to assiduously record and gather every scrap, Freud's exploratory look requires the intervention of the specialist with his expertise. In order to access the significance of the ruins, the archaeologist must—and only he can—differentiate them from the rubble.

For Freud, this means reading reluctance or disagreement as the hysteric's "resistance," which likewise he must clear away. Sabine Hake has argued that Freud's turn to archaeology relates to "his struggle for discursive mastery" over a "reading formation" centered on "the female body, which is always the hysterical body and which brings together seemingly disparate elements: the woman as archaeological site, archaeology as the paradigm of interpretation, and the problem of femininity as the test case of psychoanalysis."[65] Freud's use of archaeology also fetishizes the past as mythical site of origins and inescapable truth of identity, in a turn familiar to readers of romance.

In *Dora*, Freud's archaeological metaphor allowed him to finesse the question of methodology. He comments,

> In the face of the incompleteness of my analytic results, I had no choice but to follow the example of those discoverers whose good fortune it is to bring to the light of day after their long burial the priceless though mutilated relics of antiquity. I have restored what is missing, taking the best models known to me from other analyses; but like a conscientious archaeologist I have not omitted to mention in each case where the authentic parts end and my constructions begin. (7)

Here again, Freud gestures simultaneously toward both the work of science and imaginative work. His being "like a conscientious archaeologist" implicitly references the ideal of mechanical observation, given his anxiety to distinguish the "authentic" from his own additions. But Freud shatters that ideal by endorsing his bold, fictional "constructions" as necessary, even praiseworthy; his task would be incomplete had he not "restored what is missing." For Freud, just as mutilation is a necessary aspect of the relics (unmutilated memories would not result in hysteria) and restoration a critical task of the archaeologist, interpretation is an integral work of observation.[66] He thus articulates nineteenth-century clinical ideals of mechanical observation as well as an early version of what would become its twentieth-century successor: what Peter Galison has identified as a "judgment against objectivity" that makes room for evaluative expertise.[67]

Mapping an Unnavigable River: Freud and the Imperial Romance

In *Dora* Freud trades heavily on his role as explorer of some wild land as he describes how he explores the hysteric's narrative of her past, which he must trace to its secret source. He argues that the physician must not "rest content with the first 'No' that crosses his path" (18). He uses the term "der Forschung" (research) rather than "Pfad" or "Weg" (path), suggesting "Die Forschungsreise" (an exploring expedition), and "der Erforscher" (an investigator or explorer).[68] He figures his task as a convoluted and difficult journey, explaining,

> I begin the treatment ... by asking the patient to give me the whole story of his life and illness [but] [t]his first account may be compared to an unnavigable river whose stream is at one moment choked by masses of rock and at another divided and lost among shallows and sandbanks. (10)

By imagining himself as tracing an unnavigable river, Freud gestures toward the well-publicized efforts of explorers like the British adventurer Henry M. Stanley, who identified the source of the Congo River by traversing its length.[69] Freud repeats the river metaphor, retrieving Dora's tortuous memories in a "current," and using "Quelle" ("source" or "spring") to describe the originary trauma of hysteria.[70] His task recalls Stanley's famous story of his arduous journey to the source of the Congo in *Through the Dark Continent*, except Freud's "dark continent" is the vast terrain of the hysterical unconscious, and his Congo is the clotted stream of her reminiscence, which he and the patient must clear as they trace it back to its origin.[71] But if this river is "unnavigable," then Freud's task is fantastically difficult. Clinical observation alone cannot enable him to survey what cannot be traversed; only the spectacular abilities of the romantic hero can surmount obstacles like these. The clinical physician Thomas Laycock had also imagined the patient as a vast wilderness to be navigated, but Laycock has the help of a reference text. "[I]nstead of having to make his way, like the enterprising traveller, over a wide expanse of untrodden wilds, where no beaten track guides his steps," Laycock explains, the well-prepared student "can confidently pursue the well-accustomed road of systematic semeiology—enabled, with his map in his hand, to mark each turn and winding. What, then, is requisite for him to do in this case? That he shall mark them carefully, minutely, accurately."[72] While Laycock merely correlates the landmarks with the map in his hand, Freud is that "enterprising traveler" who must explore an "untrodden wild," and must construct the map himself.

Whether Freud is imagined as an Egyptologist or a Stanleyesque explorer, the passages above construe his textual project in reference to the late-nineteenth-century efforts to "open up"—by digging, mapping, and colonizing—both the past and the terrain of Africa, as is evident in *Dora*. When he comments, "I set myself the task of bringing to light what human beings keep hidden within them" (69), he figures the hysteric as a "dark continent" rich in resources that must be extracted to be seen—a trope in which what is mined may include not only ancient artifacts but also perhaps gold or diamonds. If earlier the hysteric represented a buried antique civilization like Schliemann's Troy, here Freud codes the hysteric as a savage continent, barbaric or primitive in opposition to his superior heroism, when he comments, "No one who, like me, conjures up the most evil of those half-tamed demons that inhabit the human breast, and seeks to wrestle with them, can expect to come through the struggle unscathed" (100).[73] The promise of treasure is conflated with the more sinister implication of what is "kept hidden"—perhaps the dark secrets and unspeakable practices that may lurk in unexplored territory, and haunt the romance. Freud's "demons" offer another version of the dragon of romance. Stanley, too, discussed the need to "[inoculate] the various untamed spirits [of his African bearers] ... with a respect for order and discipline, obedience and system" (I:55). Indeed, given Freud's figuration of what is "half-tamed," dark and "kept hidden" within her, the hysteric represents not only the damsel in distress whom he retrieves from the dark labyrinth, but also, synecdochally, the labyrinth itself: a kind of Africa primed for his exploration, conquest, and intellectual exploitation.[74] However, Freud's exploratory, mapping look is much different from the "monarch of all I survey" gaze—the iconic imperialist gaze out across a subject landscape—that Mary Louise Pratt has identified. Pratt's explorers must labor to reach their privileged perch, but once that is achieved, they may freely "take in" the view. They figure the landscape itself as falling away, laid out below their sweeping gaze, despite sporadic elements of the scene obscuring an entirely open view. Freud's look, in contrast, must remain saturated with intent and action; it requires the continual heroic, penetrating agency of the observer to tunnel through the land's resistance, winning mastery and vision only step by step.

Freud's romance of empire symbolizes two different, but related, struggles. In daily practice and in his theory, Freud battled the hysteric's "resistance" for mastery of her past and her story. Her carefully guarded sexual secrets represent the "truth" that, once brought to light, will retrospectively justify his insistent, probing pressure and his brutal willingness to get to, and get through, the "rubbish" in which it lies. And in the medical community, Freud battled skeptics to establish psychoanalysis as the dominant technique for the treatment of psychological disorders. Here the hysteric represents a fabulous resource, a buried wealth of neurotic "material" that, properly mined and interpreted, can provide capital for his intellectual project.

Because Freud articulates a romantic, archaeological, and exploratory model for the work that his case history records, it also serves as a map of that genre. Its narrative structure follows an explorer's adventures in some dark land, tracing a circuitous path deep into the heart of the continent to unearth and decipher a taboo, originary secret of great value. Although he frames his initial archaeological analogy as a link to a new science, he executes it as fiction: with an eye to its most curious and romantic possibilities and introduced with the keynote, "Imagine." It stands as Freud's implicit admission that his case history is not so much a record of clinical observation as it is a romantic tale of discovery.

Jameson argues that genres accumulate "sedimented content" based on their cultural incarnations in previous historical periods, and that this content inflects the engagement of any genre with its current historical context (99). Individual texts must negotiate not only the current incarnation of the genre, but also the active elements of its residual content. Freud's construct of the adventurous explorer, then, treads a path well-worn by popular imperial romances. Rider Haggard is perhaps the best known among Victorian examples. Inspired by the British annexation of the Transvaal in his early career, and sorely disappointed at the retrocession of the land to the Boers, Haggard's romances promote the extension of a responsible imperial power.[75] His Africa is a place of adventure and rich resources where bold and honorable men may prosper. As a 1920s critic commented, Haggard's "South African romances ... have ... aided far more than we can ever know in bringing British settlers and influence into the new country. They have helped to accomplish the dreams and aims of Rhodes."[76] Although the Austro-Hungarian Empire did not participate in the Scramble for Africa nor the Berlin Conference of 1885, members of the Viennese bourgeoisie like Freud would certainly have been aware of the global political ramifications of imperial expansion, especially given Austria-Hungary's affiliation with Germany (soon to be the third-largest colonial power in Africa) in the Dual Alliance of 1879.

Indeed, Freud might also be identified as an imperialist. Treating the hysterical psyche, he proleptically establishes mastery over an unruly foreign land. He seeks to found a new outpost of science in the unexplained territory of hysteria. And Sarah Winter notes that his plans went beyond the proper matter of psychoanalysis to attempt cultural and social analysis as well. This amounted, she argues, to a kind of "disciplinary imperialism," in which he "emphasizes the aptness of psychoanalysis for collaborations with other disciplines in terms that underline the epistemological indispensability of psychoanalytic knowledge."[77] Psychoanalysis is an imperialist science to the extent that it attempts to colonize other fields.

The parallels between Haggard's work and Freud's speak to a common cultural topos shaping their narratives of revelatory truth and discovery, despite their many differences. The structure of romance frames their heroes' mastery of unknown lands as a natural, necessary progress. Their narratives foreground an exploratory, "mapping" vision of a labyrinthine wilderness; a fascination with representation that sublimates the ideology of empire in the pleasure of the text; and a pronounced anxiety of genre, suggesting the ruptures that might threaten such an ideology.[78]

Haggard's best-selling novel *She* (1886) makes visible just how much Freud owes to the genre of imperial romance. In Haggard's most popular romances, white male narrators explore and record an African landscape that, Lindy Stiebel argues, he "compulsively, and at times, anxiously" figures as "vast Eden, as wilderness, as dream underworld, as sexualized bodyscape and finally as home to ancient white civilizations."[79] While Freud rhapsodizes over "an expanse of ruins, with remains of walls, fragments of columns, and tablets with half-effaced and unreadable inscriptions," Haggard offers "miles upon miles of ruins—columns, temples, shrines and the palaces of kings.... long since fallen into decay" and an awe-inspiring statue of Truth inscribed with "the usual Chinese-looking hieroglyphics."[80] Where Freud follows "an irregular and twisting path ... along the most roundabout paths ... from the periphery to the central nucleus," Haggard's band of seekers travel along a similarly circuitous track around the outside of a volcano. They journey through an eroticized topography approaching the cave where the mysterious "She" resides, climbing to

> a ledge, narrow enough at first, but which widened as we followed it, and sloped inwards, moreover, like the petal of a flower, so that we sank gradually into a kind of rut or fold of rock that grew deeper and deeper ... [and] suddenly ended in a cave.... [Judging the length of] this cavern ... owing to its numerous twists and turns ... was not an easy task. (203)

The vocabulary with which Freud and Haggard figure their narrative journey and its telos excuses that journey by highlighting its most curious and tantalizing aspects; and their topography makes that journey seem inevitable and its teleology sure. Because physical vision is obstructed (by darkness and the twisting tunnel), an imaginative mapping of the explorers' path is the only visual rendering of their progress. The gradually deepening enclosure of the explorers in both texts suggests that their progress into "the interior" is the only option. Stopping or returning to the surface would arrest the drive to knowledge and close off narrative itself.

Freud and Haggard also both demonstrate an outsized concern with reading, translation, transcription, duplication, interpretation, and evidence, in a convention that dominates late-century romances like *Dracula* and *Dr. Jekyll and Mr. Hyde* as well.[81] Just as Freud constructs psychoanalysis as an act of reading, traversing memories "stratified concentrically round the pathogenic nucleus," Haggard frames his novel with a series of nested texts, each referring to the next. He offers a model for these recursive texts as a ruined temple "arranged in a series of courts, each one of them enclosing another of smaller size, on the principle of a Chinese nest of boxes" (196). The six nested documents originate in a potsherd covered in Greek written by Leo's ancestor, transcribed by Leo's father and reproduced for the reader in both Greek characters and in Greek cursive. The generative, generational relation of these documents governs not only the transcriptions but also their provenance: they were purportedly given to his solicitors, then given to the narrator, then given to the editor, who published them. The story is further framed by a "Black-Letter Inscription" in Latin, also on the potsherd, with, "what is still more curious, an English version of the black-letter Latin" and a "Medieval Black-Letter Latin translation of the Uncial Inscription on the Sherd of Amenartas" (31, 33)—all of which the novel reproduces both in the original black-letter font and in a modernized text.

This remarkable, overdetermined set of documents signals the allegorical nature of the journey ahead as a series of concentric readings in different languages and fonts, each stage carrying the reader farther into the unknown and closer to his ancient goal. The novel mimics the explorer's progress through different cultures and (it was thought) back through previous stages of civilization as he forges farther from the metropole. But by imagining exploration as an extended dive into a *mise-en-abyme* of nested texts, the novel ironically reads imperial expansion as a contraction, moving not outward but in toward some kind of originary truth. Furthermore, it figures the labor of empire—the extraction and export of resources, the imposition of a Westernized government and discipline, and the reeducation of the population—as a kind of "translation," a morally benevolent, intellectually laudable project. While Haggard insists on the labor of imperial exploration as a kind of reading, then, Freud proposes (psychoanalytic) reading as a kind of imperial exploration.

Haggard also prefigures Freud by foregrounding an anxiety of genre. Many of the framing documents make the obligatory romantic gesture toward historicity, ironically rooted in the eighteenth-century experimentalist anxiety over reliable reporting. Haggard's narrative is also suspect as originating in the mind of an hysterical woman. Leo's father writes to his son, "[Y]ou will be able to judge for yourself whether or no you will choose to investigate what, if it is true, must be the greatest mystery in the world, or to put it by as an idle fable, originating in the first place in a woman's disordered brain" (23). And the narrator himself warns his editor—putatively Haggard himself—that the story is "so much more ma[r]vellous than [another book], that to tell the truth I am almost ashamed to submit it to you lest you should disbelieve my tale" (4). Indeed, it is "the most wonderful history, as distinguished from romance, that [the world's] records can show" (5). The onslaught of antirealist genres here—mystery, fable, marvel, romance—speaks more loudly of the curious tale to come than of its pretended historicity. As in Freud's admission that "the case histories I write ... lack the serious stamp of science," Haggard demonstrates just this kind of overdetermined anxiety over the skepticism (or, conversely, the excessive interest) of his readers. These intrusive assertions of evidentiary facticity draw undue attention to the mediation of the text and could not be farther from the conventions of transparency in nineteenth-century classic realism.

This concern in Freud and Haggard with questions of reading and translation, genre and narrative authority, betrays a persistent anxiety over the nature of their project. European expansion in Africa was justified by reference to philanthropy and science. The ideology of empire, like that of science, requires the assertion of serious, benevolent purpose, even as the structure of romance demands the solicitation of readerly interest through a curious sight and spectacular claim. The anxiety of genre which erupts in these texts points up the vexed question of narrative purpose: in striving to attract and hold the reader, the romance must emphasize those "curious" elements which most destabilize its scientific and imperial assertions of duty, responsibility, and distanced concern.

Given Freud's awareness of the disciplinary dichotomy between literature and science, his vision of psychoanalysis as a new science, and his acute ear for language, it is remarkable that he chooses for his central metaphor for psychoanalytic narrative, a figurative exploration so compatible with the curious, even sensational imperial romance. Graham Dawson considers how "the very form of the modern adventure tale is imbued with the imaginative resonance of colonial power relations underpinned by science and technology."[82] In fact, one could reverse this sentence without losing its accuracy, for science itself—at least Freud's science—is equally "imbued with the imaginative resonance of colonial power relations," and equally "underpinned" by "the very form of the modern adventure tale." Indeed, the theory and narrative of psychoanalysis—defined through Freud's process of discovery, exploration, and mastery—becomes visible as an imperial fiction.

FREUD AND THE END OF THE CASE HISTORY

This book has argued in part that the critical commonplace about the nineteenth-century clinical case history—that it is a realist narrative—needs to accommodate the historical heterogeneity of the form. Freud also cannot seem to forgo indulgence in these nonrealist or even antirealist genres, and this florid environment makes even his most clinical observations suspect. The specter of the novel—whether the sentimental novel, the roman à clef, the imperial romance, or even the realist novel—thus haunts Freud's aggressively "clinical" case histories.

Freud's continued, backhanded allusions to all these genres demonstrate that, despite the disadvantages to his project, he refuses the chance to revise literary work out of his text. This becomes most evident in his conclusion to *Dora*. Freud had warned his readers that "[n]othing of any importance has been altered" in the record except for the order of some of the explanations (4). Yet his decision not to revise necessitates not only the inclusion of some inaccuracies—which he corrects in footnotes—but also permits him to indulge himself in a climax worthy of the most sentimental romance:

> Dora had listened to me without any of her usual contradictions. She seemed to be moved; she said good-bye to me very warmly, with the heartiest wishes for the New Year, and—came no more.... I knew Dora would not come back again [*Sie schien ergriffen, nahm auf die liebenswürdigste Weise mit warmen Wünschen zum Jahreswechsel Abschied und—kam nie wieder*]. (100)

Freud's melodrama is undercut by his admission, ten pages later in the "Postscript," that Dora did indeed come back again, "fifteen months after the case was over and this paper drafted" (111). He does not even include a footnote on the earlier page to correct it, as he does elsewhere. His decision to leave the earlier scene entirely unrevised and uncorrected seems peculiar, given that he did not publish the case history until four years after it was written. Freud clearly wishes not only to claim scientific status for his text; he also wants to keep intact its romantic closure.

Freud carefully advertises his investment in and debt to the nineteenth-century cult of science. But each time Freud asserts the clinical, scientific purpose of his work, he reiterates what is most curious and literary about it. As a result, disavowed elements from the eighteenth-century case history effloresce in the psychoanalytic case history at the close of a clinical century. Freud's affinity for a romantic, heroic narrative of his project infects the psychoanalytic case history at the moments of his most earnest attempts to grasp the mantle of science, endangering his professional legitimacy even as he claimed it.

Freud himself believed his project to be a success: he closes the "Postscript" to his 1935 *Autobiography* with the words, "[T]he whole impression is a satisfactory one—of serious scientific work carried on at a high level."[83] But it was perhaps in part due to his inability to maintain the markings of science in his case history that he succeeded in founding psychoanalysis as a social science more than a clinical one, and that his influence, while tremendous, is as much a cultural as a scientific and medical one.[84] As a result of Freud's curious sight and his persistent skill with and pleasure in literary work, the psychoanalytic case history provides an institutionalized other for clinical medicine, safely housing these suspect methods of vision and representation at the margins of medical discourse.

More important, Freud here violates the taboo restricting the physician's field of vision to the patient and the disease. He deflects his and the reader's gaze from the patient (the proper subject of clinical observation) to the physician himself, traversing the landscape of his patient; and he substitutes for the cold and steady gaze of science, an interested eye. This book has argued that clinical observation served many purposes, not least of which was to certify professional scientific practice for Victorian physicians; so the ostentatious use of clinical methodologies is as much about the physician as it is the patient. But the ideal of mechanical observation, with the observer's self-erasure, complicated clinical physicians' relation to their own professional desires, even after the development of speculative realism. Freud's psychoanalytic case history, structured as the doubled narrative of the suffering patient and the heroic physician who explores, interprets, and finally records her story, ultimately brings to light the subterranean desires not only of the hysteric but also of the clinical case history and its author.

Freud makes central what clinical physicians had been resisting in their narratives for decades: the romance of their own insight.

Freud offers a telling vantage point on the discursive range of the case history in its relation to the novel. His case history, despite his claim to inaugurate an entirely new science, in fact both invokes the objective, professional tradition of clinical medicine and resurrects the occulted, curious literature of eighteenth-century medicine. "Curious sight" here reemerges as a sexualized and sexualizing scrutiny, so that Freud must strenuously assert his prose to be scientific rather than literary, an experimental report rather than a roman à clef, in order to avoid attracting, or appearing himself to enjoy, a prurient interest in the case. His complex imbrication of curious sight, clinical observation, and a speculative human insight both enabled his extraordinary case histories and forced him into the role of an embattled visionary, as he struggled to find a secure site of scientific narrative authority on which to found psychoanalysis. It was thus in part Freud's commitment to literary work that doomed psychoanalysis to its enduring success as a literary and cultural rather than a strictly scientific project. Graham Frankland has argued that "it is partly because Freud's hermeneutic was derived from a literary-critical paradigm that it was able to suspend the opposition between scientific positivism and irrationalism" (150). But Freud's struggle to find acknowledgment in the scientific community is testimony to the fact that, while his affinity for literary work may well be largely responsible for the remarkable power of his innovative hermeneutic, that affinity was not ultimately successful in suspending the demands of scientific medicine in opposition to its others.

"Curious sight," insight, and the recognition of medicine's narrative aspects survive today largely under erasure or in spaces disjunct from the medical case history. Although discursive meditations on medicine and its culture have become more common in recent years—in forums like the "On My Mind" column in the *Journal of the American Medical Association,* and with books by Oliver Sacks, Lewis Thomas, and other physician-authors widely read—their popularity is extracurricular, for these texts are not generally considered central to the progress of a strictly medical knowledge. Likewise, despite the valuable work of Rita Charon, Kathryn Montgomery, Anne Hunsaker Hawkins, Anne Hudson Jones, Arthur Kleinman, Janis Caldwell, and others who call for literary critics, historians, and physicians to recognize and explore the role of narrative in medical discourse, this discussion is often confined to medical humanities centers, interdisciplinary journals like *Literature and Medicine,* or the occasional medical school course (often marginalized as part of an ethics curriculum) intended to "humanize" the physician-product. Seeing Freud's work and its reception as an important node in the trajectory of the modern case history may help illuminate the vexed status of narrative medicine today.

Overall, Freud's prose shows the fault lines of a historical tension in his attempts to blend the distancing and professionalizing techniques of clinical medicine with the curious approach of an earlier practice. His at times brilliant deployment of the narrative capabilities of his case history constitutes neither a capitulation to the thoroughly novelistic, nor a synthesis of it with the clinical, but a particularly contentious installment of the case history's century-long struggle to negotiate the differing (and often conflicting) demands, benefits, and liabilities of the modes of vision and representation that are—by the end of the century—strongly associated with either scientific or literary practice.

At the opening of the twentieth century, novelists could draw upon the clinical case history as an exemplary narrative of the real, and could turn to the Freudian case history as a provocative (and increasingly influential) visualization of interiority; but the novel and its insights had become altogether unavailable as a discursive model for medical prose. That model had become suspect in a clinical age for its very success in inhabiting, and eliciting, the subjectivity of another.

Conclusion

> FATHER. Come hither, Charles; what is it that you see grazing in the meadow before you?
> CHARLES. It is a horse....
> FATHER. ...Let us see if you can tell how a horse differs from a cabbage?
> CHARLES. Very easily; a horse is alive.
> FATHER. True; and how is every thing called which is alive?
> CHARLES. I believe all things that are alive are called *animals*.
> FATHER. Right...
>
> FATHER. Now, then, observe what particulars we have got. *A horse is an animal of the quadruped kind, whole-hoofed, with short erect ears, a flowing mane, and a tail covered in every part with long hairs....* Do you know now what we have been making?...A DEFINITION.... It is a kind of chase, and resembles the manner of hunting in some countries, where they first enclose a large circle with their dogs, nets, and horses; and then, by degrees, draw their toils closer and closer, driving their game before them till it is at length brought into so narrow a compass that the sportsmen have nothing to do but to knock down their prey.[1]

John Aiken's and Anna Letitia Barbauld's aptly named "A Lesson in the Art of Distinguishing," a parable for young readers, is remarkably suggestive about both the promise and the pitfalls of genre, which (like definition) relies upon careful observation, and upon a categorization that is narrow enough to be distinctive, yet broad enough to encompass the entire population of a type. The descriptive power of such an approach is evident; its dangers, like faulty premises or a rigid, territorial notion of categorization and ownership, are also evident above.

Physicians, like young Charles, often observed in order to find difference; they worked to distinguish typhus from typhoid fever, or measles from scarlet fever. These chapters have, however, attempted to trouble the accretion of difference between novels and medical texts, by distinguishing some of their common visual and narrative strategies.

This book has focused on particular genres—the novel and the case history—and on the British context in the nineteenth century, but it also hopes to lay out a more flexible, dynamic, and relational model of genre. While I draw on Frederic Jameson's construct of genre as a nuanced response to social structures and Michel Foucault's notion of genre as archive, I propose a model of genre as contingent, strategic, and situational. The visual and representational strategies I examine here help to determine genres like the clinical case history or the sentimental novel, but they are mobile and scalable; they can be imported strategically and are shaped by context. The genre of any text is formed in a complex negotiation. While we tend to privilege the author's voice and rhetorical authority, the text is constructed and consumed under the sometimes conflicting pressures of disciplinary norms and the perceived expectations of readers. Chapter 3 demonstrates how surprisingly often physician-writers deploy a sentimental discourse momentarily, in apparent contradiction of clinical norms, but strategically, to meet a contextual demand.

Such a reading of genre will necessarily affect how we study the history of medicine. This book argues that physicians were and are writers, working in a narrative genre (the case history) with a history like any other literary genre. Moreover, physicians worked in the context of an explosion of print. The field of periodical studies demonstrates how fully physicians and novelists were reading and writing each other in the same pages. As literate workers physicians would have read and discussed novels and reviews of novels; their nonscientific reading is likely to have shaped their writing of medical narrative and their interpretation of cases.

The history of medical writing casts ripples on so-called literary writing as well, when novelists make strategic use of clinical modes of seeing and stating. I have suggested that a newly rich and varied interplay of discursive hybridity in the novel may be revealed and examined, once we consider that medical modes of seeing and stating may be useful to the novel outside their original context. While Victorian studies has long been an interdisciplinary field, with critics delving into the novel's relation to political economy, photography, and anthropology as well as medicine (to name a few examples), the recent surge in periodical studies speaks to a new interest in how many Victorian novels were written for and read in periodicals, that is to say, in the immediate context of other genres. The *Waterloo Directory* points out that the sheer volume of newspaper, periodical, and other print media in the Victorian period was more than one hundred times that of books. The Victorian novel was published in, read in, and crucially shaped by these adjacent texts, and only a more flexible model of genre will allow us to capture the nuances of their relation. The medical case history and the Victorian novel both risked much and gained much from their shared use of curious, clinical, and literary sights and insights, even as they developed toward different disciplinary goals and different truths.

Notes

Introduction

1. [Hamley], "Life and Letters," 170.
2. Brooks, *Realist Vision*, 17.
3. Beer, *Open Fields*, 149.
4. See Rothfield, *Vital Signs*.
5. See Isobel Armstrong, "Transparency" and *Victorian Glassworlds;* Nancy Armstrong, *Age of Photography;* Beer, "'Authentic Tidings'"; Flint, *Visual Imagination;* Brooks, *Realist Vision.* Recent critics discussing objectivity or disinterestedness in relation to visuality include Anderson, *Powers of Distance;* Levine, *Dying to Know.* See also Krasner, *Entangled Eye.* On the history of optics and visuality including the Victorian period, see Isobel Armstrong, "Sub-Visible World"; Crary, *Techniques;* Crary, *Suspensions of Perception;* Cartwright, *Screening the Body* (although this focuses on a postcinematic visuality).
6. See Caldwell, *Literature and Medicine;* Tougaw, *Strange Cases.*
7. Jay, "Scopic Regimes of Modernity," 4. Otter, *Victorian Eye,* 21.
8. Daston and Galison, *Objectivity,* 318.
9. See Daston and Galison, *Objectivity;* Daston and Galison, "Image of Objectivity."
10. Crary identifies an early-nineteenth-century break from naïve eighteenth-century optical theories. Whereas at first "the ... observer confronts a unified space of order, unmodified by his or her own sensory and physiological apparatus," later subjectivity unavoidably shapes and mediates perception, because "vision is always an irreducible complex of elements belonging to the observer's body and of data from an exterior world." Despite W. J. T. Mitchell's caveats, textual evidence suggests that the shift began at about 1830 in medicine and physiology. Crary, *Techniques,* 55, 70–71; Mitchell, *Picture Theory,* 19–21.

11. Ross, "*Scientist,*" 67, 82. Ross locates one watershed moment in 1620, when Bacon published the *Novum Organum* (67). Bacon argued that knowledge "must gradually evolve, using observation and experiment, by refining and clarifying its former partial truths."

12. This shift has itself been quantified by Gross. Rhetorical elements of the modern scientific report include complex noun phrases, navigational infrastructure (abstract, subheadings), detailed citation practices, and prominent visual elements (graphs, tables). See Gross et al., *Communicating Science;* Dear, "*Totius in Verba*"; Dear, "Introduction," in *Literary Structure;* Vickers, "Royal Society."

13. The word "scientist," first suggested by William Whewell in 1834, aroused vigorous debate and as late as c. 1910 was still considered "a colloquialism" inferior to the more traditional "man of science." Ross, "*Scientist,*" 75. Whereas "natural philosophy" was a gentlemanly interest, science was not considered an autonomous profession—one which could itself confer social standing—until the 1830s. Susan Cannon, *Science in Culture.*

14. I follow critics like George Levine (*Realistic Imagination*) and Harry Shaw (*Narrating Reality*), who are among the most forceful critics working to complicate our understanding of realism, countering charges that realist novels impose a totalizing vision and are deluded or deceptive in their claims of a transparent access to the real.

15. Bailin, *Sickroom*, 3.

16. Vrettos, *Somatic Fictions;* Logan, *Nerves and Narratives;* Wood, *Passion and Pathology;* Frawley, *Invalidism and Identity;* Porter, *Patients and Practitioners.*

17. Oliphant, *Doctor's Family,* 87.

18. Shapin and Schaffer in *Leviathan* discuss the scientific report as a means of replicating experiments for a wider audience, providing a virtual audience for the experimenter and a virtual experience for the reader. Although eyewitnesses were no longer crucial as testimonials to the authenticity of Victorian experiments, the scientific report remained to certify individual experiences as professional, and thus communal, knowledge.

19. These examples are drawn from Dickens, *Bleak House;* Eliot, "Brother Jacob"; and Oliphant, *Hester.*

20. Disraeli, *Sybil,* 193. He uses this phrase throughout the novel, as well as in the advertisement at the beginning.

21. Disraeli literalizes the imperative that Pamela Gilbert identifies in midcentury medical mapping: to open up and illuminate the dark spaces of poverty. See Gilbert, *Mapping,* 27–54.

22. Synochus is a continued (not remittent or intermittent) fever; the term is little used after the 1840s.

23. Poovey, *Social Body,* 58.

24. Forbes, *Inaugural Lecture on Botany,* 11.

25. Peterson, *Medical Profession,* 60. For a sense of the contentious debates over the medical curriculum, see Romano, *Making Medicine Scientific.*

26. "Literary Tastes," 413 (emphasis in original).

27. Bramwell, "Perforating Tumour."

28. Bramwell, "Diagnostic Value," 119.

29. Bramwell, "Perforating Tumour," 252; Bramwell, "Stricture of the Oesophagus," 200.

30. Bramwell, "Diagnostic Value," 115.

31. Bramwell, "Remarkable Case," 58.

32. It is rare, but humor also surfaces in the case history, as in John Elliotson's report of a single woman in her thirties with an abdominal disorder, who adamantly denied pregnancy: "She had a pulse of 80; something within her had a pulse of 128; and what that was, I left her to settle by herself. All that I could say was, that if she waited patiently, the whole of the disease would come away, to a certainty, in two or three months." Elliotson et al., *Principles and Practice,* 61.

33. Colvin, Review of *Middlemarch*, 144.
34. Hardy, *Greenwood Tree*, 24.
35. Latham, *Collected Works*, 27.
36. King, *Bloom*.
37. The great seventeenth-century physician Thomas Sydenham, for example, grounded his classificatory system on his observations of individual cases, as did Giovanni Morgagni in the eighteenth century. But the case's reference to a norm of disease did not become predominant until the nineteenth century.
38. See Kathryn Montgomery Hunter, *Doctors' Stories*, 71–73, 81–82.
39. W. B. Cannon, "Case Method"; Epstein, *Altered Conditions*, 51n84.
40. Critics who discuss the case as a model for the narrative of individual experience have focused largely on the relevance of the philosophical case. See McKeon, *Origins of the English Novel*, 82–83; J. Paul Hunter, *Before Novels*, 290–94; Starr, *Defoe and Casuistry*. Thomas Laqueur has posed the realist medical "case" as a narrative model for the humanitarian empathy that underwrites the novel ("Bodies, Details").
41. See especially McKeon, *Origins of the English Novel*.
42. Jameson, *Political Unconscious*, 138, 141.
43. Beer, *Open Fields*, 186.
44. Foucault, *Order of Things*, 128.
45. In the novel, debates over genre and style emerge in the 1830s and 1840s, with Bulwer-Lytton; the 1860s, with the sensation novel crisis; and the 1870s, with high realism. In medicine, clinical realism as a narrative technique reached a climax in the 1830s and 1840s, while debates over the use of graphing technology and statistics peak in the 1860s.
46. Nineteenth-century medicine was essentially international. British authorities seem to cite continental sources more often than American sources. But British medical treatises were often published in American editions, and British medical journal articles reappear in American journals.
47. The Royal College of Physicians of London was most prestigious and chartered in 1518. The Royal College of Surgeons of London was chartered in 1800; surgery was technically a craft rather than a profession but proved upwardly mobile. Finally, the Society of Apothecaries was chartered in 1617. Apothecaries were associated with trade because they sold medicines, but they fought to attain recognition for practicing medicine.
48. These were physicians and surgeons with hospital and teaching appointments in the metropole. Lawrence examines debates over traditional education versus a German-style continental curriculum ("Incommunicable"). Peterson identifies a rift between the London-based consultant and the provincial general practitioner. These new loyalties superseded the old tripartite divisions in both London and the provinces (*Medical Profession*).
49. Peterson, *Medical Profession*, 60, 135. See also Bynum, *Science*, 176–84.
50. Romano, *Making Medicine Scientific*, 162.
51. Christopher Lawrence, "Incommunicable," 505.
52. Quoted in Peterson, *Medical Profession*, 173.
53. See Hollinger, "Knower and Artificer."
54. Collini, "Introduction," x.
55. Huxley, "Science and Culture"; Arnold, "Literature and Science."
56. Snow, *Two Cultures*; Leavis, "Two Cultures?"
57. See Shuttleworth, *Charlotte Brontë*; Rylance, *Victorian Psychology*; Dames, *Amnesiac Selves*; Otis, *Networking*; Michael Davis, *George Eliot*.
58. Dames, *Physiology of the Novel*.
59. A few studies, especially recently, focus on the genre of the case history in relation to the novel. Small includes an extended reading of medical case histories of the "love-mad

woman." Sill argues that study of the passions contributed to the empiricism that founds both eighteenth-century medicine and the novel. Caldwell examines the "double vision" of "Romantic materialism" in pre-Darwinian British literature and medicine, which, she argues, must read the world both empirically and imaginatively. She also discusses what she sees as a bipartite structure of the case history ("history" and "physical"). And Tougaw, whose project is perhaps closest to mine in scope and its focus on the case history as a genre, argues for a dual mode of reading (diagnosis or sympathy) through which novels and case histories make sense of the conjunction of pathology and identity. Small, *Love's Madness;* Sill, *Cure of the Passions;* Caldwell, *Literature and Medicine;* Tougaw, *Strange Cases.*

For books on the case history generally, see Tougaw; Epstein. Article-length histories include Temkin, "'Sinn'-Begriff"; Reiser, "Creating Form"; Stoeckle, "History-Taking"; Hurwitz, "Form and Representation"; Gilles, "Patient History"; Laqueur, "Bodies, Details"; Rylance, "Theatre and Granary."

60. See Nancy Armstrong, *Desire and Domestic Fiction;* Lennard Davis, *Factual Fictions;* J. Paul Hunter, *Before Novels;* McKeon, *Origins of the English Novel;* Price, *Anthology.*

61. See Peterson, "Medicine," 24.

Chapter One

1. Locke, *Essay Concerning Human Understanding,* 8 (II.ix). For a discussion of Molyneux's question, and of perception in the tradition of empirical philosophy, see Law, *Rhetoric of Empiricism.*

2. Chesselden, "Account of Some Observations," 448. The name is usually spelled Cheselden.

3. Most historians of medicine perceive the eighteenth century as a period of dormancy in the development of European medicine between two significant philosophical and practical developments: the New Science of the seventeenth century, and the clinical and experimental medicine of the nineteenth. See Porter, "Laymen, Doctors," 288.

4. Shapin and Schaffer, *Leviathan and the Air-Pump,* 56.

5. Ibid., 65–69.

6. Chesselden, " Explication."

7. Although surgeons and apothecaries might keep or even publish case histories, most printed case histories are authored by physicians. Practitioners who referenced the Royal Society or adopted experimentalist methods were also more likely to be physicians.

8. The patient retained power in the relationship with his physician through the eighteenth century, as Porter has shown ("Lay Medical Knowledge").

9. Pargeter, *Observations on Maniacal Disorders,* 103; Cheyne, *English Malady;* Monro, "Remarks."

10. See Richard Foster Jones, "Science and English Prose Style"; Christensen, "John Wilkins"; and Nicolson, *Seventeenth Century.* The influential arguments of these early commentators do not account for the "Rhetorick," or even the rhetoric, which persists in Royal Society texts; their conclusions have been revised. See Vickers, "Royal Society"; Dear, "*Totius in Verba.*"

11. From C. R. Weld (1848), *A History of the Royal Society,* London, I, 146–48; quoted in Hall, "Early Royal Society," 60.

12. V:iv [1728]; quoted in Jones, "Science and English Prose Style," 84.

13. Sprat, *History,* 111, 13 (emphasis in original).

14. Royal Society member John Wilkins pursued the injunction to equate words and things with his project of creating a "Real Character" in which each thing would be represent-

ed by a single sign, legible to readers of any language. Signs would follow a logical progression, so that the sign for "dog" would incorporate the sign for "animal," and so on. Mermaids, fairies, and the like had no signs, as they did not exist and hence were not truly "things."

15. I will adopt the eighteenth-century spelling, "Rhetorick," to distinguish the Royal Society's term, with all its connotations, from our modern usage of "rhetoric": any set of stylistic rules and principles, unavoidable in any organized discourse.

16. Fairfax, "Bullet Voided by Urine," 803.

17. Daston and Park, *Wonders,* 259.

18. Law argues that empiricism accomplishes this focus on perception through an unacknowledged emphasis on rhetoric and on language (*Rhetoric of Empiricism*).

19. Barbara Stafford also examines the eighteenth-century "antimony ... between spectacle, or gawking at heaped-up goods, and observation, or the reasoned apprehension of phenomena." *Artful Science,* xxvi.

20. See especially Benedict, *Curiosity;* Tougaw, *Strange Cases.*

21. These included, besides the *Philosophical Transactions* of the Royal Society, the French *Journal des Savants* and *Histoires et Mémoires de l'Académie Royale des Science,* and the Italian *Giornale de litterati.* See Daston, "Marvelous Facts," 259.

22. Daval, "Extraordinary Rainbow"; de Vallemont, "Small Egg"; "Part of a Letter ... Account of a Double Pear"; Conny, "Shower of Fishes."

23. Molineux, "Epidemick Distempers," 105.

24. Cheyne, *English Malady,* N2.

25. McKeon, *Origins,* 47.

26. See Dennis Todd on the epistemological issues raised by physicians' response to the Mary Toft (rabbit-birth) case (*Imagining Monsters*); and Stafford on the eighteenth-century nexus between science and entertainment, truth and foolery (*Artful Science*). Terry Castle suggests that spectators might actually want to be deceived ("Culture of Travesty").

27. Pargeter, *Maniacal Disorders,* 109; Myddelton, "Extra-Uterine Conception," 337.

28. On the "physician of the mind," see Sill, *Cure of the Passions,* 13–34. The literature on eighteenth-century medicine and sensibility is considerable. See especially Van Sant, *Eighteenth-Century Sensibility,* 50–59, for a comparison of the mechanism of sensibility—as an observation of suffering, which excites a sympathetic response—in the literary context and that in the physiological one. On "sympathetic practitioners" and how the eighteenth-century John Gregory, in *Observations on the Duties and Offices of a Physician* (1770), theorized that practitioners need both "sympathy" and "composure," see Ward, *Desire and Disorder,* 30–53; Caldwell, *Literature and Medicine,* chap. 2.

29. Mandeville, *Hypochondriack and Hysterick Diseases,* 19–20.

30. Cheyne, *Health and Long Life,* xvii.

31. Pargeter, *Maniacal Disorders,* 49 (emphasis in original).

32. Although Boddington and two others write the main portion of the text, it is framed and thus "authored" by Henry Baker. See Baker et al., "Margaret Cutting," 143.

33. "Two Letters from a Gentleman," 1499–1500.

34. Watt, *Rise of the Novel,* 188, 157.

35. Dent, "Worms Found in the Tongue," 220.

36. Despite the apparent conflict with the ideal of a disinterested observation, terms like "entertainment" (as in the water-newt case) do not seem to disrupt the experimentalist's contract with witnesses. The term can indicate intellectual exercise, as in this discussion of fluid dynamics in rivers: "As it is a problem somewhat curious, though' not difficult, and its solution not generally known ... I thought it might give some entertainment to the curious in these matters, if the whole process were published." Robertson, "Water under Bridges," 493.

37. Parsons, "Hermaphrodite," 142, 143 (emphasis in original).

38. Todd comments that "the English fascination with monsters and their willingness to pay to see them were almost proverbial" (5).

39. See Byrd, "Negro-Boy"; Parsons, "White Negro"; "Of the Posture Master"; Machin, "Distempered Skin"; Baker, "Distempered Skin." Baker mentions that the patient was "shown at London by the name of the porcupine-man" (22).

40. The extended debate over the efficacy and safety of transfusion included three previous articles or notices regarding the experiments in transfusion in Paris: Denis, "Letter . . . Touching the Transfusion of Blood," briefly discussing a dog-to-dog transfusion; Denis, "Letter . . . Touching a Late Cure," an extensive account with cases and a detailed explanation of equipment arrangement for performing a transfusion; Denis, "Letter . . . Touching the Differences Risen," detailing the legal investigation into the man's death, which Denis attributes to arsenic poisoning. The *Philosophical Transactions* also publishes an anonymous article claiming British priority in the procedure: "Advertisement Concerning the Transfusion of Bloud."

41. Denis, "Letter . . . Touching a Late Cure," 617, 620. For a second transfusion, Denis lists the spectators as "several very able physicians, *Bourdelot, Lallier, Dodar, de Bourges*, and *Vaillant*" (621). He claims "that divers physitians, and other persons worthy of credit, that have seen [the patient], can render an authentick testimony to all the circumstances here advanced by me" (624).

42. Ibid., 620.

43. Stack's case is one of several on unusual lactation. In 1674 "a Person of great veracity in Germany" wrote to the editor of the *Philosophical Transactions* "concerning an aged Woman of 60 Years, giving suck to her Grandchild" (the author's own child). In 1741 Robert, Lord Bishop of Cork wrote to the Royal Society about "a Man who gave Suck to a Child." Unfortunately, the suckling had occurred long before the bishop met him, so unlike Stack he could not witness it firsthand; but "[t]he bishop looked at his breasts, which were then very large for a man; and the nipple was as large or larger than any woman's he ever saw." Stack, "Woman," 140 (emphasis in original); "Relation Written . . . Concerning an Aged Woman"; Robert, Lord Bishop of Cork, "Man Who Gave Suck," 517.

44. Manginot, "Unusual Medical Case," 756.

45. Denis, "Letter . . . Touching a Late Cure," 622.

46. Chesselden, "Young Gentleman," 450, 448.

47. See, for example, Barker-Benfield, *Culture of Sensibility*, 1–35; Mullan, *Sentiment and Sociability*, 210–40; Brissenden, *Virtue in Distress*, 35–45; Flynn, "Running out of Matter"; Rousseau, "Nerves, Spirits, and Fibres"; Van Sant, *Eighteenth-Century Sensibility*, 1–16.

48. Pye-Smith, "Medicine as a Science," 309.

49. For the lack of public confidence in establishment medicine, see Peterson, *Medical Profession*, 38, 90. Homeopathy and other peculiar practices had rapidly established colonies of support in influential patient populations. By professionalizing and regularizing care, by repudiating both quacks and "heroic medicine" as unscientific, and by distancing their work from the craft of surgery and the trade of apothecary, reformist physicians hoped to regain market share and public trust, and to secure a position in the powerful new professional class. However, as George Eliot's *Middlemarch* dramatizes, patients themselves were not sure they wanted reformist, professional physicians.

50. Medical schools affiliated with hospitals and providing intensive clinical training were rare until the latter half of the century. The Medical Reform Act of 1858 established ground rules for licensure, but there was no universal exam until 1884. Physics, chemistry, and biology were not generally required for entry into medical schools until the 1880s. See Peterson, *Medical Profession*, 5, 60, 64, 241; Warner, *Therapeutic Perspective*, 175ff.

51. The *Lancet* was the best known reformist organ, although the *London Medical and Surgical Journal* also exposed incompetent practitioners. Medical journals provided a central

force for reform. See Crawford, "Scientific Profession," esp. 223; Warner, "Idea of Science," 138–42.

52. Warner, *Therapeutic Perspective*, 182.

53. Georges Canguilhem has analyzed this shift toward perceiving pathology as a physiological state along a continuum of bodily conditions; Warner places the shift in the bodily ideal from "natural" to "normal" around the 1850s. Canguilhem, *Normal and Pathological*; Warner, *Therapeutic Perspective*, 87. See also Huet, *Monstrous Imagination*.

54. Canguilhem, *Normal and Pathological*, 69–85.

55. Gould and Pyle, *Anomalies and Curiosities*, 2, 1.

56. Barnes, *William Dempster*; Clanny, *Mary Jobson*; Millingen, *Curiosities*; Sayre, *Remarkable Case*. Thomas Renwick published in 1817 a pamphlet, *Narrative of the Case of Miss Margaret McAvoy* (with "some optical experiments" on what he later explained as "her peculiar powers of distinguishing colours, reading &c., through the medium of her fingers"). Renwick's (and Miss McAvoy's) claims invited a rebuttal by Joseph Sandars, which was itself rebutted by Renwick. See Renwick, *Narrative of the Case;* Renwick, *Continuation of the Narrative;* Sandars, *Hints to Credulity!*

57. Stafford talks about this gesture as a crucial component of the Enlightenment itself: "Most fundamentally, to enlighten meant unmasking charlatanism of every stripe by teaching the public its conning stratagems.... Fear of contaminating pristine or authentic experience reached epidemic proportions in the second half of the eighteenth century" (74). Enthusiasm for an unmasking "enlightenment" pervades the case history most strongly in the early nineteenth century.

58. Greenhow, "Concussion of the Brain," 392. The case is "reported (with a drawing) by Mr. H. M. Greenhow," but Mary K. is actually "under the care of" Mr. T. M. Greenhow (392).

59. Rick Rylance argues that the curious is not even much obscured. Analyzing two contrasting elements of the nineteenth-century case history, the "granary" (practical, methodical) and the "theatre" (spectacular, curious), he notes the persistence of the theatre in cases throughout the century, specifically in tone, narrative conventions, the diversity of journal contents, and "the sustained and substantial presence of the bizarre, the grotesque, the freakish, and the comical. "Theatre and Granary," 262–63.

Chapter Two

1. Latham, *Collected Works*, 29, 37–38.

2. Janis Caldwell complicates this trajectory by arguing that clinical medicine in fact is grounded on the same "Romantic materialism" that nurtured Romantic literature, a "dialectical hermeneutic" that "tacked back and forth between physical evidence and inner, imaginative understanding." Caldwell's readings are persuasive, but I am more interested in tracing the expression of empirical ideals in nineteenth-century case history writing, examining how and why these ideals seemed to demand the exclusion of any subjective insight, despite the impossibility of this aim. Despite the existence of the productive "Romantic materialism" that Caldwell examines, many cases demonstrate their allegiance instead to the ascendant epistemology that Lorraine Daston and Peter Galison have termed "mechanical objectivity." In chapter 5, I examine the shift at midcentury when case histories may once again acknowledge imagination and insight, now coded as "speculation" and "hypothesis." Caldwell, *Literature and Medicine*, 1.

3. Clinics (publicly funded hospitals) first arose in France, shifting the intellectual center of medicine from Edinburgh to Paris for much of the nineteenth century. See Ackerknecht,

Paris Hospital; W. F. Bynum, *Science;* Foucault, *Birth of the Clinic;* Peterson, *Medical Profession;* Shryock, *Development;* Warner, *Against the Spirit;* Warner, "Idea of Science."

4. In an 1816 casebook by a Bristol surgeon, James Bedingford, 32 of the 34 cases underwent an autopsy after death. Fissell, "Disappearance," 100.

5. Epstein, *Altered Conditions,* 51.

6. Caldwell locates the beginnings of the modern format in the 1820s, and Epstein comments that the "more or less standard order ... began to be established in the early nineteenth century and became codified in the last decade of the century." My research suggests that the modern format begins to emerge in the first decade. Gilles argues that around 1860, the "symptom" (the patient's subjective experience of disease) became distinguished from the physician's observation of the "objective signs" of disease. See Caldwell, *Literature and Medicine,* 149; Gilles, "Patient History," 493.

7. Finlayson, "Examination and Reporting," 39.

8. Ferriar, *Medical Histories* (1792), iii–iv.

9. Analogy persists in that the individual patient with phthisis was understood as an analogue of the normative patient with phthisis; but analogies between diseases, as in the old nosologies, became problematic. The physician William Osler warns in 1892,

> [T]here is a form of acute phthisis which may closely simulate ordinary pneumonia.... A healthy, robust-looking young Irishman, a cab-driver, who had been kept waiting on a cold, blustering night until three in the morning, was seized the next afternoon with a violent chill, and the following day was admitted to my wards at the University Hospital, Philadelphia. He was made the subject of a clinical lecture on the fifth day, when there was absent no single feature in history, symptoms, or physical signs of acute lobar pneumonia of the right upper lobe. It was not until ten days later, when bacilli were found in his expectoration, that we were made aware of the true nature of the case.

Here analogy is held up as an inexact science, corrected by the newer diagnostic methods of germ theory. Osler, *Principles and Practice,* 211. See also Foucault, *Birth,* 100–101.

10. Fissell, "Disappearance," 103.

11. Frawley, *Invalidism and Identity,* 5.

12. Foucault, *Birth,* 89.

13. The interest in surfaces does not contradict the clinic's interest in delving into the body (through autopsy and new technologies like the laryngoscope); these conceptually extend the surfaces visible to the clinical gaze. See also Foucault, *Birth,* 128–29.

14. Foucault, *Birth,* 113 (emphasis in original).

15. Cheyne, *English Malady,* 307–11.

16. Morgagni, *Seats and Causes,* xxxi.

17. Daston and Galison, "Image of Objectivity," 87–88.

18. Morgagni, *Seats and Causes,* 819 (XXVI:31).

19. Caldwell usefully examines a similar shift in anatomical atlases, away from the subjectivity of the "animated cadaver" and toward an aesthetic displaying "the physical body, shorn of emotion, imagination, agency, individuality, and personhood." Ironically, the human subjects in the images she discusses are all cadavers, whether animated and emotive, or unexpressive and inert. Caldwell, "Strange Death," 343.

20. Bennett, *Clinical Lectures,* iii.

21. See Reiser, *Reign of Technology.*

22. Bramwell, *Practical Medicine,* 25.

23. Peterson, *Medical Profession,* 172.

24. Holland, *Mental Physiology,* 18–19.

25. Sims, *Discourse*, 99–101.

26. Latham, *Collected Works*, 69 (emphasis in original).

27. "Empiricism" is a difficult term at about this time. While it ostensibly refers to the practice of empirical science—induction based on material observations rather than deductions from the theories of eighteenth-century and earlier medical authorities—it also was associated with quackery, because alternative practitioners ("empirics") were thought to rely on seat-of-the-pants experience rather than book learning. The difficulty is evident in James Sims's text, for example, where, in order to valorize "empiricism," he must also explicitly disassociate it from quackery.

28. Stillé, *Elements*, 34.

29. Daston and Galison, "Image of Objectivity," 82–83.

30. Daston and Galison, *Objectivity*, 123.

31. Stillé, *Elements*, 46 (emphasis in original).

32. Stillé quotes from Baglivi here. Ironically, he cites early physicians to support his empiricism.

33. Daston and Galison, *Objectivity*, 229.

34. Bramwell, "Value of Cultivating," 243; Levine, *Dying to Know*, 27.

35. See Levine's nuanced discussion of the ideal of self-abnegation in *Dying to Know*.

36. W. J. T. Mitchell, *Picture Theory*, 325.

37. Elliotson et al., *Principles and Practice*, 18, 50; Williams and Clymer, *Principles of Medicine*, 436; Laycock, *Lectures*, 34; Hartshorne, *Essentials*, 21 (emphasis in original); Bramwell, "Value of Cultivating," 237.

38. Bigelow and Holmes, "Medical Observation," 3–4; Bullitt, "Art of Observing," 399.

39. Warter, *Observation in Medicine*, vii.

40. Warner, *Against the Spirit*, 175.

41. Huet, *Monstrous Imagination*, 188. In 1920, Hilaire Belloc explains this paradox, discussing the figures at Madame Tussaud's: "it is precisely because the likeness is so great, precisely because the effect is so parallel to that of reality, that we note the minor details in which illusion is not achieved." Introduction to John Theodore Tussaud, *The Romance of Madame Tussaud's* (New York: Doran, 1920), 27, quoted in Huet, 188. Benjamin, "Work of Art," 220.

42. See Jennifer Tucker, *Nature Exposed*, for a nuanced examination of how photography both inspires and resists Victorian scientists' ideals of truth and accuracy.

43. Barbara Stafford argues for a somewhat different version of eighteenth-century visual truth: "William Cheselden, in the monumental *Osteographia* (1733), required his artists to represent bones without showing the forming hand behind the image. 'Objectivity,' or the honest conduct of the practitioner, was thus synonymous with the absence of any visible sign of manufacture. The rise of objectivity as a scientific ideal in the early modern period was facilitated by the development of measuring and distancing apparatuses. These truly 'automatic' devices seemed to preclude shady handling and phony gadgetry." But Cheselden's ideal of an absent artist in fact requires the artist to intervene by leaving out any evidence of his presence. The artist draws the skeleton, not the tripod holding it or the men steadying it: he draws truth to [what he knows to be true] nature. In contrast, the mechanical observer of the nineteenth century must include whatever data were collected, even artifacts indicating the situation and role of the observer. Stafford, *Artful Science*, 103.

44. Gallagher, *Nobody's Story*, 173–74.

45. Blanc, "Typhoid Fever," 191.

46. The case also references new medical technologies. Blanc pairs it with the case of "a young English lady" in Gogo, India, with a very high fever due to typhoid. Her "Thermometrical Register" (temperature chart) is reproduced directly underneath Mr. P——'s case (191).

47. See Fissell on the "disappearance of the patient" (as a person and a voice) from the clinical case history.

48. Pye-Smith spoke at the annual meeting of the British Medical Association held at Ipswich on August 1, 1900. Cheever, "Value of Statistics," 449; Bennett, *Clinical Lectures,* 28; Bramwell, *Practical Medicine,* 23; Pye-Smith, "Medicine as Science," 309. See also Foucault, *Birth,* 120–22.

49. Porter, "Lay Medical Knowledge."

50. Rothfield, *Vital Signs,* 99. Examples of recent research into popular science culture include the Science in the Nineteenth-Century Periodical project and the Science Index of the Athenaeum Projects, especially the Index of Reviews and Reviewers, which indexes the book reviews in the *Athenaeum* between 1828 and 1870. Gillian Beer has discussed the "wonderful inclusiveness of generalist journals at that time." Rick Rylance also briefly examines the inclusion of medical cases in general-circulation periodicals, as well as the "literary" character of the specialized medical periodicals. Beer, *Open Fields,* 202–3; Rylance, "Theatre and Granary."

51. Latham, *Collected Works,* 44.

52. Frawley, *Invalidism and Identity,* 18.

53. Hills, *Instructions to Patients,* 7, 4, 2. Hills largely reprints this series of questions from homeopathic treatises dating back to mid-century.

54. Peterson, "Medicine," 256.

55. Topham, "Bridgewater Treatises," 249.

56. [Lankester], review of Bennett. Texts that were considered appropriate for a popular readership include Beale (9 February 1856); *Poor Man's Guide* (26 January 1856); J. L. Levinson's *Obscure Nervous Diseases,* popularly explained (12 April 1856, 1485); T. Wharton Jones, *Defects of Sight* (1 August 1857, 973); Spencer Thomson, *The Structure and Functions of the Eye* (5 December 1857, 1517); Benjamin Ridge, *Health and Disease* (5 March 1859, 324); Forbes Winslow, *On Obscure Disease of the Mind and Disorders of the Mind* (22 September 1860, 388); James Wylde, *The Magic of Science: A Manual of Easy and Instructive Scientific Experiments* (12 January 1861, 48).

57. [Lankester], review of Johnson.

58. [St. John], "Life of Cullen."

59. [Lankester], review of Hall.

60. [Lankester], review of Churchill.

61. [Lankester], review of Lobb.

62. [Lankester], review of Johnson.

63. [Lankester], review of Taylor.

64. [Lankester], review of Ferguson; review of Burgess.

65. [Lankester], review of Ross; [Noble], review of Neilson; [Lankester], review of Ridge.

66. Cooley, "Inverted Vision."

67. [Lankester], review of Ramsbotham; [Lankester], review of Barker; [Lankester], review of Fermer, 36.

68. Holland, "Wellcome Index."

69. Thackeray, letter to G. H. Lewes (November 1, 1859), quoted in Smith, "Our Birth," 7.

70. Altick, *English Common Reader,* 359, 95.

71. Dawson, *"Cornhill Magazine,"* 147.

72. [Thompson], "Under Chloroform," 499.

73. Anstie, "On Physical Pain," 458, 459

74. Dawson discusses the possible adverse effects from Herschel's use of a remarkably professional level of discourse for the *Cornhill*'s "Notes on Science." Dawson, *"Cornhill Magazine,"* 147–48.

75. MacLaren, "Management," 515–16. MacLaren had some medical training, but he made his living as a proponent of physical fitness.

76. Macmillan, "Human Vegetation," 461, 462.
77. Anstie, "Corpulence," 458.
78. Anstie, "Medical Etiquette," 163.
79. Whitehead, "Broad Street Pump," 113.

Chapter Three

1. Dickens, *Dombey and Son*, chap. 4, 36. Further references to this novel will give chapter and page number from this edition.

2. Jude V. Nixon argues that Dickens "believed that science and the imagination, troped as fact and fancy, head and heart, should operate dialectically." While this is true, this chapter argues that this dialectic functions within, not between, the different genres of scientific and literary narrative ("Dickens and Science," 267).

3. Kaplan, *Sacred Tears*, 5, 37.

4. Bailin, *Sickroom*, 79.

5. Indeed, Kaplan, among others, connects it to the "moral sentiments." I will, however, be using "sentiment" in a more modern and restricted sense, referring to the force animating sentimentalism rather than to "emotion" generally. And although eighteenth-century commentators do contemplate humankind's "sympathy" with the rich and prosperous, my concern here is with "sympathy" in its more common modern relation to sorrow and suffering.

6. Kaplan, *Sacred Tears*, 37.

7. Stephen, in the *Cornhill*, defines sentimentality as the use of "tender emotions in an improper manner," and affiliates it with what is "theatrical and affected." A sentimental author has "begun to think about himself, and how cleverly he could describe the sources of tender emotion, and how pleasant it was to stimulate their action." Sterne, he says, "likes to make himself and some of his readers cry" ("Sentimentalism," 69, 71).

8. Lerner, *Angels and Absences*, 183. Adam Smith makes a similar distinction in discussing "extreme sympathy with misfortunes which we know nothing about," calling it "a certain affected and sentimental sadness, which, without reaching the heart, serves only to render the countenance and conversation impertinently dismal and disagreeable." Smith, *Moral Sentiments*, 197 (pt. III, chap. 3). Further references to this text will give part, section (if relevant) and chapter number, along with page number.

9. Hume, *Treatise*, 368 (bk. III, pt. iii, sec. 1) (emphasis in original). Further references to this text will give book, part, and section number, along with page number.

10. Smith, *Moral Sentiments*, 162 (III.1).

11. Jaffe, *Scenes of Sympathy*, 32. Other critics discussing this association include Amit Rai, who links sympathy and spectacle; and Laura Hinton, who discusses Hume and sympathy as a spectacle, and Smith and sympathy as spectatorship. Hinton also discusses how the sympathetic spectator acts as fetishist and voyeur (3). See Rai, *Rule of Sympathy*, xiv; Hinton, *Perverse Gaze*, 2, 23.

12. Other critics have examined the power relation inherent to, but never fully acknowledged by, sympathy's benevolent relation to the sufferer. Roberts emphasizes the unequal power relationship in sympathy and its need to both consume and inhabit another's suffering (*Schools of Sympathy*, 9). Rai discusses how sympathy is implicated in colonialism not just despite but through its expressed interest in humanitarianism (*Rule of Sympathy*, xiii).

13. Hume, *Treatise*, 368 (III. iii.1).

14. Smith, *Moral Sentiments*, 201 (III.3).

15. Hume, *Treatise*, 207–8 (II.i.11).

16. Smith, *Moral Sentiments*, 4–5 (I.i.1).

17. Especially Gallagher, *Nobody's Story*; Roberts, *Schools of Sympathy*; Lenard, *Preaching Pity*; Lowe, *Insights of Sympathy*. See also Jaffe, Hinton, Rai, and Stoddart, "Tracking the Sentimental Eye."

18. Literary critics have also examined the role of visuality in producing sentimental readers. My understanding of the sentimental gaze in Dickens's narrators differs from that of Stoddart, who argues that "[t]he sentimental eye ... attempts to stabilize [the] oscillating perspective" between a fixed, stable perspective or a fluctuating series of individual, embodied, "particularized acts of viewing" ("Tracking the Sentimental Eye," 196). The sentimental eye in the texts I examine here offers, I would say, rather a supplement to or an alternate vision than an attempt to consolidate multiple perspectives.

19. [Stephen], "Sentimentalism," 74–75.

20. Stoddart, "Tracking the Sentimental Eye," 195, 196.

21. Critics of sympathy have examined how it relies on and produces difference, but I am interested in what sympathy claims to do more than how it may actually operate. See, for example, Gallagher, *Nobody's Story*, xvii–xviii; Jaffe, *Scenes of Sympathy*, 32; Rai, *Rule of Sympathy*, xix, 22.

22. Kneeland, "Contagiousness," 4.

23. Isham and Keyt, "Editors' Preface," iii.

24. Sansom, *Manual*, 5–6.

25. Hope, *Treatise*, 401. The false hope on the deathbed is a common trope of sentimental medicine. John Ferriar explains, "[T]he patient appears better ... and hopes of recovery are given. In the height of this security, the fatal stroke arrives: every one is astonished; and an event which ought to have been foreseen and foretold, passes for sudden death." Ferriar, *Medical Histories*, 92.

26. See Kennedy, "'Poor Hoo Loo'"; Thrailkill, "Killing Them Softly."

27. Ferriar, *Medical Histories* (1810), 193–94.

28. Williams, *Authentic Narrative*, 20.

29. Williams and Clymer, *Principles of Medicine*, 440. This passage does not seem to appear in later editions.

30. "A London Curiosity," 95.

31. See Holmes, *Fictions of Affliction*.

32. Carpenter, *Principles of Human Physiology* (1868), 533, 545.

33. Swain, "Diseased Conditions," 542.

34. Occasionally such identification with the patient can backfire, as when John Elliotson discusses cretins in the Swiss Alps. "Some females have a great number of these children," he says. "They have desires, like other people; and they fall in love with each other, and marry." To this point, a sympathetic identification helps to clarify the context of this medical problem. But he continues, "Certainly *nobody else* would marry them." This offhand comment at once destroys the fragile insight linking the physician to his patient and retrospectively casts all affective response as likewise unprofessional and unhelpful (*Principles and Practice*, 545–46; emphasis in original).

35. Stoddart, *Anecdote Biographies*, 124–25.

36. Miriam Bailin identifies the sentimental as a force sublimating the frictions of social ambition ("'Dismal Pleasure'"). This anecdote about Thackeray suggests that perhaps his focus on the sentimental as a measure of writerly success similarly deflects professional judgments into aesthetic ones.

37. See Lerner, *Angels and Absences*, 177.

38. Dickens, *Dombey and Son*, 14.156, 158–59, 160, 164–65.

39. Similar romanticized deaths occur with adults: see the deaths of Paul's mother and Alice.

40. For the lack of clear diagnoses in sentimental child deaths in the Victorian novel, see Lerner, *Angels and Absences*, 154ff.

41. For a sampling of readers' sentimental responses to Nell's death, see Lerner, *Angels and Absences*, 174–77, 179.

42. Dickens, *Old Curiosity Shop*, chap. 72, 539–40. Further references to this novel will give chapter and page number from this edition.

43. Huxley, "Vulgarity of Little Nell." The quotations from Dostoevsky are from bk. 10, chap. 5.

44. See Lerner, *Angels and Absences*, 180–83. Evangelical contemporaries of Dickens also critiqued his deathbeds as shallow; see Lerner, *Angels and Absences*, 202–4. Henry Hallam critiqued Paul's death as "pure business"; see Kaplan, *Sacred Tears*, 47.

45. This pattern obtains also in less-celebrated deaths in Dickens, such as those of little Johnny and Betty Higden in *Our Mutual Friend*.

46. Jalland, *Death*, chaps. 1–3, esp. 52, 59.

47. Taylor, *Manual*, 42.

48. Dyson, *Inimitable Dickens*, 44.

49. Dickens, *Old Curiosity Shop*, 43.324, 327; 44.330–31; 45.338, 340–41.

50. Dickens's process of "taking the histories" of fallen women admitted to Urania Cottage demonstrates a number of similarities with the system of "case-taking" in clinical medicine, including the anxiety over inadvertently prompting misleading or fallacious responses from the patient. Anderson, *Tainted Souls*, 73–74.

51. Anderson, *Tainted Souls*, 10.

52. Lerner discusses the term "old-fashioned" in reference to its dialect meaning, "precocious, knowing" (*Angels and Absences*, 89). While this meaning of the term may provide an overtone to Paul's character, Dickens clearly uses it here as a kind of diagnosis, to suggest his unearthliness, his being not long for this world. Thus, Paul's increasing delicacy means he "grows more and more old-fashioned" (the title of chapter 14); and his death is not the moment when he "loses his old-fashionedness," as Lerner suggests (90), but when he becomes more old-fashioned than ever, as is clear in Dickens's apostrophe, "The old, old fashion—Death!" (16.191).

53. *The Old Curiosity Shop* was followed (in *Master Humphrey's Clock*) by *Barnaby Rudge*, after which the frame story was brought to a close.

54. Trodd et al. note that the tradition of "cabinets of curiosities" and antiquarian collection extends into the nineteenth century, with texts like Thomas Wright's *A History of Caricature and Grotesque in Literature* (1865) and William Fairholt's *Eccentric and Remarkable Characters* (1849). Collections of medical curiosities were published as late as 1897, with George Gould and Walter Pyle's *Anomalies and Curiosities of Medicine*. But these were primarily eighteenth-century projects, and Dickens signals that his tale is modeled on eighteenth-century literature by referencing, in his three prefaces, Sheridan, Goldsmith, Fielding, and Sterne.

55. Kaplan analyzes the relation between Dickens's sentimentality and the tradition of the "moral sentiments" of the eighteenth century (*Sacred Tears*, 39–70).

56. Dickens comments in letters to this effect: "I am breaking my heart over this story," "Old wounds bleed afresh when I only think of the way of doing it.... Dear Mary died yesterday, when I think of this sad story" (*Letters* II, 170 [to Cattermole] and II, 181–82). Qtd. in MacPike, "Old Curiosity Shop," 35.

57. Dickens, *Letters*, 188 (to John Forster, [?17] January 1841).

58. Dickens's Edinburgh speech, delivered on 25 June 1841. Dickens, *Speeches*, 10. Qtd. in MacPike, "Old Curiosity Shop," 35.

59. Kaplan, *Dickens*, 268.

60. Vrettos, *Somatic Fictions*, 1.

61. Gaskell, *Ruth*, 346.
62. Osler, *Principles and Practice*, 40.
63. Ferriar, *Medical Histories and Reflections* (1792), 74–75.
64. Haley, *Healthy Body*, 6, 7.
65. d'Albertis, *Dissembling Fictions*, 93, 92.
66. Jaffe, *Scenes of Sympathy*, 78.
67. Buchan, *Domestic Medicine*, 135.
68. Elliotson et al., *Principles and Practice*, 188–89.
69. Buchan, *Domestic Medicine*, 113, 136.
70. Elliotson et al., *Principles and Practice*, 194.
71. Yonge, *Heir of Redclyffe*, 429.
72. Jalland, *Death*, 26.
73. An important exception to this might be the death of the protagonist's mother, which so often (as in *Dombey*) instead propels the newly orphaned protagonist into both action and agency.

Chapter Four

1. Imraad Coovadia similarly argues, "[b]ecause George Eliot is acutely conscious of the distorting power of figurative language, she employs metaphors rather carefully—and so we can place considerable interpretive pressure upon those she does use" ("George Eliot's Realism," 824).
2. See Yeo, "Scientific Method," 282ff; Yeo, *Defining Science*, 102–6.
3. Helmholtz, "Theory of Vision," 147; Watson, *Lectures*, 15.
4. See, for example, J. Hillis Miller, countered by Levine and D. A. Miller, among others. For a critique of George Eliot's realism, see, for example, MacCabe, countered by Lodge, Beer, and Shaw, among others. Coovadia also references this debate (820–21). J. Hillis Miller, "Optic and Semiotic"; Levine, "Hypothesis of Reality"; Levine, *Realistic Imagination*; D. A. Miller, *Narrative and Its Discontents*; MacCabe, *Revolution of the Word*; MacCabe, "Realism and the Cinema"; Lodge, "Classic Realist Text"; Beer, *Darwin's Plots*; Shaw, *Narrating Reality*.
5. Shuttleworth, *George Eliot*, 206.
6. Colvin, review of *Middlemarch*, 144.
7. See Levine, *Realistic Imagination*, 252–74; Shuttleworth, *George Eliot*; Beer, *Darwin's Plots*, 137–68; Rothfield, *Vital Signs*, 84–119; Logan, *Nerves and Narratives*, 166–96, Mason, "*Middlemarch* and Science"; Tambling, "*Middlemarch*, Realism"; Wormald, "Microscopy and Semiotic"; Menke, "Fiction as Vivisection."
8. Deanna Kreisel also directs critical attention to the importance of medical discourse, particularly obstetric rhetoric, in this early novel ("Incognito").
9. Shuttleworth reads *Adam Bede* in relation to natural history and a passive observer who reflects the world. King places George Eliot in the context of natural history when she started to write fiction. Mason places George Eliot and Lewes in relation to the competing empiricisms of John Stuart Mill, William Whewell, and Herbert Spencer, and Levine points to her friendships with T. H. Huxley, John Tyndall, and W. K. Clifford. Shuttleworth, *George Eliot*, 23–50; King, *Bloom*, 166–72, 79–86; Mason, "*Middlemarch* and Science"; Levine, *Realistic Imagination*, 253. In addition, the character Charles Meunier, in George Eliot's short story "The Lifted Veil" (1859), suggests the physiologist Charles-Edouard Brown-Séquard. See Eliot, *Lifted Veil*; Flint, *Visual Imagination*, 102–5.
10. Eliot, *Quarry for Middlemarch*; Kitchel, "Introduction," 8; Gray, "Pseudoscience," 413.
11. Thomson, *Recollections and Reflections*, 282.

12. See O'Connor, *Founders of British Physiology*, 116–17.
13. See, for example, Coovadia, "George Eliot's Realism and Adam Smith"; Logan, "Fetish of Realism."
14. Spencer, "Genesis of Science."
15. Williams and Clymer, *Principles of Medicine*, 371; Holland, *Medical Notes and Reflections*, 28; Bennett, *Clinical Lectures*, 4.
16. Watson, *Lectures*, 15 (emphasis in original); Forbes, *Inaugural Lecture on Botany*, 8 (emphasis in original); Holland, *Medical Notes and Reflections*, 28.
17. This concern reflected the difficulties of using such instruments. Bennett warns that "[t]he art of observation is at all times difficult, but is especially so with a microscope, which presents us with forms and structures concerning which we had no previous idea. Rigid and exact investigation, therefore, should be methodically cultivated from the first" (*Clinical Lectures*, 69).
18. George Eliot, *Adam Bede*, ed. Valentine Cunningham (New York: Oxford University Press, 1996), 175, 177. In the 1867 Blackwood edition, George Eliot strengthens her emphasis on the importance of the "faithful account" by amending the text to read, "my strongest effort is to avoid any such arbitrary picture." She also removes the 1859 reference to the "clever novelist," stating instead, "Certainly I could [romanticize my characters], if I held it the highest vocation of the novelist to represent things as they never have been and never will be." This allows for the possibility of realist novelists; the previous version could imply that all novelists are "clever [e.g., romantic] novelists." George Eliot, *Adam Bede*, ed. Gordon S. Haight (New York: Holt, Rinehart, and Winston, 1965). All further references will be to the Cunningham edition, based on the 1859 edition of the novel. See also "The Sad Fortunes of the Reverend Amos Barton" for a similar passage disdaining "fertile imagination." It prefers "faithfulness" to "the humble experience of an ordinary fellow-mortal," which produces sympathy. Eliot, *Scenes of Clerical Life*, 59.
19. Gunn, "Dutch Painting," 368.
20. Eliot, review of Ruskin, 626; Ruskin, *Modern Painters*, IV.7.16.
21. Ruskin also used the trope of deformed or distorted reflections, in *Stones of Venice*, although somewhat differently. He disdains optical devices, thinking a culture steeped in such experience would be coarsened to true aesthetic experience. Without them, an ideally artistic vision is possible. See Isobel Armstrong, "Transparency," 144; Isobel Armstrong, "Microscope," 43–46.
22. In "The Sad Fortunes of the Reverend Amos Barton" and "Mr. Gilfil's Love Story," the narrators similarly defend realist texts against romantic readers. Eliot, *Scenes of Clerical Life*, 59, 87.
23. Gillian Beer suggests that this kind of pleasure is an important commonality between scientists and authors. Beer, *Open Fields*, 152.
24. George Eliot knew how hard it is to make a flawless mirror. While visiting Munich in 1858, she and Lewes met Baron Justus von Liebig, a professor of chemistry there. "He is now occupied with a new invention, that of silver mirrors," wrote Lewes to the publisher John William Parker Jr., "and he has gone over the whole process with us, explaining each detail, and finally presenting Marian with a mirror of remembrance." Eliot, *Letters*, I, 276 [12 May 1858].
25. She shared these concerns with Lewes; see Isobel Armstrong, "Microscope," 40–43.
26. For a different articulation of this philosophy, see an early letter to John Blackwood (Eliot, *Letters* II, 362 [12 July 1857]).
27. Daston and Galison, *Objectivity*, 121, 185.
28. Daston and Galison, *Objectivity*, 174, 176, 197, 203.
29. Levine, *Dying to Know*. See Charles Babbage in 1830 on both "minute precision" and

the "*occasional discordance from the mean*, which attends *even the most careful observations*"; or John Herschel, also in 1830, on "the erroneous judgments we unconsciously form from" sensory experience and the "illusion which the senses practice on us." Babbage, *Decline of Science*, 168 (emphasis in original); Herschel, *Preliminary Discourse*, 81–82; Daston and Galison, "Image of Objectivity," 82–83.

30. Amy King also notices this suggestion of the botanist. King, *Bloom*, 169.

31. Amanda Anderson also notes the "active, vigilant self-suppression ... which paradoxically required stringent personal practices" to attain self-regulation. Anderson, *Powers of Distance*, 11.

32. Anderson surveys some critiques and defenses of detachment along these lines. Ibid., 23–33.

33. Daston, "Moral Economy of Science," 21, 23. Janis Caldwell nods to this concept but recasts "morality" as "affect" when she observes, "Nineteenth-century objectivity was, despite its rhetoric, not at all free of affect, but rather reached toward a different kind of affect, that of faithfulness to the object, careful craft, precision, and self-restraint." Caldwell, "Strange Death," 350. While I concur with her description of the objective aesthetic, I might term its aim not a "kind of affect" but a "kind of subjectivity" or perhaps Anderson's term, a "lived relation" (178). These, to me, suggest the conundrum of mechanical observation; that it is designed to specifically not hold or channel feeling, but that it is inescapably in relation to the self and its affect.

34. Andrew H. Miller, "Bruising," 302. Anderson's discussion of George Eliot also places her realism in the context of mechanical objectivity, as I do, but my interest is specifically in the visual structure of the realist ideal.

35. Logan, *Nerves and Narratives*, 170.

36. See especially Lewes's *Principles of Success in Literature*, a series of essays published in the *Fortnightly Review* in 1865.

37. Skilton, *Early and Mid-Victorian Novel*, 159. The *Westminster Review*, similarly, thought Trollope should "refrain from striking off more copies of an idea than the plate will bear." "Contemporary Literatures: Belles Lettres," 134.

38. The quotation appears in a letter Blackwood wrote to George Eliot (*Letters* II, 291 [30 January 1857]).

39. Stillé, *Elements of General Pathology*, 46 (emphasis in original).

40. Ibid., 36, 39, 42. Eliot, *Adam Bede*, 42.

41. Daston and Galison, *Objectivity*, 120.

42. This trope reappears at the end of the book, when Mr. Irwine realizes the enormity of Arthur's offense, and how very close he had come to disclosing it. He muses, "[I]t was cruel to think how thin a film had shut out rescue from all this guilt and misery. He saw the whole history now by that terrible illumination which the present sheds back upon the past" (407).

43. See Horton, 104, 121.

44. Crary contends that "[n]oninstrumental descriptions of the camera obscura are pervasive" during the nineteenth century, but George Eliot clearly turns to it as a means to an end: producing a humanist realism. Crary, *Techniques*, 33.

45. Helmholtz famously concludes his lecture, "[I]f an optician wanted to sell me an instrument which had all these defects [that are in the human eye], I should think myself quite justified in blaming his carelessness in the strongest terms, and giving him back his instrument." Helmholtz, "Recent Progress," 141; Helmholtz, *Description of Ophthalmoscope*, 8, 9.

46. Descartes had famously explained how to create a camera obscura using a human or bovine eye as the lens (Crary, *Techniques*, 47, quoting from *La Dioptrique* [1637]), and another seventeenth-century scholar, Kaspar Schott, revised the experiment (Hammond, *Camera*

Obscura? 31). Helmholtz, *Description of an Ophthalmoscope,* 8, 9; [Noble], review of Wilson. Interestingly, given George Eliot's defense of color blindness in 1857 in "Janet's Repentance" (265), the notice of Wilson's camera obscura book immediately followed the notice for his *Researches on Colour-Blindness.*

47. Hammond, *Camera Obscura,* 132, citing *Photographic News,* December 1859. Spiller credits Allan B. Dick as coauthor.

48. Ward, *Microscope Teachings,* 82, 85.

49. Crary offers a lengthy examination of this break. Isobel Armstrong associates it not only with the "collapse" of the "connection between veridical correspondence and the viewing subject as a privileged form of knowing," but also with the rise of a "consumer-observer, whose body became codified and fragmented into multiple areas of sensory experience as a consequence of the arbitrary relation between stimulus and sensation." Armstrong insists that critics account for "rival epistemologies of seeing" and "the uncomfortable interventions of mediation" ("Microscope," 34–35).

50. Crary points to "the texts of Marx, Bergson, Freud, and others," where "the very apparatus that a century earlier was the site of truth becomes a model for procedures and forces that conceal, invert, and mystify truth." See also Kofman on the deceptive nature of the camera obscura in Marx, Freud, Nietzsche, and Descartes; and Mitchell on the double meaning of the camera obscura. Crary, *Techniques,* 29, 32, 33; Kofman, *Camera Obscura of Ideology;* W. J. T. Mitchell, *Iconology,* 171, 178.

51. Bennett, *Clinical Lectures,* 69.

52. See Beer, *Darwin's Plots;* Shuttleworth, *George Eliot.* Jane Wood comments that "Bernard's work on pathology and physiology was a major influence on the ideas of G. H. Lewes, whose copy of *Leçons sur la physiologie et la pathologie du système nerveux* (1858) is extensively annotated" (*Passion and Pathology,* 93).

53. Bernard, *Experimental Medicine,* 148, 21–22.

54. See Daston and Galison, "Image of Objectivity," 98, and Crary, *Techniques,* 16–17. These reject the notion that the advent of photography hastened the development of a theory of mechanical observation. Rather, photography provided scientists with an important trope for figuring mechanical observation through a familiar and culturally authoritative reference.

55. The camera is simply a camera obscura with a photographic plate in place of the mirror. The *Magazine of Science* featured a camera obscura on the cover of its first issue, in 1839, noting Talbot's and Daguerre's "newly discovered invention of Photogenic Drawing," "which is the natural property of the camera obscura, made permanent." See Hammond, *Camera Obscura,* 128. While the camera does combine the observing and recording functions of the camera obscura, Bernard does not acknowledge that it still requires agency and intervention on the part of the operator.

56. Daston and Galison, examining scientific atlases, perceive a midcentury scientific optimism (like Stillé's or Bernard's) about the possibility of evicting subjectivity altogether. Flint, however, surveying scientists, writers, and artists more generally, concludes that "[o]bservation, however careful, is—and this came to be well recognized by Victorians—never removed from the exercise of subjectivity." Flint, *Visual Imagination,* 30.

57. My reading differs somewhat from that of Amanda Anderson, who also examines this conflux of ideas in George Eliot. Anderson discusses the close observation as one with what it produces, thus referring to "Eliot's ... sympathetic observation." She argues that "Eliot shows how the stance of detached analysis undermines the individual's moral character and responsiveness" (*Powers of Distance,* 12). I consider, instead, how Eliot's early work carefully separates the steps of observation, representation, and sympathy even as it argues that realism can *produce* sympathy. Clinical realist vision in *Middlemarch,* by contrast, does involve sympathy and imagination from the outset.

58. Ruskin, *The Stones of Venice*, II, 161; Ruskin, *Modern Painters*, IV.1.17. Mansell points out that George Eliot attempts to fix this problem by making her realism represent the (mediated) reflection of reality in the artist's mind, not reality directly. But while Mansell discusses art as a mirror, George Eliot figures the observer's mind as the mirror, and the artwork as a representation of it. Mansell, "Ruskin," 205.

59. Eliot, "Janet's Repentance," in *Scenes of Clerical Life*, 268.

60. Eliot, letter, 18 February 1857. See also a letter to William Blackwood (*Letters* [18 February 1857]) and to Sara Hennell (*Letters* III, 90 [24 June 1859]), and her essay "The Natural History of German Life" (*Westminster Review*, July 1856). An 1853 review in the *Spectator*, "My Novel," called for just such a conception of authorship. George Brimley describes a mirroring realism that, informed by the imagination of the poet, would call forth sympathy for the common worker: "Would such a work of art be possible? A mirror that should show to a nation of workers ... its own life ... as it might reflect itself upon the imagination of a great poet, who to masculine understanding trained by observation and study should add the large heart and the clear eye to which nothing human is uninteresting or blank?" Reprinted in Brimley, *Essays*, 286.

61. Ironically, the moments at which the narrator clearly solicits readerly sympathy often accompany not the glimpses of a "monotonous homely existence" valorized in chapter 17, but rather scenes perilously close to the extremities of "indigence" or "wretchedness," although perhaps not the "picturesque sentimental" variety the narrator excoriates (177, 178).

62. Eliot, *Letters* III, 110–11 (5 July 1859) (emphasis in original).

63. Daston, "Escape from Perspective," 603.

64. Ibid., 616.

65. Daston, "Moral Economy of Science," 20.

Chapter Five

1. George Eliot elsewhere similarly aligns polished surfaces with reflection and egoistic distortion: in *Adam Bede* the vain Hetty Sorel "often took the opportunity, when her aunt's back was turned, of looking at the pleasing reflection of herself in those polished surfaces, for the oak-table was usually turned up like a screen ... and she could see herself sometimes in the great round pewter dishes that were ranged on the shelves above the long deal dinner table, or in the hobs of the grate, which always shone like jasper." Like the more deliberate "mirror" scene in her bedroom, this passage signals the vanity and superficiality of character that will condemn Hetty. Eliot, *Adam Bede*, ed. Cunningham, 73.

2. Eliot, *Middlemarch*, 248 (bk. III, chap. 27). All further references to this novel will be given with book, chapter, and page number.

3. Other mirrors in the novel all suggest distorted vision, self-deception, and vanity: "'[Mr. Casaubon] thinks with me,' said Dorothea to herself, 'or rather, he thinks a whole world of which my thought is but a poor twopenny mirror'" (I.3.23); "This was not the first time that Mr. Bulstrode had begun by admonishing Mr. Vincy, and had ended by seeing a very unsatisfactory reflection of himself in the coarse unflattering mirror which that manufacturer's mind presented to the subtler lights and shadows of his fellow-men ..." (II.13.123); and, in reference to the townspeoples' low estimation of Casaubon, "I am not sure that the greatest man of his age, if ever that solitary superlative existed, could escape these unfavourable reflections of himself in various small mirrors; and even Milton, looking for his portrait in a spoon, must submit to have the facial angle of a bumpkin" (I.10.77–78).

4. Feltes, "Eliot's 'Pier-Glass.'"

5. Bernard, *Experimental Medicine*, 16.

NOTES TO CHAPTER FIVE

6. Crary, *Techniques*, 92 (emphasis in original). See also Müller, "'Subjective' Phenomena of Vision," in *Elements of Physiology*, 740–44.

7. Wormald, "Microscopy and Semiotic," 517. George Eliot writes at a watershed moment for microscopists, due to the work of Ernst Abbé on resolution and the development of aniline dyes. Although British instrument makers resisted Abbé's innovations, the aniline dyes alone allowed much better visualization of the object, making the microscope a much more powerful tool than previously. On Abbé, see Hacking, *Representing and Intervening*, 194.

8. MacCabe, "Realism and the Cinema," 39.

9. One of Abbé's improvements to the microscope in the 1870s was that he devised a way to increase the light collected in an objective, improving resolution without magnification.

10. Wormald, too, notes that "the narrator's own project of representation is compromised" in this passage and contrasts the narrator's skepticism with Lydgate's naïve enthusiasm (519).

11. Bennett, *Clinical Lectures*, 69; Laycock, *Lectures*, 74; Quekett, *Practical Treatise*, 208. The "specters" quotation is from Thomas Williams, "On the Pathology of Cells," *Guy's Hospital Reports* 1 (1843), 424; quoted in Reiser, *Reign of Technology*, 79.

12. Wormald points out that the rainbow of light surrounding Rosamond, in the "gossamer web" passage, represents "the symptoms of chromatic aberration" which flawed early microscope lenses. Pritchard notes that "the great and sensible dispersion, which envelopes every object seen through [ordinary compound microscopes] in a false prismatic halo, and utterly obliterates all its delicate markings and structure, renders this instrument almost useless for investigation." However, achromatic microscopes were available by the mid-1820s, when Lydgate would have been studying medicine. Wormald, "Microscopy and Semiotic," 523; Pritchard, *Microscopic Cabinet*, 105–6; Carpenter, *Microscope* (1901), 148–50. Interestingly, the problem of spherical aberration is caused by "the fact that you polish a lens by random rubbing" (producing a spherical surface)—the same process that renders the pier-glass an unreliable source of information about the world. Hacking, *Representing and Intervening*, 193.

13. Bennett, *Clinical Lectures*, 65. See also Reiser, *Reign of Technology*, 80.

14. Bernard valorized, as a necessary "mastery," this engagement with the flaws of the instrument. Shuttleworth argues for the shift from *Adam Bede* to *Daniel Deronda* as a shift from passive to active, and from natural history to experimental science. Shuttleworth, *George Eliot*, xii, 24–50, 175–200.

15. MacCabe, "Realism and the Cinema," 44, 43 (emphasis in original).

16. J. Hillis Miller perceives a "strict homogeneity" between different scales in *Middlemarch*, but the passage emphasizes the same dispersal of truths that Miller perceives elsewhere in the novel ("Optic and Semiotic," 69).

17. Beer, "'Authentic Tidings,'" 90–91.

18. Improvements to the instrument in the 1860s had made it possible to turn a turret with multiple objectives on it, which greatly facilitated the process George Eliot describes.

19. Carpenter, *Microscope* (1891), 62 (emphasis in original). Isobel Armstrong discusses the incommensurability of vision inside and outside the microscope. Hacking considers whether or not we even do "see . . . with a microscope." Armstrong, "Microscope," 31; Hacking, *Representing and Intervening*, 187.

20. MacCabe, "Realism and the Cinema," 49.

21. Lydgate had hoped to combine medical practice with intellectual inquiry "in the hope that the two purposes would illuminate each other: the careful observation and inference which was his daily work, the use of the lens to further his judgment in special cases, would further his thought as an instrument of larger inquiry" (100).

22. Lawrence Rothfield also notes that in *Middlemarch* "the medical perspective . . . is supplemented by other equally valid perspectives with other narrative possibilities" (*Vital Signs*, 89).

23. See Shuttleworth, *George Eliot*, 22–23, 145; Levine, "Hypothesis of Reality," 12; Mason, "*Middlemarch* and Science," 60.

24. For Lewes's defense of science, in *Problems of Life and Mind* (1874), as an "Ideal Construction," see Shuttleworth, *George Eliot*, 22–23; Levine, *Realistic Imagination*, 252–90; Levine, "Hypothesis of Reality," 11–14; Rylance, *Victorian Psychology*, 259–60. Shuttleworth also examines experimental science and physiology in *Middlemarch* (*George Eliot*, 143–74). Mason identifies the mid-1860s as the period when Lewes started to consider the scientific imagination. Logan examines Tyndall's 1870 "Scientific Use of the Imagination" in relation to *Middlemarch*. Beer discusses imagination in Darwin and *Middlemarch*. Flint examines the scientific imagination in Tyndall and Lewes. See also Yeo on the development of the scientific method in the nineteenth century. Mason, "*Middlemarch* and Science," 152, 60, 65; Logan, *Nerves and Narratives*, 181–82; Beer, *Darwin's Plots*, 141–42, 48–55, 49–80; Flint, *Visual Imagination*, 62–63, 113–15, 307–8; Yeo, "Scientific Method."

25. Bernard, *Experimental Medicine*, 24. In discussing experiment, Bernard moves away from the extreme automatism he requires of observation and offers a role for imagination. Shuttleworth points out that Lewes, too, "extending these premises, argues that the processes of fiction are indispensable to the Experimental Method, for science is 'Ideal Construction'" (*George Eliot*, 22–23). However, Bernard cautions that once the experiment is in train, "the experimenter must now disappear or rather change himself instantly into an observer" by setting his hypothesis aside lest it color his observations (22).

26. Lewes makes this explicit in his *Problems of Life and Mind*, explaining, "The grandest discoveries, and the grandest applications to practice ... have revealed by the telescope of Imagination what the microscope of Observation could never have seen" (315–17 [bk. I]).

27. This shift resembles what Peter Galison identifies as a "judgment against objectivity," where the product of mechanical observation is thought less reliable than the image interpreted through a holistic cognitive process that only an expert can perform. The "objectivity, facticity, and scientific management" of mechanical observation, that is, "yielded to a new world of sorting nature in which judgment, subjectivity, artisanal practice, and theory were heralded as vital to the scientific project of visual classification." However, he sees the "judgment against objectivity" as occurring much later, in the twentieth century; and the shift he observes does not center on speculation. Galison, "Judgment against Objectivity," 343.

28. Generally, American physicians were more vehement converts to empirical methods early in the century, and British physicians seem more accepting of speculation later. On the importation of empirical methods to America and the growing resistance to theory-based medicine, see Warner, *Spirit of System*, especially 239–45.

29. Stillé, *Elements of General Pathology*, 46 (emphasis in original)..

30. Review of Robertson, *The Nature and Treatment of Gout*, 20; Stillé, *Elements of General Pathology*, 31, 28–29 (emphasis in original).

31. Crampton, "Diseased Appearance," 301–2; Lawrence, *Lectures*, 34; Watson, *Lectures*. For Eliot's knowledge of Watson, see Eliot, *Quarry for Middlemarch*, I, 17; Kitchel, "Introduction," 40n66. Watson's phrase is repeated through at least the fourth (1857) edition. The "advertisement to the first edition" comments that the text derives, with almost no revision, from lecture notes first prepared in 1836–37; and the "advertisement to the fourth edition" suggests that no further revision has taken place since then; so that Watson's suspicion of speculation in 1857 is likely a holdover from an 1830s perspective.

32. Meryon, *History of Medicine*, 5; Carpenter, *Principles of Human Physiology* (1855), 736; Carpenter, *Principles of Human Physiology* (1876), 791. Carpenter's comment about speculation as a "stimulus" appears in earlier editions as well.

33. Laycock, *Lectures*, 34; Guy, *Forensic Medicine*, 205; Holland, *Medical Notes and Reflections*, 24, 25.

NOTES TO CHAPTER SIX

34. Brinton, "Alimentary Canal," 11.
35. Laycock, *Lectures*, 39; Russell, *History and Heroes*, 115. Although Russell had his degree from Edinburgh and a practice on Harley Street, his comments come in a sense from the margins, since he was an advocate of homeopathy.
36. Laycock, *Lectures*, 38; Holland, *Medical Notes and Reflections*, 26.
37. Quoted in "Minutes of the Twenty-third Annual Session," 556.
38. Huxley, "Progress of Science," 64–65.
39. Bramwell, *Practical Medicine*, 8 (emphasis in original).
40. Bramwell, "Minute Observation," 238, 240, 243.
41. Bramwell, *Practical Medicine*, 43. Bramwell in this last passage quotes Gairdner, "Physiognomy of Disease," 8.
42. See Yeo, "Scientific Method," 269.
43. Lewes, *Problems*, I, 289. Lewes started writing this text in the late 1860s (although it was not published until 1874). See Levine, "Hypothesis," and Flint, *Visual Imagination*.
44. Isobel Armstrong has discussed a similar phenomenon, deriving from a very different kind of visuality, the "optical illusions available in street and pleasure garden" that may "suggest experiments with different subject positions, control, displacement, obliteration, power, centrality, powerlessness" ("Transparency," 143). Unlike George Eliot's imagined speculative shifts (and like the magic lantern Mr. Irwine suggests to Arthur in *Adam Bede*), however, these instruments embrace the "pleasure of deception."
45. Isobel Armstrong examines how glass allows the gaze to both move through it and be arrested by how "one's body can be, glancingly, inadvertently, and in discontinuous fragments, reflected back from the environment," although she is focusing here on plate glass in the spectacular urban environment (*Victorian Glassworlds*, 99).
46. Hogg, *Microscope*, 75–76 (emphasis in original).
47. James, "Preface," 84.
48. Beer, *Open Fields*, 164.

Chapter Six

1. Marcus, "Freud and Dora," 65.
2. Frankland, *Freud's Literary Culture*, 203.
3. Freud, *History*, 3.
4. A shortened version of Marcus, "Freud and Dora," appears in Bernheimer and Kahane, *In Dora's Case*. Classic discussions also appear in Mahony, *Freud's Dora*; Jacobus, *Reading Woman*; Showalter, *Hystories*; Moi, "Representation of Patriarchy"; Hertz, "Dora's Secrets, Freud's Techniques." *Dora* achieved canonical status not only due to its rich suggestiveness as a text, but also because it punctuates important developments in Freud's thought. It follows Freud's theories of hysteria and of dreams and coincided with his theories of sexuality, all major elements of his work, readily popularized into the cultural imaginary. *Dora* also dramatizes the crucial psychoanalytic principle of resistance, as only a "failed" case history can (Dora breaks off her analysis); and it forced Freud to take account of transference, another crucial element of psychoanalytic theory.
5. Breuer and Freud, *Studies on Hysteria*, xxxi. The "true" origin of psychoanalysis is disputed. See Strachey, "Editor's Introduction," 57. Breuer commented that the patient Anna O. herself had pioneered the "talking cure" (29–30). For a feminist argument promoting Anna O.'s contribution, see Hunter, "Hysteria, Psychoanalysis, and Feminism."
6. Wood, *Passion and Pathology*, 107.
7. Gilman, *Freud, Race, and Gender*, 115.

8. Winter, *Freud*, 132–41, 149–52. She also discusses Freud's efforts to distinguish psychoanalysis from the two most relevant medical fields, psychiatry and neurology.

9. Winter, *Freud*, 123.

10. Freud, "Aetiology," 220.

11. As chapter 5 noted, the validity of microscopic findings was debated due to many variables: the unreliable performance of the human eye, the flawed technology, the need for a skilled operator, the variability of reports even from reliable microscopists, and the changing standardization of the instrument itself. See Reiser, *Reign of Technology*; Schickore, *Microscope and Eye*.

12. Freud, *Dora*, 5. All further references to this text will be to this edition.

13. Holland, *Medical Notes and Reflections*, 20.

14. Freud had been trained in the mechanistic model of empirical science influenced by Hermann von Helmholtz, together with its strictures against speculative insight. See Frankland, *Freud's Literary Culture*, 35. Valerie Greenberg argues that "[p]hysics [rather than biology] becomes ... the ultimate provider of legitimacy for the new science: physics lends psychoanalysis its prestige." However, medicine was the community where Freud had to gain acceptance. Greenberg, "Freud and Physics," 246.

15. Breuer and Freud, *Studies on Hysteria*, 166.

16. Breuer and Freud, *Studies on Hysteria*, 135.

17. Freud, "Aetiology of Hysteria," 220.

18. Freud, *Dora*, 18.

19. Stern, *Zeitschrift für Psychologie und Physiologie der Sinnesorgane*, XXVI (1901), 133; and "Professor" Liepmann [Jones does not further identify the author], *Monatschrift für Psychiatrie und Neurologie*, 1901, 237; cited in Ernest Jones, *Sigmund Freud*, 361.

20. Webster, *Freud Was Wrong*, 257.

21. Bullough, *Science in the Bedroom*, 91.

22. Marcus, "Freud and Dora," 83.

23. Reidel-Schrewe, "Freud's Début," 8.

24. Breuer and Freud, *Studies on Hysteria*, 144.

25. Literary texts Freud discusses include Schreber's memoir, Dostoevsky, Empedocles' poems, Hebbel's *Judith*, Jensen's *Gradiva*, and Hoffmann's *The Sandman*. For Connolly's cases in *An Inquiry Concerning the Indications of Insanity* (1830), or psychiatrists' readings of *Hamlet* at midcentury, see Small, *Love's Madness*, 48–57.

26. Breuer and Freud, *Studies on Hysteria*, 265.

27. "Professor Freud and Hysteria," 103.

28. Breuer and Freud, *Studies on Hysteria*, 49.

29. See footnote to the case of Fräulein Elisabeth von R. (*Studies on Hysteria*, 169–70).

30. Breuer and Freud, *Studies on Hysteria*, 25–26.

31. "Curious," *Oxford English Dictionary*.

32. Freud, "Aetiology of Hysteria," 199.

33. "Professor Freud and Hysteria," 103–4.

34. Jameson, *Political Unconscious*, 106–7.

35. Critics who have focused on the centrality of reading, writing, and translation to his work include Bernheimer, "Introduction, Part 1," 10–11; Gallop, "Keys to Dora"; Ramas, "Freud's Dora, Dora's Hysteria," 149; van den Berg, "Reading Dora Reading"; Gilman, "Preface"; Kofman, *Freud and Fiction;* Mahony, *Freud as a Writer;* Marcus, "Freud and Dora"; Rieff, "Introduction," ix. Reidel-Schrewe, "Freud's Début in the Sciences," 1–2, 2–15. Frankland offers an extensive discussion in *Freud's Literary Culture*.

36. Mahony, *Freud as a Writer*, 9–12.

37. Frankland examines how Freud's methodology is grounded in literary work, especially

in *Interpretation of Dreams* (117–61). He discusses free association, condensation, and displacement, for example, and compares elements of analysis to styles of literary criticism. I focus here on the earliest elements of psychoanalysis and on the dialogic figuration and interpretation that is central to it. I agree with Frankland that "literary criticism is ... the mother of psychoanalysis, vitally procreative and yet taboo" (117).

38. Breuer and Freud, *Studies on Hysteria*, 280.

39. Although Freud discusses the limits of the "cathartic method" in *Studies on Hysteria*, he uses a version of it in most of his full-length case histories (261).

40. Freud, *Complete Letters*, 212. Quoted in Showalter, *Hystories*, 40.

41. See Mahony, *Freud as a Writer*, 23, 241, for example.

42. Breuer and Freud, *Studies on Hysteria*, 290; Freud, "Aetiology of Hysteria," 205.

43. Freud, *Dora*, 34–35. This involvement of the body differentiates hysteria from other neuroses (*Dora*, 35). Occasionally the hysteric's symptoms do indicate "merely" a physical problem (*Dora*, 10).

44. Freud, *Dora*, 76.

45. Ironically, Freud uses nonorganic objects—sand, wire—rather than organic ones—seed, skeleton—to represent organic (bodily) injury.

46. Freud, *Dora*, 46. The word "simultaneously" is in italics in the English version but not stressed in the original German. Freud, "Bruchstück Einer Hysterie-Analyse."

47. The "clues" can be nonphysical: Frau Cäcilie also suffers from hallucinations, "the explanation of which often called for much ingenuity." The vision of Freud and Breuer hanging from two trees in the garden follows a disagreement with her doctors; she had decided that "'[t]here's nothing to choose between the two of them; one's the *pendant* [match] of the other'" (181). This tenuous association, offered in a footnote, provides Freud's very last word in the case of "Frau Elisabeth von R."

48. Symonds, *Letters*, 821.

49. Frau Cäcilie M., in *Studies on Hysteria*, 180.

50. Freud's anxious eagerness to disavow the roman à clef recalls the efforts of eighteenth-century authors who "stressed their renunciation of personal satire and slander." However, unlike Freud, they reference the roman à clef in order to claim fictionality rather than factuality: "the explicit fictionality of their works initially recommended them as wholesome goods." Gallagher, *Nobody's Story*, xvii.

51. Freud differs from his predecessors in the eighteenth century in that his sly promise of "intimacies" attempts to deny the vulgar gaze of the crowd, while inviting select readers to consider and share his privileged view.

52. Beer, *Open Fields*, 156. See also 181–82.

53. See Frankland, *Freud's Literary Culture*.

54. Auerbach, "Magi and Maidens," 297–98.

55. Katz provides an extended discussion of "The Politics of Romance" (*Rider Haggard*).

56. Likewise, in the sentence describing the "quota of affect" cited earlier, Freud offers a mathematical model—"If we ... try to represent the ideational mechanism in a kind of algebraical picture"—but never follows through with a picture or equation.

57. Frye, *Anatomy of Criticism*, 193, 195.

58. Frankland also discusses Freud's self-positioning as hero, but he focuses on Freud's interest in the "classical hero" or in a specific literary hero like Faust (10, 206–7).

59. Frankland, *Freud's Literary Culture*, 32; Richard Armstrong, *Compulsion for Antiquity*, 114–20; Rudnytsky, "Freud's Pompeiian Fantasy," 228.

60. Freud, *Interpretation of Dreams*, 490 (emphasis in original).

61. Freud, "Aetiology of Hysteria," 192.

62. See, for example, Levine's comments on Bacon (*Dying to Know*, 22).

63. Freud, "History of Psycho-Analytic Movement," 23.
64. Breuer and Freud, *Studies on Hysteria*, 128, 139.
65. Hake, "Saxa Loquuntur," 148.
66. Freud's describing the antiquities as "priceless though mutilated" recalls Frye's comment that "[m]utilation . . . is often the price of unusual . . . power" in romance (193).
67. Galison, "Judgment against Objectivity."
68. Freud, "Bruchstück Einer Hysterie-Analyse," 18.
69. Stanley followed the Congo from Lake Tanganyika to the Atlantic Ocean, proving that the Congo, not the Nile, originates at the lake. He also identified the source of the Nile, by circumnavigating Lake Victoria rather than traveling up the river to its origin. Soon after, Stanley was hired by Belgium's King Leopold II to advise his notorious colonial projects in the Congo.
70. See Freud, *Dora*, 44, 46, 110.
71. Stanley's *Through the Dark Continent* was first published in London in 1878. The text included a foldout map of his journeys. Freud was certainly aware of Stanley's journeys, whether in English or German. There were at least sixteen books by or about Stanley's explorations published in German in the late nineteenth century, including two editions of *Durch den dunkeln Weltheil* in 1878 and 1881.
72. Laycock, *Lectures*, 65.
73. Frankland notes a possible allusion to Faust here (*Freud's Literary Culture*, 207). Freud persistently codes the hysteric as "other" despite symptoms of hysteria in his own narrative.
74. In 1906 Freud listed, as one of "ten good books," Kipling's *Jungle Book*. He had recommended other Kipling stories to Fliess. See Gay, *Reading Freud*, 98, 104. Richard Armstrong also briefly discusses Freud as an imperialist (*Compulsion for Antiquity*, 121–26).
75. The fifteen-month rush of composition (January 1885 to March 1886) that produced *King Solomon's Mines, Allan Quatermain, Jess*, and *She* occurred only four years after his disgruntled departure from Africa, feeling "betrayed" by "Gladstone's treachery" in ceding British rule of the Transvaal. Katz, *Rider Haggard*, 11; Monsman, *Rider Haggard*, 37–40.
76. Horace G. Hutchinson, "Sir Rider Haggard's Autobiography," rev. of *The Days of My Life. Edinburgh Review*, 244 [October 1926]), 344; quoted in Katz, *Rider Haggard*, 1.
77. Winter, *Freud*, 210.
78. Bruce Mazlish also reads Freud alongside Haggard. He notes their shared interest in "the buried past," "the eternal feminine," Darwinian race theory, and "the Dark Continent of the mind," although he identifies Haggard as "embracing" the unconscious, while Freud seeks to master it ("Triptych," 741–43).
79. Stiebel, *Imagining Africa*, viii.
80. Haggard, *She*, 195, 199.
81. Unlike Bruce Mazlish, I place this as a convention of romance, not a nod to realism in Haggard's text. Mazlish, "Triptych," 732.
82. Graham Dawson, *Soldier Heroes*, 59.
83. Freud, *Autobiography*, 153.
84. Winter also examines Freud's "mixed results" in the scientific and the cultural realms (207).

Conclusion

1. Aiken and Barbauld, "Evenings," 138–39, 143.

Works Cited

Primary Texts

[Hamley, E. B.]. "The Life and Letters of George Eliot." Review of *George Eliot's Life, as Related in Her Letters and Journals*. *Blackwood's Edinburgh Magazine* 137, no. 832 (1885): 155–76.

[Lankester, Edwin]. Review of *Atlas of Human Anatomy and Physiology*, by William Fermer. *Athenaeum* 1585 (1858): 36.

———. Review of *The Climate of Pau*, by Alexander Taylor. *Athenaeum*, no. 1514 (1856): 1337.

———. Review of *The Immediate Cause and the Specific Treatment of Pulmonary Phthisis and Tuberculous Diseases*, by J. Francis Churchill. *Athenaeum* 1588 (1858): 434.

———. Review of *The Microscope*, by John Ferguson. *Athenaeum* 1606 (1858): 168.

———. Review of *Observations on the Life, Disease, and Death of John Hunter*, by Joseph Ridge. *Athenaeum* 1474 (1856): 105.

———. Review of *On Epidemic Diarrhea and Cholera*, by George Johnson. *Athenaeum* 1474 (1856): 105.

———. Review of *On Some of the More Obscure Forms of Nervous Affections*, by Henry W. Lobb. *Athenaeum* 1632 (1859): 192.

———. Review of *On the Hygienic Management of Infants and Children*, by T. Herbert Barker. *Athenaeum* 1656 (1859): 119.

———. Review of *Outlines of Physiology*, by John Hughes Bennett. *Athenaeum* 1656 (1859): 118.

———. Review of *The Physiology of the Senses*, by A. B. Johnson. *Athenaeum* 1514 (1856): 1337.

———. Review of *Stray Leaves of a Naturalist*, by David Ross. *Athenaeum* 1670 (1859): 564.

———. Review of *Suggestions in Reference to the Means of Advancing Medical Science*, by Francis Ramsbotham. *Athenaeum* 1551 (1857): 910.

———. Review of *Torquay in Its Medical Aspect*, by C. Radcliffe Hall. *Athenaeum* 1553 (1857): 973.

[Noble, Daniel]. Review of *Mesmerism in Its Relation to Health and Disease*, by William Neilson. *Athenaeum* 1483 (1856): 394.

———. Review of *On the Extent to Which the Received Theory of Vision Requires, as to Regard the Eye as a Camera Obscura*, by George Wilson. *Athenaeum* 1476 (1856): 171.

[St. John, Horace Stebbing]. "An Account of the Life, Lectures and Writings of William Cullen, M.D." *Athenaeum* (1859): 498.

[Stephen, Fitzjames]. "Sentimentalism." *Cornhill Magazine* 10 (1864): 65–75.

[Thompson, Henry]. "Under Chloroform." *Cornhill Magazine* 1 (1860): 499–504.

"Advertisement Concerning the Transfusion of Bloud, An." *Philosophical Transactions* 2, no. 27 (1667): 489–90.

"Literary Tastes and Habits of the Irish." *Dublin Medical Press* 15 (1846): 413–14.

"London Curiosity of Medical Literature, A." *Dublin Medical Press* 16, no. 396 (1846): 95.

"Of the Posture Master, or a Man Having an Absolute Command of His Joints and Muscles." *Philosophical Transactions* 20, no. 242 (1698): 262.

"Part of a Letter to Dr Sloane, Wherein. Is an Account of a Double Pear." *Philosophical Transactions* 22 (1700): 470.

"Professor Freud and Hysteria." *British Medical Journal* (11 January 1908): 103–4.

"Relation Written to the Editor from a Person of Great Veracity in Germany, Concerning an Aged Woman of 60 Years, Giving Suck to Her Grandchild, A." *Philosophical Transactions* 9, no. 105 (1674): 100–101.

Review of *Can You Forgive Her?* by Anthony Trollope. *Westminster Review* (1865): 284–85.

Review of *The Medical and Legal Relations of Madness*, by Joshua Burgess. *Athenaeum* (1859): 192.

Review of *The Nature and Treatment of Gout*, by William Henry Robertson (London, 1845). *Dublin Medical Press* 16, no. 392 (1846): 20–21.

Aiken, [John] and [Anna Letitia] Barbauld. *Evenings at Home; or, The Juvenile Budget Opened.* Rev. ed. New York: Harper and Brothers, 1868.

Anstie, Francis Edmund. "Corpulence." *Cornhill Magazine* 7 (1863): 457–68.

———. "Medical Etiquette." *Cornhill Magazine* 8 (1863): 154–63.

———. "On Physical Pain." *Macmillan's Magazine* 8 (1863): 457–63.

Arnold, Matthew. "Literature and Science." In *The Complete Prose Works of Matthew Arnold*, ed. R. H. Super. Ann Arbor: University of Michigan Press, 1974.

Babbage, Charles. *Reflections on the Decline of Science in England, and on Some of its Causes.* London: B. Fellowes, 1830.

Baker, Henry, Benjamin Boddington, William Notcutt, and William Hammond. "Account of Margaret Cutting, a Young Woman, Now Living at Wickham Market in Suffolk, Who Speaks Readily and Intelligibly, Though She Has Lost Her Tongue." *Philosophical Transactions* 42, no. 464 (1742): 143–52.

———. "Supplement to the Account of a Distempered Skin, Published in the 42th Number of the Philosophical Transactions." *Philosophical Transactions* 49 (1755): 21–24.

Barnes, Thomas. *Account of William Dempster, Who Swallowed a Table-Knife Nine Inches Long with a Notice of a Similar Case in a Prussian Knife-Eater.* Edinburgh: A. Constable, 1824.

Bennett, John Hughes. *Clinical Lectures on the Principles and Practice of Medicine.* New York: Samuel and William Wood, 1860.

Bernard, Claude. *An Introduction to the Study of Experimental Medicine.* New York: Schuman, 1947.

Bernheimer, Charles. "Introduction, Part 1." In *In Dora's Case: Freud—Hysteria—Feminism,*

ed. Charles Bernheimer and Claire Kahane, 1–18. New York: Columbia University Press, 1990.
Bernheimer, Charles, and Claire Kahane, eds. *In Dora's Case: Freud—Hysteria—Feminism.* 2d ed. New York: Columbia University Press, 1990.
Bigelow, Jacob, and Oliver Wendell Holmes. "Medical Observation." In *Principles of the Theory and Practice of Medicine,* 3–20. Boston: C. C. Little and J. Brown, 1839.
Blanc, Henry. "On the Cold-Water and Antiseptic Treatment of Typhoid Fever." *Lancet* 1 (6 February 1875): 190–91.
Bramwell, Byrom. "Case Illustrative of the Diagnostic Value of the Sphygmograph." *Studies in Clinical Medicine* I (1890): 115–19.
———. "Case of So-Called Perforating Tumour of the Skull." *Studies in Clinical Medicine* I, no. 15 (1890): 249–52.
———. *Practical Medicine and Medical Diagnosis.* Edinburgh: Pentland, 1887.
———. "Remarkable Case of Euphoria." *Studies in Clinical Medicine* I, no. 3 (1889): 57–58.
———. "Stricture of the Oesophagus, the Result of Swallowing Caustic Soda; Diseased Conditions Resembling Acute Irritant Poisoning." *Studies in Clinical Medicine* I, no. 11 (1890): 195–200.
———. "The Value of Cultivating the Habit of Minute Observation...." In *Studies in Clinical Medicine,* 235–46. Edinburgh and London: Pentland, 1890.
Breuer, Josef, and Sigmund Freud. *Studies on Hysteria.* Trans. James Strachey. Ed. James Strachey. 23 vols. Vol. 2 (1893–1895). New York: Basic Books, 1955.
Brimley, George. *Essays.* Ed. William George Clark. Cambridge: Macmillan, 1858.
Brinton, William. "Contributions to the Physiology of the Alimentary Canal: Part II.B., on the Physiology of Intestinal Obstructions." *London Medical Gazette,* n.s., 9 (1849): 9–13.
Buchan, William. *Domestic Medicine.* London: A. Strahan, 1800.
Bullitt, H. M. "The Art of Observing, or the Proper Method of Examining Patients, with a View to Correct Diagnosis." *Western Lancet* 3, no. 3 (1845): 397–409.
Byrd, William. "An Account of a Negro-Boy That Is Dappel'd in Several Places of His Body with White Spots." *Philosophical Transactions* 19 (1697): 781–82.
C, Mr. "Two Letters from a Gentleman in the Country...." *Philosophical Transactions* 23 (1702–1703): 1494–1501.
Carpenter, William B. *The Microscope and Its Revelations.* 7th ed. Ed. W. H. Dallinger. Philadelphia: P. Blakiston, Son, 1891.
———. *The Microscope and Its Revelations.* 8th ed. Philadelphia: P. Blakiston's Son, 1901.
———. *Principles of Human Physiology. With Their Chief Applications to Pathology, Hygiène, and Forensic Medicine.* London: John Churchill, 1846.
———. *Principles of Human Physiology. With Their Chief Applications to Pathology, Hygiène, and Forensic Medicine.* 4th Am. ed. Philadelphia: Lea & Blanchard, 1850.
———. *Principles of Human Physiology. With Their Chief Applications to Psychology, Pathology, Therapeutics, Hygiène, and Forensic Medicine.* 5th ed. London: John Churchill, 1855.
———. *Principles of Human Physiology and Forensic Medicine, with their Chief Applications to Psychology, Therapeutics, Hygienes, and Forensic Medicine.* Ed. Francis Gurney Smith. Philadelphia: Henry C. Lea, 1868.
———. *Principles of Human Physiology.* Ed. Francis G. Smith and Henry Power. Philadelphia: Henry C. Lea, 1876.
Cheever, David W. "The Value and the Fallacy of Statistics in the Observation of Disease." *Boston Medical and Surgical Journal* 63, no. 23 (1861): 449–56.
Chesselden, William. "An Account of Some Observations Made by a Young Gentleman, Who Was Born Blind, or Lost His Sight So Early, That He Had No Remembrance of Ever

Having Seen, and Was Couched between 13 and 14 Years of Age." *Philosophical Transactions* 35, no. 402 (1728): 447–50.

———. "An Explication of the Instruments Used, in a New Operation on the Eyes." *Philosophical Transactions* 35, no. 402 (1728): 451–52.

Cheyne, George. *The English Malady*. London and New York: Tavistock/Routledge, 1976.

———. *An Essay of Health and Long Life*. London: Strahan and Leake, 1724.

Clanny, William Reid. *A Faithful Record of the Miraculous Case of Mary Jobson*. 2d ed. Newcastle-upon-Tyne: M. A. Richardson, 1841.

Colvin, Sidney. Review of *Middlemarch*. *Fortnightly Review* 13 (1873): 142–47.

Conny, Rob. "A Letter from Dr. Rob. Conny ... Concerning a Shower of Fishes." *Philosophical Transactions* 20 (1698): 289–90.

"Contemporary Literature: Belles Lettres." *Westminster Review* 115 (July 1865): 133–44.

Cooley, W. Desborough. "The Mystery of Inverted Vision." *Athenaeum* 1525 (1857).

Cowley, Abraham. "To the Royal Society." In Thomas Sprat, *The History of the Royal Society of London*, n.pag. London: J. Martyn and J. Allestry, 1667.

Crampton, John. "Account of a Diseased Appearance in the Intestines of Children." In *Dublin Hospital Reports and Communications in Medicine and Surgery*, 286–302. Dublin: Hodges and M'Arthur, 1818.

Daval, Peter. "A Description of an Extraordinary Rainbow Observed July 15, 1748." *Philosophical Transactions* 46 (1749): 193–95.

Denis, [J.]. "An Extract of a Letter of M. Denis ... to M.*** Touching the Transfusion of Blood." *Philosophical Transactions* 2 (1667): 453.

———. "Extract of a Letter Written by J. Denis ... Touching a Late Cure of an Inveterate Phrensy by the Transfusion of Blood." *Philosophical Transactions* 2, no. 32 (1667): 617–23.

———. "An Extract of a Printed Letter, Addressed to the Publisher, by M. Jean Denis ... Touching the Differences Risen about the Transfusion of Bloud." *Philosophical Transactions* 2, no. 36 (1668): 710–15.

Dent, Thomas. "A Letter from the Reverend Mr. Thomas Dent ... Concerning a Sort of Worms Found in the Tongue, and Other Parts of the Body, Etc." *Philosophical Transactions* 18 (1694): 219–21.

Dickens, Charles. *Bleak House*. New York: Signet, 1964.

———. *Dombey and Son*. Oxford: Oxford University Press, 1999.

———. *The Letters of Charles Dickens*. Ed. Madeline House, Graham Storey, and Kathleen Tillottson. 11 vols. Vol. 2. Oxford: Clarendon, 1969.

———. *The Old Curiosity Shop*. Oxford: Oxford University Press, 1999.

———. *Speeches of Charles Dickens*. Ed. K. J. Fielding. Oxford: Oxford University Press, 1960.

Disraeli, Benjamin. *Sybil*. Oxford: Oxford University Press, 1998.

Eliot, George. *Adam Bede*. Ed. Gordon S. Haight. New York: Holt, Rinehart, and Winston, 1965.

———. *Adam Bede*. Ed. Valentine Cunningham. New York: Oxford University Press, 1996.

———. *The George Eliot Letters*. Ed. Gordon S. Haight. 9 vols. New Haven, CT: Yale University Press, 1954–78.

———. *The Lifted Veil. Brother Jacob*. Ed. Sally Shuttleworth. New York: Penguin, 2001.

———. *Middlemarch*. Oxford: Oxford University Press, 1997.

———. *Quarry for Middlemarch*. Ed. Anna Theresa Kitchel. Supplement to *Nineteenth-Century Fiction* IV (1950). Berkeley: University California Press, 1950.

———. Review of John Ruskin, *Modern Painters*, Vol. III. *Westminster Review* 65 (1856).

———. *Scenes of Clerical Life*. Ed. Jennifer Gribble. New York: Penguin, 1998.

Elliotson, John, Nathaniel Rogers, Alexander Cooper Lee, and Thomas Stewardson. *The Principles and Practice of Medicine.* 1st Am. ed. Philadelphia: Carey and Hart, 1844.
Epstein, Julia. *Altered Conditions: Disease, Medicine, and Storytelling.* New York: Routledge, 1995.
Feltes, N. N. "George Eliot's 'Pier-Glass': The Development of a Metaphor." *Modern Philology* 67 (1969): 69–71.
Ferriar, John. *Medical Histories and Reflections.* Warrington: T. Cadell, 1792.
———. *Medical Histories and Reflections.* London: Cadelle and Davies, 1795.
———. *Medical Histories and Reflections.* London: Cadell and Davies, 1810.
Finlayson, James. "Examination and Reporting of Medical Cases." In *Clinical Manual for the Study of Medical Cases,* ed. James Finlayson, 33–49. London: Smith, Elder, 1878.
Forbes, Edward. *An Inaugural Lecture on Botany, Considered as a Science, and as a Branch of Medical Education.* London: John Van Voorst, [1843].
Freud, Sigmund. "The Aetiology of Hysteria." In *The Standard Edition of the Complete Psychological Works of Sigmund Freud,* ed. James Strachey, 190–221. London: Hogarth Press, 1962.
———. *Autobiography.* Trans. James Strachey. New York: W. W. Norton, 1935.
———. "Bruchstück Einer Hysterie-Analyse." In *Sammlung Kleiner Schriften Zur Neurosenlehre Aus Den Jahren 1893–1906,* 1–110. Leipzig: Franz Deuticke, 1921.
———. *Complete Letters of Sigmund Freud to Wilhelm Fliess, 1887–1904.* Ed. Jeffrey Moussaif Masson. Cambridge, MA: Harvard University Press, 1985.
———. *Dora: An Analysis of a Case of Hysteria.* New York: Collier Books, 1963.
———. *The Interpretation of Dreams.* Trans. and ed. James Strachey. New York: Avon, 1965.
———. *On the History of the Psycho-Analytic Movement.* From *The Standard Edition of the Complete Psychological Works of Sigmund Freud,* ed. James Strachey. New York: Norton, 1990.
Gairdner, W. T. "On the Physiognomy of Disease." In *Clinical Manual for the Study of Medical Cases,* ed. James Finlayson, 1–32. London: Smith, Elder, 1878.
Gaskell, Elizabeth. *Ruth.* New York: Penguin, 1997.
Gould, George M., and Walter M. Pyle. *Anomalies and Curiosities of Medicine; Being an Encyclopedic Collection of Rare and Extraordinary Cases....* Philadelphia: W. B. Saunders, 1897.
Greenhow, H. M. "Case of Concussion of the Brain, with Displacement of the Vertebrae." *Lancet* II (1850): 392.
Guy, William A. *Principles of Forensic Medicine.* 2d ed. London: Henry Renshaw, 1861.
Haggard, H. Rider. *She.* In *Three Adventure Novels: She, King Solomon's Mines, Allan Quatermain,* 2–238. New York: Dover, 1951.
Hardy, Thomas. *Under the Greenwood Tree.* Oxford: Oxford University Press, 1999.
Hartshorne, Henry. *Essentials of the Principles and Practice of Medicine: A Handy-Book for Students and Practitioners.* Philadelphia: Henry C. Lea, 1867.
Helmholtz, [Hermann] von. *The Description of an Ophthalmoscope [Beschreibung Eines Augenspiegels].* Trans. Thomas Hall Shastid. Chicago: Cleveland Press, 1916.
———. "The Recent Progress of the Theory of Vision." In *Science and Culture: Popular and Philosophical Essays,* 127–203. Chicago: University of Chicago Press, 1995.
Herschel, John Frederick William. *Preliminary Discourse on the Study of Natural Philosophy.* London: Longman, Rees, Orme, Brown, & Green, 1840.
Hills, Alfred K. *Instructions to Patients for Communicating with Physicians.* New York: Henry M. Smith, [1870].
Hogg, Jabez. *The Microscope: Its History, Construction, and Application.* 7th ed. London: Routledge and Sons, 1869.
Holland, Henry. *Chapters on Mental Physiology.* London: Longman, Brown, Green, and Longmans, 1852.

———. *Medical Notes and Reflections.* Philadelphia: Blanchard and Lea, 1857.
Hope, J[ames]. *A Treatise of the Diseases of the Heart and Great Vessels.* 3d ed. London: John Churchill, 1839.
Hume, David. *A Treatise of Human Nature.* Ed. David Fate Norton and Mary J. Norton. Oxford: Clarendon, 2007.
———. *Enquiries Concerning the Human Understanding and Concerning the Principles of Morals.* 2d. ed. Eds. Lewis A. Selby-Bigge and P. H. Nidditch. Oxford: Oxford University Press, 1978.
Huxley, Thomas Henry. "The Progress of Science." In *Method and Result: Essays,* 42–87. New York: D. Appleton, 1898.
———. "Science and Culture." In *Science and Education,* 134–59. New York: D. Appleton, 1896.
Isham, Asa B., and M. H. Keyt. "Editors' Preface." In *Sphygmography and Cardiography, Physiological and Clinical,* ed. Alonzo T. Keyt, iii. New York and London: G. P. Putnam's Sons, 1887.
James, Henry. *The Art of the Novel: Critical Prefaces.* New York: Scribner's Sons, 1934.
Kneeland, Samuel, Jr. "On the Contagiousness of Puerperal Fever." *American Journal of Medical Sciences* 11 (January 1846): 45–63.
Latham, Peter Mere. *The Collected Works of Dr. P.M. Latham.* Ed. Robert Martin. 2 vols. Vol. II. London: New Sydenham Society, 1878.
Lawrence, William. *Lectures on Physiology, Zoology, and the Natural History of Man.* Salem: Foote and Brown, 1828.
Laycock, Thomas. *Lectures on the Principles and Methods of Medical Observation and Research, for the Use of Advanced Students and Junior Practitioners.* Philadelphia: Blanchard and Lea, 1857.
Lee, Robert. "On Puerperal Fever and Crural Phlebitis." In *The History, Pathology, and Treatment of Puerperal Fever and Crural Phlebitis,* ed. Charles D. Meigs, 221–335. Philadelphia: Barrington & Haswell, 1842.
Lewes, George Henry. *Principles of Success in Literature.* Boston: Allyn and Bacon, 1891.
———. *Problems of Life and Mind.* 2 vols. London: Trübner, 1874.
Locke, John. *An Essay Concerning Human Understanding.* Ed. Kenneth P. Winkler. Abridged ed. Indianapolis, IN: Hackett, 1996.
Machin, John. "An Extract from the Minutes of the Royal Society, March 16, 1731, Containing an Uncommon Case of a Distempered Skin." *Philosophical Transactions* 37 (1731): 299–301.
MacKenzie, Colin. *MacKenzie's Ten Thousand Receipts in All the Useful and Domestic Arts.* Philadelphia: T. Ellwood Zell, 1867.
MacLaren, Archibald. "Management of the Nursery (Part I)." *Macmillan's Magazine* 5 (1862): 514–23.
Macmillan, Hugh. "Human Vegetation." *Macmillan's Magazine* 6 (1862): 459–67.
Mandeville, Bernard. *Treatise of the Hypochondriack and Hysterick Diseases.* 2d ed. Delmar, NY: Scholars' Facsimiles and Reprints, 1976.
Manginot, Francis. "Account of an Unusual Medical Case." *Philosophical Transactions* 22, no. 268 (1700–1701): 756–58.
Meryon, Edward. *The History of Medicine, Comprising a Narrative of Its Progress from the Earliest Ages to the Present Time and of the Delusions Incidental to Its Advance from Empiricism to the Dignity of a Science.* Vol. I. London: Longman, Green, Longman, and Roberts, 1861.
Millingen, J. G. *Curiosities of Medical Experience.* Philadelphia: Haswell, Barrington, and Haswell, 1838.
"Minutes of the Twenty-third Annual Session of the Medical Society of the State of Pennsylvania." *Medical and Surgical Reporter* 26 (22 June 1872): 555–63.

Molineux, Dr. "Dr. Molineux's Historical Account of the Late General Coughs and Colds; with Some Observations on Other Epidemick Distempers." *Philosophical Transactions* 18 (1694): 105–11.

Monro, John, M.D. "Remarks on Dr. Battie's Treatise on Madness." In *A Treatise on Madness, by William Battie, M.D., and Remarks on Dr. Battie's Treatise on Madness, by John Monro, M.D.: A Psychiatric Controversy of the Eighteenth Century*, ed. Richard Hunter and Ida Macalpine, 1–23. London: Dawsons, 1962.

Morel, C[harles]. *Compendium of Human Histology*. Ed. and trans. W. H. Van Buren. New York: Ballière Brothers, 1861.

Morgagni, Giovanni. *Seats and Causes of Disease, Investigated by Anatomy*. London: Longman, Hurst, Rees, Orme, and Brown, 1822.

Mullan, John. *Sentiment and Sociability: The Language of Feeling in the Eighteenth Century*. Oxford: Clarendon, 1988.

Müller, J[ohannes]. *Elements of Physiology*. Trans.William Baly. Ed. John Bell. Philadelphia: Lea and Blanchard, 1843.

Myddelton, Starkey. "An Account of an Extra-Uterine Conception." *Philosophical Transactions* 43 (1744–45): 336–40.

Oliphant, Margaret. *Hester*. Oxford: Oxford University Press, 2003.

———. *The Rector and the Doctor's Family*. New York: Penguin (Virago), 1986.

Osler, William. *The Principles and Practice of Medicine, Designed for the Use of Practitioners and Students of Medicine*. New York: D. Appleton, 1892.

Pargeter, William. *Observations on Maniacal Disorders*. Ed. W. F. Bynum and Roy Porter. New York: Routledge, 1988.

Parsons, James. "An Account of the White Negro Shewn before the Royal Society." *Philosophical Transactions* 55 (1765): 45–53.

———. "A Letter to the President, Concerning the Hermaphrodite Shewn in London." *Philosophical Transactions* 47 (1751–52): 142–45.

Pinney, Joel. *An Exposure of the Causes of the Present Deteriorated Condition of Health*. London: Longman, Rees, Orme, Brown, and Green, 1830.

Pritchard, Andrew. *The Microscopic Cabinet of Select Animated Objects*. London: Whittaker, Treacher, and Arnot, 1832.

"Professor Freud and Hysteria," *British Medical Journal* (11 January 1908): 103.

Pye-Smith, Philip Henry. "Medicine as a Science and Medicine as an Art." *Lancet* II (4 August 1900): 309–12.

Quekett, John. *Practical Treatise on the Microscope, Including the Different Methods of Preparing and Examining Animal, Vegetable, and Mineral Structures*. 2d ed. London: H. Bailliere, 1852.

Renwick, Thomas. *The Continuation of the Narrative of Miss Margaret M'avoy's Case. With General Observations Upon the Case Itself; Upon Her Peculiar Powers of Distinguishing Colours, Reading &c. Through the Medium of Her Fingers*. London: Baldwin, Cradock, and Joy, 1820.

———. *A Narrative of the Case of Miss Margaret Mcavoy; with an Account of Some Optical Experiments Connected with It*. London: Baldwin, Cradock, and Joy, 1817.

Review of *The Nature and Treatment of Gout*, by William Henry Robertson (London, 1845). *Dublin Medical Press* 16, no. 392 (1846): 20

Robert, Lord Bishop of Cork. "Concerning an Extraordinary Skeleton, and of a Man Who Gave Suck to a Child." *Philosophical Transactions* 41, no. 461 (1741): 810–14.

Robertson, J. "Concerning the Fall of Water under Bridges." *Philosophical Transactions* 50 (1758): 492–99.

Ruskin, John. *Modern Painters*. Ed. David Barrie. Abridged ed. New York: Knopf, 1987.

———. *The Stones of Venice*. London: Smith, Elder, 1867.

Russell, John Rutherford. *The History and Heroes of the Art of Medicine.* London: John Murray, 1861.
Sandars, Joseph. *Hints to Credulity! Or, an Examination of the Pretensions of Miss M. M'avoy, Occasioned by Dr. Renwick's "Narrative" Of Her Case.* Liverpool, England: J. & J. Smith, 1817.
Sansom, Arthur Ernest. *Manual of the Physical Diagnosis of the Diseases of the Heart: Including the Use of the Sphygmograph and Cardiograph.* 3d ed. London: J. & A. Churchill, 1881.
Sayre, Lewis Albert. *Remarkable Case of Deception: A Woman Professing to Secrete Nothing but Charcoal and Stones for a Number of Years, All the Natural Functions Being Arrested, and the Deception Unmasked.* Albany, NY: Steam Press of C. Van Benthuysen, 1863.
Sims, James. *Discourse on the Best Method of Prosecuting Medical Enquiries.* London: J. Johnson, 1774.
Smith, Adam. *The Theory of Moral Sentiments.* London: Henry G. Bohn, 1853.
Smith, George M. "Our Birth and Parentage." *Cornhill Magazine* n.s. x, no. 1 (January 1901): 4–17.
Spencer, Herbert. "The Genesis of Science." *British Quarterly Review* 20 (1854): 108–62.
Sprat, Thomas. *The History of the Royal Society.* Ed. Jackson I. Cope and Harold Whitmore Jones. St. Louis, MO: Washington University Press, 1958.
Stack, Thomas. "A Letter from Tho. Stack, M.D. . . . Containing an Account of a Woman Sixty-Eight Years of Age, Who Gave Suck to Two of Her Grand-Children." *Philosophical Transactions* 41, no. 453 (1739): 140–42.
Stillé, Alfred. *Elements of General Pathology.* Philadelphia: Lindsay & Blakiston, 1848.
Stoddard, Richard Henry, ed. *Anecdote Biographies of Thackeray and Dickens.* New York: Scribner, Armstrong, 1874.
Swain, William Paul. "On Diseased Conditions of the Knee-Joint." *British Medical Journal* 2 (1866): 540–44.
Sydenham, Thomas. *The Works of Thomas Sydenham, M.D. . . .* Ed. R. G. Latham. 2 vols. Vol. 1. London: Sydenham Society, 1850.
Symonds, John Addington. *The Letters of John Addington Symonds.* Ed. Herbert M. Schueller and Robert L. Peters. 3 vols. Detroit: Wayne State University Press, 1969.
Taylor, Frederick. *A Manual of the Practice of Medicine.* 5th ed. London: J. and A. Churchill, 1898.
Thomson, Joseph John. *Recollections and Reflections.* New York: Macmillan, 1937.
Vallemont, de. "Extract of a Letter from Mr. De Vallemont, Etc. Concerning a Small Egg Being Found within an Ordinary One. . . ." *Philosophical Transactions* 19 (1695): 632.
Ward, The Hon. Mrs. [Mary]. *Microscope Teachings: Descriptions of Various Objects of Especial Interest and Beauty Adapted for Microscopic Observation.* London: Groombridge and Sons, 1866.
Warren, Samuel. *Passages from the Diary of a Late Physician.* 2 vols. Vol. I. Leipzig: Bernhard Tauchnitz, 1844.
Warter, John Southey. *Observation in Medicine, or the Art of Case-Taking: Including a Special Description of the Most Common Thoracic Diseases, and Abnormal States of the Blood and Urine.* London: Longmans, Green, 1865.
Watson, Thomas. *Lectures on the Principles and Practice of Physic: Delivered at King's College, London.* Philadelphia: Lea and Blanchard, 1844.
Whitehead, H. "The Broad Street Pump: An Episode in the Cholera Epidemic of 1854." *Macmillan's Magazine* 13 (1866): 113–.
Williams, Charles J. B. *Authentic Narrative of the Case of the Late Earl St. Maur.* London: Longmans, Green, 1870.
Williams, Charles J. B., and Meredith Clymer. *Principles of Medicine: Comprising General Pathology and Therapeutics. . . .* 3rd Am. ed. Philadelphia: Lea and Blanchard, 1848.

Yonge, Charlotte Mary. *The Clever Woman of the Family*. Ed. Claire A. Simmons. Peterborough, ON: Broadview, 2001.
———. *The Heir of Redclyffe*. Oxford: Oxford University Press, 1997.

SECONDARY TEXTS

Ackerknecht, Erwin H. *Medicine at the Paris Hospital, 1794–1848*. Baltimore and London: Johns Hopkins University Press, 1967.
Altick, Richard D. *The English Common Reader: A Social History of the Mass Reading Public, 1800–1900*. 2d ed. Columbus: The Ohio State University Press, 1998.
Anderson, Amanda. *The Powers of Distance: Cosmopolitanism and the Cultivation of Detachment*. Princeton, NJ: Princeton University Press, 2001.
———. *Tainted Souls and Painted Faces: The Rhetoric of Fallenness in Victorian Culture*. Ithaca, NY: Cornell University Press, 1993.
Armstrong, Isobel. "The Microscope: Mediations of the Sub-Visible World." In *Transactions and Encounters: Science and Culture in the Nineteenth Century*, ed. Roger Luckhurst and Josephine McDonagh, 30–54. Manchester: Manchester University Press, 2002.
———. "Transparency: Towards a Poetics of Glass in the Nineteenth Century." In *Cultural Babbage: Technology, Time and Invention*, ed. Francis Spufford and Jenny Uglow, 123–48. London: Faber and Faber, 1996.
———. *Victorian Glassworlds: Glass Culture and the Imagination 1830–1880*. Oxford: Oxford University Press, 2008.
Armstrong, Nancy. *Desire and Domestic Fiction: A Political History of the Novel*. Oxford: Oxford University Press, 1987.
———. *Fiction in the Age of Photography: The Legacy of British Realism*. Cambridge, MA: Harvard University Press, 1999.
Armstrong, Richard. *A Compulsion for Antiquity: Freud and the Ancient World*. Ithaca, NY: Cornell University Press, 2005.
Auerbach, Nina. "Magi and Maidens: The Romance of the Victorian Freud." *Critical Inquiry* 8, no. 2 (1981): 281–300.
Bailin, Miriam. "'Dismal Pleasure': Victorian Sentimentality and the Pathos of the Parvenu." *ELH* 66, no. 4 (1999): 1015–32.
———. *The Sickroom in Victorian Fiction*. New York: Cambridge University Press, 1994.
Barker-Benfield, G. J. *The Culture of Sensibility: Sex and Society in Eighteenth-Century Britain*. Chicago: University of Chicago Press, 1992.
Beer, Gillian. "'Authentic Tidings of Invisible Things': Vision and the Invisible in the Later Nineteenth Century." In *Vision in Context: Historical and Contemporary Perspectives on Sight*, ed. Teresa Brennan and Martin Jay, 85–98. New York: Routledge, 1996.
———. *Darwin's Plots: Evolutionary Narrative in Darwin, George Eliot, and Nineteenth-Century Fiction*. 2d ed. Cambridge: Cambridge University Press, 2000.
———. *Open Fields: Science in Cultural Encounter*. Oxford: Clarendon Press, 1996.
Benedict, Barbara. *Curiosity: A Cultural History of Early Modern Inquiry*. Chicago: University Chicago Press, 2001.
Benjamin, Walter. "The Work of Art in the Age of Mechanical Reproduction." In *Illuminations*, ed. Hannah Arendt, 217–51. New York: Schocken Books, 1968.
Brissenden, R. F. *Virtue in Distress: Studies in the Novel of Sentiment from Richardson to Sade*. New York: Harper & Row, 1974.
Brooks, Peter. *Realist Vision*. New Haven, CT: Yale University Press, 2005.
Bullough, Vern L. *Science in the Bedroom: A History of Sex Research*. New York: Basic Books, 1994.

Bynum, W. F. *Science and the Practice of Medicine in the Nineteenth Century.* Cambridge: Cambridge University Press, 1994.
Caldwell, Janis McLarren. *Literature and Medicine in Nineteenth-Century Britain: From Mary Shelley to George Eliot.* Cambridge: Cambridge University Press, 2004.
———. "The Strange Death of the Animated Cadaver: Changing Conventions in Nineteenth-Century British Anatomical Illustration." *Literature and Medicine* 25, no. 2 (2006): 325–57.
Canguilhem, Georges. *On the Normal and the Pathological.* Trans. Carolyn Fawcett. Ed. Robert S. Cohen. London: D. Reidel, 1978.
Cannon, Susan Faye. *Science in Culture: The Early Victorian Period.* New York: Dawson and Science History Publications, 1978.
Cannon, W. B. "The Case Method of Teaching Systematic Medicine." *Boston Medical and Surgical Journal* 142, no. 2 (1900): 31–36.
Carroll, David, ed. *George Eliot: The Critical Heritage.* London: Routledge & Kegan Paul, 1971.
Cartwright, Lisa. *Screening the Body: Tracing Medicine's Visual Culture.* Minneapolis: University of Minnesota Press, 1995.
Castle, Terry. "The Culture of Travesty: Sexuality and Masquerade in Eighteenth-Century England." In *Sexual Underworlds of the Enlightenment,* ed. George S. Rousseau and Roy Porter, 156–80. Chapel Hill: University of North Carolina Press, 1988.
Christensen, Francis. "John Wilkins and the Royal Society's Reform of Prose Style." *MLQ* 7 (1946): 179–87, 279–90.
Clayborough, Arthur. *The Grotesque in English Literature.* Oxford: Oxford University Press, 1965.
Collini, Stefan. "Introduction." In *The Two Cultures,* ed. C. P. Snow, vii–lxxi. Cambridge: Cambridge University Press (Canto), 1993.
Coovadia, Imraan. "George Eliot's Realism and Adam Smith." *Studies in English Literature (SEL)* 42, no. 4 (2002): 819–35.
Crary, Jonathan. *Suspensions of Perception: Attention, Spectacle, and Modern Culture.* Cambridge, MA: MIT Press, 1999.
———. *Techniques of the Observer: On Vision and Modernity in the Nineteenth Century.* Cambridge, MA: MIT Press, 1990.
Crawford, Catherine. "A Scientific Profession: Medical Reform and Forensic Medicine in British Periodicals of the Early Nineteenth Century." In *British Medicine in an Age of Reform,* ed. Roger French and Andrew Wear, 203–30. London: Routledge, 1991.
"Curious," *Oxford English Dictionary,* https://proxy.stg.brown.edu:443/cgi-bin/oed/oed.pl?mode=entry&type=entry&byte=.
d'Albertis, Deirdre. *Dissembling Fictions: Elizabeth Gaskell and the Victorian Social Text.* New York: St. Martin's Press, 1997.
Dames, Nicholas. *Amnesiac Selves: Nostalgia, Forgetting, and British Fiction, 1810–1870.* Oxford: Oxford University Press, 2001.
———. *Physiology of the Novel: Reading, Neural Science, and the Form of Victorian Fiction.* Oxford: Oxford University Press, 2007.
Daston, Lorraine. "Marvelous Facts and Miraculous Evidence in Early Modern Europe." In *Questions of Evidence: Proof, Practice, and Persuasion across the Disciplines,* ed. James Chandler, Arnold I. Davidson, and Harry Harootunian, 243–74. Chicago: University of Chicago Press, 1994.
———. "The Moral Economy of Science." *Osiris* 10 (1995): 3–24.
———. "Objectivity and the Escape from Perspective." *Social Studies of Science* 22, no. 4 (1992): 597–618.
Daston, Lorraine, and Katherine Park. *Wonders and the Order of Nature, 1150–1750.* New York: Zone Books [Cambridge, MA: Distributed by MIT Press], 1998.

Daston, Lorraine, and Peter Galison. "The Image of Objectivity." *Representations* 40 (1992): 81–128.
———. *Objectivity*. New York: Zone, 2007.
Davis, Lennard. *Factual Fictions: The Origins of the English Novel*. Philadelphia: University of Pennsylvania Press, 1997.
Davis, Michael. *George Eliot and Nineteenth-Century Psychology: Exploring the Unmapped Country*. Aldershot, England and Burlington, VT: Ashgate, 2006.
Dawson, Gowan. "The *Cornhill Magazine* and Shilling Monthlies in Mid-Victorian Britain." In *Science in the Nineteenth-Century Periodical: Reading the Magazine of Nature*, ed. Geoffrey Cantor et al., 123–50. Cambridge: Cambridge University Press, 2004.
Dawson, Graham. *Soldier Heroes: British Adventure, Empire, and the Imagining of Masculinities*. New York: Routledge, 1994.
Dear, Peter. "Introduction." In *The Literary Structure of Scientific Argument: Historical Studies*, ed. Peter Dear, 1–9. Philadelphia: University of Pennsylvania Press, 1991.
———. "*Totius in Verba*: Rhetoric and Authority in the Early Royal Society." *Isis* 76 (1985): 145–61.
Dyson, A. E. *The Inimitable Dickens: A Reading of the Novels*. New York: St. Martin's, 1970.
Fairfax, Nathan. "Extract of a Letter Written by Dr. Nathan Fairfax to the Publisher, About a Bullet Voided by Urine." *Philosophical Transactions* 2, no. 40 (1668): 803–5.
Fissell, Mary E. "The Disappearance of the Patient's Narrative and the Invention of Hospital Medicine." In *British Medicine in an Age of Reform*, ed. Roger French and Andrew Wear, 92–109. London: Routledge, 1991.
Flint, Kate. *The Victorians and the Visual Imagination*. Cambridge: Cambridge University Press, 2000.
Flynn, Carol Houlihan. "Running out of Matter: The Body Exercised in Eighteenth-Century Fiction." In *The Languages of Psyche: Mind and Body in Enlightenment Thought*, ed. G. S. Rousseau, 147–85. Berkeley: University of California Press, 1990.
Foucault, Michel. *The Birth of the Clinic: An Archaeology of Medical Perception*. Translated by A. M. Sheridan Smith. New York: Vintage, 1973.
———. *The Order of Things: An Archaeology of the Human Sciences*. New York: Vintage, 1970.
Frankland, Graham. *Freud's Literary Culture*. Cambridge: Cambridge University Press, 2000.
Frawley, Maria H. *Invalidism and Identity in Nineteenth-Century Britain*. Chicago: University of Chicago Press, 2004.
Frye, Northrop. *Anatomy of Criticism*. Princeton, NJ: Princeton University Press, 1957.
Galison, Peter L. "Judgment against Objectivity." In *Picturing Science, Producing Art*, ed. Caroline A. Jones and Peter Louis Galison, 327–59. New York: Routledge, 1998.
Gallagher, Catherine. *Nobody's Story: Women Writers in the Marketplace*. Berkeley: University of California Press, 1995.
Gallop, Jane. "Keys to Dora." In *In Dora's Case: Freud—Hysteria—Feminism*, ed. Charles Bernheimer and Claire Kahane, 200–20. New York: Columbia University Press, 1990.
Gay, Peter. *Reading Freud: Explorations and Entertainments*. New Haven, CT: Yale University Press, 1990.
Gilbert, Pamela K. *Mapping the Victorian Social Body*. Albany: SUNY Press, 2004.
Gilles, Jonathan. "The History of the Patient History since 1850." *Bulletin of the History of Medicine* 80 (2006): 490–512.
Gilman, Sander L. *Freud, Race, and Gender*. Princeton, NJ: Princeton University Press, 1993.
———. "Preface." In *Reading Freud's Reading*, ed. Sander L. Gilman, Jutta Birmele, Jay Geller, and Valerie D. Greenberg, xiii–xvi. New York: New York University Press, 1994.
Gray, B. M. "Pseudoscience and George Eliot's 'The Lifted Veil.'" *Nineteenth-Century Fiction* 36, no. 4 (March 1982): 407–23.

Greenberg, Valerie D. "'A Piece of the Logical Thread...': Freud and Physics." In *Reading Freud's Reading*, ed. Sander L. Gilman, Jutta Birmele, Jay Geller, and Valerie D. Greenberg, 232–51. New York: New York University Press, 1994.
Gross, Alan G., Joseph E. Harmon, and Michael Reidy. *Communicating Science: The Scientific Article from the 17th Century to the Present.* Oxford: Oxford University Press, 2002.
Gunn, Daniel. "Dutch Painting and the Simple Truth in *Adam Bede.*" *Studies in the Novel* 24 (1992): 366–80.
Hacking, Ian. *Representing and Intervening: Introductory Topics in the Philosophy of Natural Science.* Cambridge: Cambridge University Press, 1983.
Hake, Sabine. "Saxa Loquuntur: Freud's Archaeology of the Text." *boundary 2* 20, no. 1 (1993): 146–73.
Haley, Bruce. *The Healthy Body and Victorian Culture.* Cambridge, MA: Harvard University Press, 1978.
Hall, M. B. "Science in the Early Royal Society." In *The Emergence of Science in Western Europe*, ed. Maurice Crosland, 57–77. New York: Science History Publishing, 1976.
Hammond, John H. *The Camera Obscura: A Chronicle.* Bristol: Adam Hilger, 1981.
Hertz, Neil. "Dora's Secrets, Freud's Techniques." In *In Dora's Case: Freud—Hysteria—Feminism*, ed. Charles Bernheimer and Claire Kahane, 221–42. New York: Columbia University Press, 1990.
Hinton, Laura. *The Perverse Gaze of Sympathy: Sadomasochistic Sentiments from Clarissa to Rescue 911.* Albany: SUNY Press, 1999.
Holland, Susan. "Wellcome Index of Science and Medicine in the Athenaeum: Project Progress Report." athenaeum.soi.city.ac.uk/scientific/athrep.ps.
Hollinger, David A. "The Knower and the Artificer." *American Quarterly* 39, no. 1 (1987): 37–56.
Holmes, Martha Stoddard. *Fictions of Affliction: Physical Disability in Victorian Culture.* Ann Arbor: University of Michigan Press, 2004.
Horton, Susan R. "Were they Having Fun Yet? Victorian Optical Gadgetry, Modernist Selves." In *Victorian Literature and the Victorian Visual Imagination.* Eds. Carol T. Christ and John O. Jordan. Berkeley: University of California Press, 1995.
Huet, Marie-Hélène. *Monstrous Imagination.* Cambridge, MA: Harvard University Press, 1993.
Hunter, Dianne. "Hysteria, Psychoanalysis, and Feminism: The Case of Anna O." *Feminist Studies* 9, no. 3 (1983): 465–88.
Hunter, J. Paul. *Before Novels: The Cultural Contexts of Eighteenth-Century English Fiction.* New York: W. W. Norton, 1990.
Hunter, Kathryn Montgomery. *Doctors' Stories: The Narrative Structure of Medical Knowledge.* Princeton, NJ: Princeton University Press, 1991.
Hurwitz, Brian. "Form and Representation in Clinical Case Reports." *Literature and Medicine* 25, no. 2 (2006): 216–40.
Huxley, Aldous. "The Vulgarity of Little Nell." In *The Dickens Critics*, ed. George H. Ford and Lauriat Lane, 153–56. Ithaca, NY: Cornell University Press, 1961.
Jacobus, Mary. *Reading Woman: Essays in Feminist Criticism.* New York: Columbia University Press, 1986.
Jaffe, Audrey. *Scenes of Sympathy: Identity and Representation in Victorian Fiction.* Ithaca, NY: Cornell University Press, 2000.
Jalland, Pat. *Death in the Victorian Family.* Oxford: Oxford University Press, 1996.
Jameson, Fredric. *The Political Unconscious: Narrative as a Socially Symbolic Act.* Ithaca, NY: Cornell University Press, 1981.
Jay, Martin. "Scopic Regimes of Modernity." In *Vision and Visuality*, ed. Hal Foster, 3–23. Seattle: Bay Press, 1988.

Jones, Ernest. *The Life and Work of Sigmund Freud.* Vol. 1, *The Formative Years and the Great Discoveries, 1856–1900.* New York: Basic Books, 1953.

Jones, Richard Foster. "Science and English Prose Style in the Third Quarter of the Seventeenth Century." In *The Seventeenth Century: Studies in the History of English Thought and Literature from Bacon to Pope,* ed. Marjorie Nicolson, 75–110. Stanford, CA: Stanford University Press, 1951.

Kaplan, Fred. *Dickens: A Biography.* Baltimore: Johns Hopkins University Press, 1988.

———. *Sacred Tears: Sentimentality in Victorian Literature.* Princeton, NJ: Princeton University Press, 1987.

Katz, Wendy R. *Rider Haggard and the Fiction of Empire: A Critical Study of British Imperial Fiction.* Cambridge: Cambridge University Press, 1987.

Kennedy, Meegan. "The Ghost in the Clinic: Gothic Medicine and Curious Fiction in Samuel Warren's Diary of a Late Physician." *Victorian Literature and Culture* 32, no. 2 (2004): 327–51.

———. "'Poor Hoo Loo': Sentiment, Stoicism, and the Grotesque in British Imperial Medicine." In *Victorian Freaks,* ed. Marlene Tromp, 79–113. Columbus: The Ohio State University Press, 2008.

King, Amy M. *Bloom: The Botanical Vernacular in the English Novel.* Oxford: Oxford University Press, 2003.

Kitchel, Anna Theresa. "Introduction." In *Quarry for Middlemarch,* ed. George Eliot, 1–19. Berkeley: University of California Press, 1950.

Kofman, Sarah. *Camera Obscura of Ideology.* Trans. Will Straw. Ithaca, NY: Cornell University Press, 1998.

———. *Freud and Fiction [Quatre Romans Analytiques].* Trans. Sarah Wykes. Boston: Northeastern University Press, 1991.

Krasner, James. *The Entangled Eye: Visual Perception and the Representation of Nature in Post-Darwinian Narrative.* Oxford: Oxford University Press, 1992.

Kreisel, Deanna K. "Incognito, Intervention, and Dismemberment in *Adam Bede*." *ELH* 70 (2003): 541–74.

Kuhn, Thomas S. *The Structure of Scientific Revolutions.* 3d ed. Chicago: University of Chicago Press, 1997.

Laqueur, Thomas. "Bodies, Details, and the Humanitarian Narrative." In *The New Cultural History,* ed. Lynn Hunt, 176–204. Berkeley: University of California Press, 1989.

Law, Jules David. *The Rhetoric of Empiricism: Language and Perception from Locke to I. A. Richards.* Ithaca, NY: Cornell University Press, 1993.

Lawrence, Christopher. "Incommunicable Knowledge: Science, Technology and the Clinical Art in Britain 1850–1914." *Journal of Contemporary History* 20 (1985): 503–20.

Leavis, F. R. "Two Cultures? The Significance of Lord Snow." In *Nor Shall My Sword: Discourses on Pluralism, Compassion and Social Hope,* 41–74. London: Chatto and Windus, 1972.

Lenard, Mary. *Preaching Pity: Dickens, Gaskell, and Sentimentalism in Victorian Culture.* New York: Peter Lang, 1999.

Lerner, Laurence. *Angels and Absences: Child Deaths in the Nineteenth Century.* Nashville, TN: Vanderbilt University Press, 1997.

Levine, George. *Dying to Know: Scientific Epistemology and Narrative in Victorian England.* Chicago: University of Chicago Press, 2002.

———. "George Eliot's Hypothesis of Reality." *Nineteenth-Century Fiction* 35 (1980): 1–28.

———. *The Realistic Imagination: English Fiction from Frankenstein to Lady Chatterley.* Chicago: University of Chicago Press, 1981.

Lodge, David. "*Middlemarch* and the Idea of the Classic Realist Text." In *The Nineteenth-Century Novel: Critical Essays and Documents,* ed. Arnold Kettle, 218–38. London: Heinemann, 1981.

Logan, Peter Melville. "George Eliot and the Fetish of Realism." *Studies in the Literary Imagination* 35, no. 2 (2002): 27–51.

———. *Nerves and Narratives: A Cultural History of Hysteria in Nineteenth-Century British Prose.* Berkeley: University of California Press, 1997.

Lowe, Brigid. *Victorian Fiction and the Insights of Sympathy: An Alternative to the Hermeneutics of Suspicion.* London: Anthem, 2007.

MacCabe, Colin. *James Joyce and the Revolution of the Word.* London: Macmillan, 1978.

———. "Realism and the Cinema: Notes on Some Brechtian Theses." In *Tracking the Signifier: Theoretical Essays: Film, Linguistics, Literature,* 33–57. Minneapolis: University of Minnesota Press, 1985.

MacPike, Loralee. "The Old Curiosity Shop: Changing Views of Little Nell." *Dickens Studies Newsletter* 12, no. 2; 3 (1981): 33–38; 70–76.

Mahony, Patrick J. *Freud as a Writer.* 2d ed. New Haven, CT: Yale University Press, 1987.

———. *Freud's Dora: A Psychoanalytic, Historical, and Textual Study.* New Haven, CT: Yale University Press, 1996.

Mansell, Darrel, Jr. "Ruskin and George Eliot's 'Realism.'" *Criticism* 7 (1965): 205–14.

Marcus, Steven. "Freud and Dora: Story, History, Case History." In *In Dora's Case: Freud—Hysteria—Feminism,* ed. Charles Bernheimer and Claire Kahane, 56–91. New York: Columbia University Press, 1990.

———. "Freud and Dora: Story, History, Case History." In *Representations,* 247–309. New York: Random House, 1975.

Mason, Michael York. "*Middlemarch* and Science: Problems of Life and Mind." *Review of English Studies,* n.s., 22, no. 86 (1971): 151–69.

Mazlish, Bruce. "A Triptych: Freud's *The Interpretation of Dreams,* Rider Haggard's *She,* and Bulwer-Lytton's *The Coming Race.*" *Comparative Studies in Society and History* 35 (1993): 726–45.

McCarthy, Patrick. "The Curious Road to Death's Nell." *Dickens Studies Annual* 29 (1991): 35–56.

McKeon, Michael. *The Origins of the English Novel 1600–1740.* Baltimore: Johns Hopkins University Press, 1987.

Menke, Richard. "Fiction as Vivisection: G. H. Lewes and George Eliot." *ELH* 67, no. 2 (2000): 617–53.

Miller, Andrew H. "Bruising, Laceration, and Lifelong Maiming: Or, How We Encourage Research." *ELH* 70 (2003): 301–18.

Miller, D. A. *Narrative and Its Discontents: Problems of Closure in the Traditional Novel.* Princeton, NJ: Princeton University Press, 1981.

Miller, J. Hillis. "Optic and Semiotic in *Middlemarch.*" In *The Worlds of Victorian Fiction,* ed. Jerome H. Buckley, 125–45. Cambridge, MA: Harvard University Press, 1975.

Mitchell, W. J. T. *Iconology: Image, Text, Ideology.* Chicago: University of Chicago Press, 1986.

———. *Picture Theory: Essays on Verbal and Visual Representation.* Chicago: University of Chicago Press, 1994.

Moi, Toril. "Representation of Patriarchy: Sexuality and Epistemology in Freud's Dora." In *In Dora's Case: Freud—Hysteria—Feminism,* ed. Charles Bernheimer and Claire Kahane, 181–99. New York: Columbia University Press, 1990.

Monsman, Gerald. *H. Rider Haggard on the Imperial Frontier.* Greensboro, NC: ELT, 2006.

Nixon, Jude V. "'Lost in the Vast Worlds of Wonder': Dickens and Science." *Dickens Studies Annual* 35 (2005): 267–333.

O'Connor, W. J. *Founders of British Physiology: A Biographical Dictionary, 1820–1885.* Manchester: Manchester University Press, 1988.

Otis, Laura. *Networking: Communicating with Bodies and Machines in the Nineteenth Century.* Ann Arbor: University of Michigan Press, 2001.

Otter, Chris. *The Victorian Eye: A Political History of Light and Vision in Britain, 1800–1910.* Chicago: University of Chicago Press, 2008.

Peterson, M. Jeanne. *The Medical Profession in Mid-Victorian London.* Berkeley: University of California Press, 1978.

———. "Medicine." In *Victorian Periodicals and Victorian Society,* ed. J. Don Vann and Rosemary T. VanArsdel, 22–44. Toronto: University of Toronto Press, 1994.

Poovey, Mary. *Making a Social Body: British Cultural Formation, 1830–1865.* Chicago: University of Chicago Press, 1995.

Porter, Roy, ed. "Lay Medical Knowledge in the Eighteenth Century: The Evidence of the *Gentleman's Magazine.*" *Medical History* 29 (1985): 138–68.

———. "Laymen, Doctors and Medical Knowledge in the Eighteenth Century: The Evidence of the 'Gentleman's Magazine.'" In *Patients and Practitioners: Lay Perceptions of Medicine in Pre-Industrial Society,* ed. Roy Porter, 283–314. Cambridge: Cambridge University Press, 1985.

———, ed. *Patients and Practitioners: Lay Perceptions of Medicine in Pre-Industrial Society.* Cambridge: Cambridge University Press, 1985.

Pratt, Mary Louise. *Imperial Eyes: Studies in Travel Writing and Transculturalism.* New York: Routledge, 1992.

Price, Leah. *The Anthology and the Rise of the Novel: From Richardson to George Eliot.* Cambridge: Cambridge University Press, 2000.

Rai, Amit. *Rule of Sympathy: Sentiment, Race, and Power 1750–1850.* New York: Palgrave, 2002.

Ramas, Maria. "Freud's Dora, Dora's Hysteria." In *In Dora's Case: Freud—Hysteria—Feminism,* ed. Charles Bernheimer and Claire Kahane, 149–80. New York: Columbia University Press, 1990.

Reidel-Schrewe, Ursula. "Freud's Début in the Sciences." In *Reading Freud's Reading,* ed. Sander L. Gilman, Jutta Birmele, Jay Geller, and Valerie D. Greenberg, 1–22. New York: New York University Press, 1994.

Reiser, Stanley Joel. "Creating Form out of Mass: The Development of the Medical Record." In *Transformation and Tradition in the Sciences: Essays in Honor of I. Bernard Cohen,* ed. Everett Mendelsohn, 303–16. Cambridge: Cambridge University Press, 1984.

———. *Medicine and the Reign of Technology.* Cambridge: Cambridge University Press, 1978.

Rieff, Philip. "Introduction." In *Dora: An Analysis of a Case of Hysteria,* ed. Sigmund Freud, vii–xix. New York: Collier Books, 1963.

Roberts, Nancy. *Schools of Sympathy: Gender and Identification through the Novel.* Montreal: University of British Columbia Academic Women's Association/McGill-Queen's University Press, 1997.

Romano, Terrie M. *Making Medicine Scientific: John Burdon Sanderson and the Culture of Victorian Science.* Baltimore: Johns Hopkins University Press, 2002.

Ross, Sydney. "*Scientist:* The Story of a Word." *Annals of Science* 18, no. 2 (1962): 65–85.

Rothfield, Lawrence. *Vital Signs: Medical Realism in Nineteenth-Century Fiction.* Princeton, NJ: Princeton University Press, 1992.

Rousseau, G. S. "Nerves, Spirits, and Fibres: Towards Defining the Origins of Sensibility." In *Studies in the Eighteenth Century: Papers...,* ed. R. F. Brissenden and J. C. Eade, 137–57. Toronto: University of Toronto Press, 1976.

Rudnytsky, Peter. "Freud's Pompeiian Fantasy." In *Reading Freud's Reading,* ed. Sander L. Gilman, Jutta Birmele, Jay Geller, and Valerie D. Greenberg, 211–31. New York: New York University Press, 1994.

Rylance, Rick. "The Theatre and the Granary: Observations on Nineteenth-Century Medical Narratives." *Literature and Medicine* 25, no. 2 (2006): 255–76.

———. *Victorian Psychology and British Culture, 1850–1880.* Oxford: Oxford University Press, 2000.
Schickore, Jutta. *The Microscope and the Eye.* Chicago: University of Chicago Press, 2007.
Shapin, Steven, and Simon Schaffer. *Leviathan and the Air-Pump: Hobbes, Boyle, and the Experimental Life.* Princeton, NJ: Princeton University Press, 1985.
Shaw, Harry E. *Narrating Reality: Austen, Scott, Eliot.* Ithaca, NY: Cornell University Press, 1999.
Showalter, Elaine. *Hystories: Hysterical Epidemics and Modern Media.* New York: Columbia University Press, 1997.
Shryock, Richard Harrison. *The Development of Modern Medicine: An Interpretation of the Social and Scientific Factors Involved.* New York: Knopf, 1947.
Shuttleworth, Sally. *Charlotte Brontë and Victorian Psychology.* Cambridge: Cambridge University Press, 1996.
———. *George Eliot and Nineteenth-Century Science: The Make-Believe of a Beginning.* Cambridge: Cambridge University Press, 1984.
Sill, Geoffrey. *The Cure of the Passions and the Origins of the English Novel.* Cambridge: Cambridge University Press, 2001.
Skilton, David, ed. *The Early and Mid-Victorian Novel.* New York: Routledge, 1993.
Small, Helen. *Love's Madness: Medicine, the Novel, and Female Insanity, 1800–1865.* Oxford: Clarendon, 1996.
Snow, C. P. *The Two Cultures and a Second Look.* Cambridge: Cambridge University Press, 1969.
Stafford, Barbara Maria. *Artful Science: Enlightenment, Entertainment, and the Eclipse of Visual Education.* Cambridge, MA: MIT Press, 1994.
Starr, George. *Defoe and Casuistry.* Princeton, NJ: Princeton University Press, 1971.
Stiebel, Lindy. *Imagining Africa: Landscape in H. Rider Haggard's African Romances.* Westport, CT: Greenwood, 2001.
Stoddart, Judith. "Tracking the Sentimental Eye." In *Knowing the Past: Victorian Literature and Culture,* ed. Suzy Anger, 192–211. Ithaca, NY: Cornell University Press, 2001.
Stoeckle, John D., and J. Andrew Billings. "A History of History-Taking: The Medical Interview." *Journal of General Internal Medicine* 2, no. 2 (1987): 119–27.
Strachey, James. "Editor's Introduction." In Sigmund Freud, *The Standard Edition of the Complete Psychological Works of Sigmund Freud,* ed. James Strachey, ix–xxviii. London: Hogarth Press, 1955.
Tambling, Jeremy. "*Middlemarch,* Realism and the Birth of the Clinic." *ELH* 57, no. 4 (1990): 939–60.
Temkin, Owsei. "Studien Zum 'Sinn'-Begriff in Der Medizin." *Kyklos* 2 (1929): 21–105.
Thrailkill, Jane F. "Killing Them Softly: Childbed Fever and the Novel." *American Literature* 71, no. 4 (1999): 679–707.
Todd, Dennis. *Imagining Monsters: Miscreations of the Self in Eighteenth-Century England.* Chicago: University of Chicago Press, 1995.
Topham, Jonathan R. "Beyond the 'Common Context': The Production and Reading of the Bridgewater Treatises." *Isis* 89 (1998): 233–62.
Tougaw, Jason Daniel. *Strange Cases: The Medical Case History and the British Novel.* New York and London: Routledge, 2006.
Trodd, Colin, Paul Barlow, and David Amigoni, eds. *Victorian Culture and the Idea of the Grotesque.* Aldershot and Brookfield, VT: Ashgate Press, 1999.
Tucker, Jennifer. *Nature Exposed: Photography as Eyewitness in Victorian Science.* Baltimore: Johns Hopkins University Press, 2005.
van den Berg, Sara. "Reading Dora Reading: Freud's 'Fragment of an Analysis of a Case of

Hysteria.'" In *In Dora's Case: Freud—Hysteria—Feminism,* ed. Charles Bernheimer and Claire Kahane, 294–304. New York: Columbia University Press, 1990.

Van Sant, Ann Jessie. *Eighteenth-Century Sensibility and the Novel.* Cambridge: Cambridge University Press, 1993.

Vickers, Brian. "The Royal Society and English Prose Style: A Reassessment." In *Rhetoric and the Pursuit of Truth: Language Change in the Seventeenth and Eighteenth Centuries,* ed. Brian Vickers and Nancy S. Struever, 3–76. Los Angeles: Clark Memorial Library, 1985.

Vrettos, Athena. *Somatic Fictions: Imagining Illness in Victorian Culture.* Stanford, CA: Stanford University Press, 1995.

Ward, Candace. *Desire and Disorder: Fevers, Fictions, and Feeling in English Georgian Culture.* Lewisburg, PA: Bucknell University Press, 2007.

Warner, John Harley. *Against the Spirit of System: The French Impulse in Nineteenth-Century American Medicine.* Baltimore: Johns Hopkins University Press, 1998.

———. "The Idea of Science in English Medicine: The 'Decline of Science' and the Rhetoric of Reform, 1815–45." In *British Medicine in an Age of Reform,* ed. Roger French and Andrew Wear, 136–64. London: Routledge, 1991.

———. *The Therapeutic Perspective: Medical Practice, Knowledge, and Identity in America, 1820–1885.* Cambridge, MA: Harvard University Press, 1986.

Watt, Ian. *The Rise of the Novel: Studies in Defoe, Richardson, and Fielding.* Berkeley: University of California Press, 1957.

Webster, Richard. *Why Freud Was Wrong: Sin, Science, and Psychoanalysis.* New York: Basic Books, 1997.

Winter, Sarah. *Freud and the Institution of Psychoanalytic Knowledge.* Stanford, CA: Stanford University Press, 1999.

Wood, Jane. *Passion and Pathology in Victorian Fiction.* Oxford: Oxford University Press, 2001.

Wormald, Mark. "Microscopy and Semiotic in *Middlemarch.*" *Nineteenth-Century Literature* 50, no. 4 (1996): 501–24.

Yeo, Richard R. *Defining Science: William Whewell, Natural Knowledge, and Public Debates in Early Victorian Britain.* Cambridge: Cambridge University Press, 1993.

———. "Scientific Method and the Rhetoric of Science in Britain, 1830–1917." In *The Politics and Rhetoric of Scientific Method: Historical Studies,* ed. John A. Schuster and Richard R. Yeo, 259–97. Boston: D. Reidel, 1986.

Index

Abbé, Ernst, 224n7, 224n9
"absent presence," 61, 65, 67, 128. *See also* mechanical observation
"Account of an Unusual Medical Case" (Manginot), 44–45
"Account of a Woman . . . Who Gave Suck" (Stack), 42–45
"Account of some Observations Made by a Young Gentleman" (Cheselden), 30–31
"Account of William Dempster" (Barnes), 52
Adam Bede (Eliot), 120–22, 124–47, 164
"Aetiology of Hysteria, The" (Freud), 172–73, 184, 190–92
"A Faithful Record of the Miraculous Case of Mary Jobson" (Clanny), 52
affect. *See also* emotion; interest; subjectivity
Africa, 193–99, 229n69, 229n71
agency: of experimenter, 154, 156; of narrator, 129, 137; of observer, 63–66, 126–29, 148, 154. *See also* mechanical observation; subjectivity, suppression of; of physician, 129

Aiken, John, 203–4
"A Lesson in the Art of Distinguishing" (Aiken, Barbauld), 203–4
"A Letter to the President, Concerning the Hermaphrodite Shewn in London" (Parsons), 40
allegory, 19
allopathic medicine. *See* clinical medicine
All the Year Round, 73–74
alternative medicine. *See* sectarian medicine
amputation, 81–83
analogy, 57, 179, 191, 213n9
Anderson, Amanda, 106, 130, 221n31, 221n34
aneurysm, 59–61, 97–98
Anomalies and Curiosities of Medicine (Gould and Pyle), 51
Anstie, Francis, 80, 82, 84, 84–85
antibiotics, 10
antiquarianism, 106–7
antirealism, 6. *See also* curious; romance; sensationalism; sentiment
archaeologist, physician as, 187–99
archaeology, 190–92

• 247 •

INDEX

archive, 22–23
Armstrong, Isobel, 222n49, 224n19, 226n44, 226n45
Arnold, Matthew, 24
ars medica, 5, 13, 66, 70, 98–99. *See also* insight; analogy to realist novel, 123–24
art: Dutch realist, 125, 140; medicine as (see *ars medica*); not mechanical reproduction, 130, 221n37; opposed to science, 123–24, 158, 162–63, 178, 184
Athenaeum, 73–79, 134–35, 215n50
Atlas of Human Anatomy and Physiology (Fermer), 79
Auerbach, Nina, 187
Aurora Leigh (Browning), 148
authorities, citation of: in case history, 32–33, 57
authority: in 18th-century novel, 48; in 19th-century novel, 122; of periodicals, 73–74
authority, medical: in 18th century, 31–32, 39; in 19th century, 63, 65; in 19th-century novel, 17–21, 109–16; challenges to, 19–20, 97–99; female, 112–13; of physician, 59
Autobiography (Freud), 200
autopsy, 55–61, 61, 213n4, 213n13
autopsy report, 57–61

Babbage, Charles, 220–21n29
Bacon, Francis, 31, 207n11
Bailin, Miriam, 8, 88, 107–8, 217n36
Baker, Thomas Herbert: review of, 79
Barbauld, Anna Letitia, 203–4
Barnes, Thomas, 52
Bartlett, Elisha, 66–67
Battie, William, 33
beautiful: as a term, 16
Bedingford, James, 213n4
Beer, Gillian, 2, 186, 215n50, 225n24
Belloc, Hilaire, 214n41
Benjamin, Walter, 67
Bennett, John Hughes, 61, 70, 123–24, 137; review of, 75
Bennett, John Hughes, 219n9, 220n17
Bernard, Claude: on the camera, 222n55; on hypothesis, 156–59, 225n25; influence on G. H. Lewes, 222n52; on mechanical observation, 138–39; on the microscope, 224n14; on observation/experiment distinction, 150, 154
Bigelow, Jacob, 66
Blackwood, John, 140
Blackwood's Edinburgh Magazine, 1
Blake, William, 24, 25
Blanc, Henry, 68–70, 214n46
Bleak House (Dickens), 20
blind boy, case of, 30–31, 46–50
blindness, color, 221–22n46
"Blue Devils, The" (Cruikshank), 71–72
Boddington, Benjamin, 38
botany, 20
Boys' Own Paper, 79
Bramwell, Byrom: on case-taking, 62; on labor, 65, 163; literary techniques in, 14–17; on observation, 66; on sensibility, 70; on speculation, 162–63
Breuer, Josef, 170, 178
Brimley, George, 223n60
Brinton, William, 160
British Medical Journal, 177
"Broad Street Pump" (Whitehead), 85–86
Brooks, Peter, 2
Browning, Elizabeth Barrett, 148
Brugsch, Heinrich Karl, 191
Buchan, William, 71, 109, 112–13
Bullitt, H. M., 66
Bullough, Vern L., 173

C., Mr., 38–39
cadaver, 142, 144. *See also* autopsy
Caldwell, Janis: on affect, 221n33; on case history format, 56, 213n6; on medical humanities, 201; on medical illustration, 213n19; on "Romantic materialism," 3, 212n2
camera, 138–39, 166–67, 222n55
camera obscura, 221n44; double valence of, 136; eye as, 134–35, 221–22n46; metaphor of, 120, 135–38; mirror in, 134; relation to camera, 222n55
Canguilhem, Georges, 212n53
cardiac disease, 94–97
Carpenter, William, 75, 100, 155, 159
case: as typical, 21
"case" as a term, 21–23, 208n40
"Case-Book Fiction," 27
case history: analogy in, 57; causality in,

INDEX

57; citation in, 32–33, 57; clinical. *See* clinical case history; criticism on, 208–9n59; curious (*see* curious case); as genre, 26, 56, 168, 171; history of, 169; humor in, 207n32; and industrialization, 27–28; "interesting" in, 94–97; irony in, 17; Latin in, 32–33, 57; as literary text, 25–26; as means of professionalization, 27, 51; as narrative, 25–26, 131, 170–71, 202; patient's voice in, 56, 175; and the production of knowledge, 49–50; sensibility in, 37–38; sentiment in, 93–100; as social record, 26–28; standardization of, 56–58; statistics in, 57, 208n45; taking of. *See* case-taking; technology in, 56–57; use for classification, 208n37; why read, 25–29
"Case Illustrative of the Diagnostic Value of the Sphygmograph" (Bramwell), 15–16
case method of teaching, 21
"Case of Concussion of the Brain" (Greenhow), 52–53
"Case of So-called Perforating Tumor of the Skull" (Bramwell), 14–15
case-taking, 54, 58, 61–68, 70, 178; in Dickens, 218n50
Castle, Terry, 210n26
casuistry, 21
"cathartic method," 178–83, 226n5, 228n39
Cavanagh, William, case of, 96–97
Chadwick, Edwin, 11–13
Chapman, Nathaniel, 64
character, diagnosis of, 17–21
Charon, Rita, 201
Cheever, David, 70
Cheselden, William: on blind boy, 30–31, 46–50; on medical illustration, 214n43
Cheyne, George, 32–33, 33, 36, 37, 58–59
children, illnesses of, 96
cholera, 85–86, 110
Churchill, J. Francis: review of, 76
circulation of affect: in 18th-century medicine, 32, 36, 38–49; in 18th-century philosophy, 90–93; in 19th-century medicine, 87, 117; in Dickens, 88–89, 107, 117; in Eliot, 89, 121, 138–44; in Freud, 191; in Gaskell, 89–90, 117

Clanny, William Reid, 52
class status, of physicians, 13–14, 24
Clever Woman of the Family, The (Yonge), 116
climatology, 75, 108–9
clinical case history, 54–70. *See also* clinical observation; mechanical observation; and autopsy, 55–61; compared to psychoanalytic case history, 170–71; definition of, 55, 69; after Freud, 171; heterogeneity of, 199; opposed to curious case history, 93–94; resistance to, 55; sentiment in, 87–88
clinical gaze, 3, 58; compared to clinical observation, 9; compared to mechanical observation, 65
clinical medicine, 5; and autopsy, 55–61; compared to experimental medicine, 148–49; compared to psychoanalysis, 169, 179–80, 182, 193; opposed to 18th-century medicine, 93–94; resistance to, 24, 59, 211n49; rise of, 50–53, 54–70, 59, 93–94
clinical observation, 4, 9–10, 32. *See also* clinical case history; in Dickens, 20, 102–5; in Disraeli, 11–13; in Eliot, 141; in Freud, 172–74; in Gaskell, 89, 108–16; in Hardy, 17–21; novelists' use of, 12, 88–89, 204; rise of, 54–70, 200; and sentiment, 89–93; as unrealized ideal, 55
clinical realism, 2, 4, 6, 7, 120–22; compared to classic realism, 129–30, 138, 149, 152, 156; in medicine, 208n45; rise of, 56–70
clinical voice: definition of, 58, 59; in literary periodicals, 82
"Cold-Water and Antiseptic Treatment of Typhoid Fever, The" (Blanc), 68–70
Coleridge, Samuel Taylor, 25
Collins, Wilkie, 71
Colonel Townshend, 58–59
Colvin, Sidney, 122
"commons," literary, 74, 80–86. *See also* physician, as author; physician, as reader
community, human, 139, 141–43
community, literary. *See* "commons," literary
community, medical, 31–34. *See also* disci-

· 249 ·

pline; professionalism; Royal College of Physicians; Royal Society for the Promotion of Natural Knowledge
concussion, 52–53
Connolly, John, 175
consumption, 96, 101, 105, 213n9
contagion, theories of, 108–9
Cooley, W. Desborough, 77–78
Coovadia, Imraad, 219n1
Cornhill Magazine, 73, 80–86, 215n74
corporations, medical, 13–14, 23. *See also* Royal College of Physicians; Royal College of Surgeons; Society of Apothecaries
"Corpulence" (Anstie), 84
Cowley, Abraham, 39
Crampton, Dr., 158
Crary, Jonathan, 26–27, 136, 151, 206n10, 221n44, 222n49, 222n50, 222n54
Crawford, Robert, 161
Cruikshank, George, 71–72
Cullen, William: review of, 75
cultural studies of medicine, 28–29
curiosity. *See* curious
curious, 1, 4, 7; as a term, 52, 62. *See also* "interesting"
curious case, 17, 36, 41–42, 42–45, 218n54; in 18th-century medicine, 31; in 19th century, 83–84; and circulation of affect, 38; decline of, 62; in Dickens, 106–7; in Freud, 175; as normative, 52–53, 54, 57; as science, 36–37; as spectacle, 53
curious discourse, 34–35, 43–45; in 18th-century novel, 45; suppression of, 54–55
curious observation, 7, 37, 41–42; in 18th-century medicine, 31–32, 35–37, 45, 46–50, 49–50; in 19th-century medicine, 50, 58; compared to psychoanalysis, 179
curious sight, 36, 38–46, 43–45, 52, 58–59, 176; in 18th-century medicine, 31–32, 45, 46–50, 49–50; in 19th-century medicine, 50, 58, 87–88, 92–93; in 19th-century novel, 92–93, 100; and circulation of affect, 36, 38–39; in Dickens, 88–89; in Freud, 175–76, 178, 2001; in literature, 39; rejection of, 93–94

d'Albertis, Deirdre, 112
Dames, Nicholas, 25
Darwin, Charles, 123; review of, 80
Daston, Lorraine: on curious cases, 35–36; on genius, 64–65; on mechanical objectivity, 3, 128, 222n56; on morality of science, 130; on perspectivalism, 144–47; on photography, 222n54; on the "working object," 59
Dawson, Gowan, 81, 215n74
Dawson, Graham, 198–99
deathbed: in 19th-century medicine, 95–99, 217n25; clinical observation of, 88–89, 104; in Dickens, 100–107, 217n39; in Gaskell, 115–18
deception, in case history, 210n26
"Delusions and Dreams in Jensen's *Gradiva*" (Freud), 190
Denis, J., 41–42, 45
Dent, Thomas, 40
depression, 113
depth of focus, 156, 166–67
Descartes, René, 221–22n46
Description of an Opthlamoscope, The (Helmholtz), 134
De Sedibus et Causis Morborum per Anatomen Indagatis (Morgagni), 58–61
detail. *See* clinical observation; mechanical observation; realism
diagnosis: in Dickens, 20, 218n52; in Hardy, 17–21; novelists' use of, 12, 17–21; in Oliphant, 9–10; as performance, 15
dialogue, 14–15
Dickens, Charles: *Bleak House,* 20; clinical observation in, 20; compared to Eliot, 143; *Dombey and Son,* 87–89, 100–107; on Gaskell, 108; and medical knowledge, 88; and mesmerism, 88; *Old Curiosity Shop, The,* 88–89, 101–7; periodicals of, 73–74; sentiment in, 87–89, 100–107; and spontaneous combustion, 25; use of 18th-century culture, 88, 106–7
differentiation, 141–43, 203–4
digestion, 73
"dilatation of the heart," 96–97
Dilke, Charles Wentworth, 74
disability, 28, 99–100
disciplinary difference, 22, 48, 204–5

discursive hybridity: in 18th-century medicine, 45–46, 46–50; in 19th-century medicine, 46, 98; in 19th-century novel, 88, 105–6; in 19th-century periodicals, 83–84; in Freud, 5, 170–71, 199; in the novel, 25, 204; novelists' use of, 17–21
disinterestedness. *See also* clinical observation: in 18th-century medicine, 31–32, 38, 43; in autopsy, 61; in curious case, 45, 48; in curious observation, 35–36; in Dickens, 104; in Eliot, 120, 139, 144–47; and ethics, 130; in Gaskell, 115; in mechanical observation, 61–70; in Oliphant, 9; in physician, 58; and "plain speech," 33–35
Disraeli, Benjamin, 11–13
Dombey and Son (Dickens), 87–89, 100–107
domestic medicine, 71–74, 109, 112–13. *See also* popular science
Domestic Medicine (Buchan), 71, 109, 112–13
Dora: An Analysis of a Case of Hysteria (Freud), 170, 172–73, 176–78, 180–81, 184–86, 185–86, 192–94, 196–200, 226n4
Dublin Medical Press, 14, 99, 158
Dyson, A. E., 105

Eclectic Magazine, The, 80
education, medical, 23–24, 55–56, 208n48, 211n50; and *ars medica*, 123–24; and case method, 21; and Eliot, 123; literary subjects in, 13; as a metaphor, 17–21; in observation, 121, 128. *See also* case-taking
egoism, 148, 150–51
E.H., case of, 97
Elements of General Pathology (Stillé), 63–68
Elements of Physiology (Müller), 151
Eliot, George, 119–47, 148–57, 159; *Adam Bede*, 120–22, 124–47, 164; animal magnetism in, 25; and G. H. Lewes, 80; *Lifted Veil, The*, 25, 132; and medical reform, 211n49; *Middlemarch*, 122, 132, 137–38, 146, 148–57, 163–67, 211n49; observation in, 1; review of, 1, 122; *Scenes of Clerical Life*, 122; and sympathy, 89; use of 18th-century philosophy, 141
Elliotson, John, 217n34; and Dickens, 88; and Eliot, 123; and emotional susceptibility to illness, 113–14; on precision, 65–66
Ellis, Havelock, 183
emotion, 88–89. *See also* circulation of affect; interest; reader, solicitation of; subjectivity; in Eliot, 138–44; infectious quality of, 114; of patient, 46–49; of physician, 38–46; and susceptibility to illness, 85–86, 92, 113–16
empire, 28. *See also* romance, imperial
empiricism, 121, 173, 210n18, 225n28; in 18th-century medicine, 31–32, 34; in 19th-century medicine, 50, 61–63, 149, 157–58; definition of, 214n27; in Freud, 175; in literary periodicals, 84–85; and mechanical observation, 63–70; opposed to theory, 62, 157–58
English Malady (Cheyne), 32–33
Englishwoman's Domestic Magazine, 79
Enquiry Concerning the Principles of Morals (Hume), 90–93
epidemics, 85–86, 108–10, 114
Epstein, Julia, 56
Erman, Adolf, 191
Essay on the Philosophy of Medical Science (Bartlett), 67
exactitude. *See* mechanical observation
excess, 45, 67, 210n19
experimentalist medicine (18th century), 31–46, 43, 48–50, 189. *See also* Royal Society for the Promotion of Natural Knowledge; and "plain speech," 33–35
experimental medicine (19th century), 5, 148–50, 156–63. *See also* speculation; compared to clinical medicine, 148–49; in literary periodicals, 77; resistance to, 24
experimental philosophy. *See* experimentalist medicine
expertise. *See* professionalism
exploration, 161, 170, 187, 190–95

fact, medical: importance in case history, 62; opposed to speculation, 162;

patient as, 69; production of, 55, 59, 61, 173
factory work, 99
Ferguson, John: review of, 77
Fermer, William: review of, 79
Ferriar, John, 35, 57, 96–97, 109, 217n25
fever, 108–11, 113–16
Finlayson, James, 56
Fissell, Mary E., 214n46
Fliess, Wilhelm, 179
Flint, Kate, 26–27, 222n56, 225n24
Forbes, Edward, 13, 124
formalism, 28–29
Fortnightly Review, 130
Foster, Michael, 123
Foucault, Michel, 3, 9, 58, 65, 140, 204
framing of text. *See* recursive (nested) texts
Frankland, Graham, 169, 178, 201, 227–28n37, 228n58, 229n73
Frawley, Maria, 57, 73
free indirect discourse, 143, 146
Freud, Sigmund, 5, 7, 168–205; "Aetiology of Hysteria, The," 172–73, 184, 190–92; as archaeologist, 187–99, 229n66; *Autobiography,* 200; *Dora: An Analysis of a Case of Hysteria,* 170, 172–73, 176–78, 180–81, 184–86, 192–94, 196–200, 226n4; as explorer, 161, 170, 187, 190–92; genre problems of, 184–86; *On the History of the Psycho-Analytic Movement,* 171; and imperialism, 169, 170, 187–99; *Interpretation of Dreams,* 173, 190; literary style of, 170; as "man of letters," 169, 175, 177–78, 184–85, 200–202; as "man of science," 24, 171, 200–202, 227n14; as "medical man," 184–85; professional opposition to, 171–73, 177, 195; as romantic hero, 187–99; suffering of, 175; use of 18th-century literature, 189; use of 18th-century medicine, 170, 175–76, 179, 189, 191, 200–202, 228n51; use of 19th-century literature, 187–92, 189–90, 227n25; use of 19th-century medicine, 171–77, 200–202; use of clinical observation, 172–74, 175; use of literary techniques, 177–83
Frye, Northrup, 189
functionalist language, 34, 95, 183, 209–10n14

Galison, Peter, 192, 225n27; on "genius," 64–65; on mechanical objectivity, 3, 128, 222n56; on photography, 222n54; on the "working object," 59
Gallagher, Catherine, 67–68, 117, 228n50
Galton, Francis, 80
Gaskell, Elizabeth, 107–16; clinical observation in, 89, 108–16; Dickens on, 108; and medical knowledge, 110, 113; *Ruth,* 89–90, 107–16; sentiment in, 88–89
gaze: clinical. *See* clinical gaze
genius: opposition to, 64–65; physician as, 162–63, 182–83; practical, 64–65, 131
genre, 187, 189, 203–5; anxiety of, 184–86, 197; in the case history, 168, 171; conflicts of, 22, 26; definition of, 22; history of, 46, 49; in the novel, 208n45; relation to discipline, 22; theories of, 3, 203–5
gentleman. *See* class status
germ theory, 10, 94
Gilman, Sander, 171
Gothic, 8, 35, 104
Gould, George, 51
graphs, 27, 57
Grapow, Hermann, 191
Greenberg, Valerie, 227n14
Greenhow, H. M., 52–53
Gulliver's Travels (Swift), 45
Gunn, Daniel, 125
Guy, William A., 160

Hacking, Ian, 224n19
Haggard, H. Rider, 187, 190, 195–99, 229n75
Hake, Sabine, 192
Hall, C. Radclyffe: review of, 76
Hallam, Henry, 218n44
Hamilton, Sir W., 82
Hamley, E. B., 1
Hammond, Elizabeth, 112
Hardy, Thomas, 17–21
Hartshorne, Henry, 66
Hawkins, Anne Hunsaker, 201
heart, diseases of the, 94–95
Heir of Redclyffe, The (Yonge), 116
Helmholtz, Hermann von, 121, 134, 155, 221n45

INDEX

hermaphrodite, 40–41
heroic medicine, 10, 50
Herschel, John F. W., 6, 215n74, 220–21n29
heterogeneity, of genre, 22
Hills, Alfred K., 73
Hinton, Laura, 216n11
historicity. *See* "true history"
history. case as, 21–23. *See also* "true history"
"history and physical," 58. *See also* case history; in case history, 56–57
"History of the Psycho-Analytic Movement" (Freud), 171
Hogarth, Mary, 102, 218n56
Hogg, Jabez, 166
Holland, Henry, 62, 123–24, 160–61, 172
Holland, Susan, 79
Holmes, Martha Stoddard, 28
Holmes, Oliver Wendell, 66
homeopathy. *See* sectarian medicine
Hooke, Robert, 32–33
Hooker, Worthington, 119–20, 121
Hope, James, 96
hospital, 55–56, 56, 212n3
Household Words, 73–74
humanism, 123–24, 139–40, 142, 151
"Human Vegetation," 83–84
Hume, David, 90–93, 141, 144–45
Hunter, John, 119–20
Hunter, Kathryn Montgomery, 201
Hutchinson, Horace G., 229n76
Huxley, Aldous, 102, 105
Huxley, Thomas Henry, 24, 80, 123, 161–62
hypothesis, 6, 121, 156–57. *See also* experimental medicine; speculation
hysteria, 5, 174–83, 187–92, 192–94, 197

identification: with the patient, 89–93, 217n34; through sympathy, 89–93, 117; through the novel, 100, 103, 140–41, 146–47
"illusionism," 65
imagination, 5. *See also* speculation; in 19th-century medicine, 121, 156–63; in Eliot, 156; in Freud, 190, 195; rejection of, 4. *See also* mechanical observation

imperial medicine: in case history, 28
imperial romance. *See* romance, imperial
individuality, 9, 16, 21, 231n19. *See also* "curious case"; typicality
industrialization, 27–28, 99
insight, 7. *See also* sensibility; sentiment; speculation; sympathy; in 18th-century medicine, 36, 37–38; in 19th-century medicine, 15–16, 38, 58, 87–88, 92–93, 157–63; in 19th-century novel, 92–93, 100; in Dickens, 107; in Eliot, 148, 156, 163–67; in Gaskell, 108; in Hardy, 19; in Oliphant, 9–10
"Instructions to Patients" (Hills), 73
instruments, medical. *See* technology, medical
interest. *See also* emotion: of observer, 1; of physician, 38–46, 61, 63–70; of reader, 23, 51, 139; suppression of, 63–70
"interesting": as link to 18th-century medicine, 94; and sensibility, 94; in sentimental novel, 94; as solicitation of reader, 94; as a term, 62, 94–97. *See also* "curious"
interpretation, as psychoanalytic tool, 178–83, 192, 228n47
Interpretation of Dreams (Freud), 190; review of, 173
Introduction to Experimental Medicine (Bernard), 138–39, 158
invalid culture, 73
"Irish fever." *See* typhus
irony, 17, 132
irregular medicine. *See* sectarian medicine

Jaffe, Audrey, 91, 114, 117
James, Henry, 167
Jameson, Frederic, 22, 62, 187, 195, 204
"Janet's Repentance" (Eliot), 137, 145–47, 221–22n46
Jay, Martin, 3
Jensen, William, 190
Johnson, A. B.: review of, 75
Johnson, George: review of, 76
Jones, Anne Hudson, 201
Jones, Ernest, 173
Journal of the American Medical Association, 201
journals, medical, 27. See also *British*

• 253 •

Medical Journal; Dublin Medical Press; Lancet; Philosophical Transactions of the Royal Society; in 18th century, 36; in 19th century, 57; rise of, 70–71; specialization in, 71
judgment, 147. *See also* diagnosis
"judgment against objectivity," 192, 225n27

Kaplan, Fred, 89, 216n5, 218n55
Katz, Wendy R., 228n55
Kay, James Phillips, 12
Keyt, Alonzo T., 94–95
King, Amy, 20, 219n9
Kleinman, Arthur, 201
knowledge: expansion of general, 75, 78–79, 81; unmediated, 67, 209–10n14
knowledge, medical: limits of, 15, 17, 36–37, 44–45, 51, 70, 87–88, 94, 106, 107–10, 117; novelists' use of, 17–21; production of, 10, 31–32, 49–50, 58, 63; transcendence of, 89
Kofman, Sarah, 173
Kreisel, Deanna, 219n8

labor: in mechanical observation, 64–65, 120, 128–31; of novelist, 128
laboratory findings, 56
labyrinth tracing, in Freud, 5, 188–90, 193–97
lactation, 42–44, 211n43
"Laid Up in Lodgings" (Collins), 71
Lancet, 52, 68; and literature, 24; and medical reform, 27, 50–51, 56, 211–12n51
Lankester, Edwin, 74–79, 85
Latham, Peter Mere, 18, 54, 57, 62, 65, 71
Latin, in case history, 32–33, 57
Law, Jules David, 210n18
Lawrence, Sir William, 159
Laycock, Thomas, 153, 161, 193
Leavis, F. R., 24
lens, smoked glass, 132–33
Lerner, Lawrence, 89, 218n52
"Letter ... Touching a Late Cure" (Denis), 41–42
Levine, George, 65, 128, 219n9, 228n62
Lewes, George Henry: as editor of *Cornhill,* 80; on experiment, 154; on imagination in science, 156, 164, 225n24, 225n26, 226n43; as physiologist, 123, 222n52; and professionalism, 27; and spontaneous combustion, 25
"Life and Letters" (Hamley), 1
Lifted Veil, The (Eliot), 25, 132
literary periodicals. *See* periodicals, literary
Literature and Medicine, 201–2
literature and medicine, 2, 201–2
literature and science. *See also* art, opposed to science: debates over, 24–25
Littell's Living Age, 80
"live object," 61
Lobb, Henry: review of, 76
Locke, John, 30–31
Logan, Peter Melville, 108, 130, 225n24
London Medical and Surgical Journal, 211–12n51
Louis, Pierre Charles Alexandre, 66–67. *See also* statistics
Löwy, Emanuel, 190

Mackenzie, Colin, 110–11
Mackenzie's Ten Thousand Receipts (Mackenzie), 110–11
MacLaren, Archibald, 83, 215n75
Macmillan, Rev. Hugh, 83–84
Macmillan's Magazine, 73, 80–86
Magazine of Science, The, 222n55
magic lantern. *See* transparency (magic lantern slide)
Mahony, Peter, 178
"Management of the Nursery" (MacLaren), 83
Mandeville, Bernard, 37
Manginot, Francis, 44–45
"man of letters," 25–26, 86, 169, 175, 184–85
"man of science," 24, 130, 171
Mansell, Darrel, Jr., 223n58
Manual of the Physical Diagnosis of the Diseases of the Heart (Sansom), 95–96
mapping, 169–70, 187–89, 190, 193–97
Marcus, Steven, 168, 173, 178
Mason, Michael York, 219n9, 225n24
Master Humphrey's Clock (Dickens), 106–7
"matter of fact," 4, 31–32, 34, 36, 45
Mazlish, Bruce, 229n78, 229n81
McKeon, Michael, 37, 121

mechanical objectivity, 59, 63, 128. *See also* mechanical observation
mechanical observation, 4, 6, 7, 61–70, 212n2; in Bernard, 138–39; compared to psychoanalysis, 191; compared to speculation, 149, 159–63; definition of, 63; and disinterestedness, 64–67, 200; Eliot's revision of, 120–47, 122, 142, 152, 164–67; in Freud, 173; and labor, 64–65, 120; opposition to, 66; and statistics, 63; and technology, 64; as an unrealized ideal, 66–67
mediation, 197–98. *See also* recursive (nested) texts; avoiding, 125, 139; in camera obscura, 134, 137; inevitability of, 139; problem of, 121, 129–30
medical authority. *See* authority, medical
medical community. *See* community, medical
medical education. *See* education, medical
"Medical Etiquette" (Anstie), 84–85
Medical Gazette, 71
medical humanities, 2, 28, 201–2
medical instruments. *See* technology, medical
medical knowledge. *See* knowledge, medical
medical realism. *See* clinical realism
Medical Reform Act of 1858, 13–14, 23, 211n50. *See also* reform, medical
medicine, clinical. *See* clinical medicine
medicine, domestic. *See* domestic medicine
medicine, experimental. *See* experimental medicine
medicine as an art. See *ars medica*
"Medicine as a Science" (Pye-Smith), 50
melodrama, 82, 106; in 19th-century medicine, 95–96; in Freud, 199–200; and sentiment, 89, 99–100
Meryon, Edward, 159
mesmerism, 88
Mesmerism in Its Relation to Health and Disease (Neilson): review of, 77
metaphor. *See also* metonymy; synecdoche: as argument, 119–20, 219n1; in Freud, 174, 188, 198–99, 228n45, 228n56; and hysteria, 180–82, 191; mind-as-blank-page, 120–21; mind-as-mirror, 120–22, 125–30, 135–37; novelists' use of, 12; as psychoanalytic tool, 178–79

metonym, 180
microscope, 27, 124, 227n11; and depth of focus, 166–67; difficulty of using, 154–55, 220n17; in Eliot, 163–67, 224n21; in Freud, 172; history of, 224n7, 224n9, 224n12, 224n18; mirror in, 148, 152–53; problems with, 153–57, 224n12
Middlemarch (Eliot), 122, 132, 137–38, 146, 148–57, 163–67, 211n49
Miller, Andrew, 130
Miller, J. Hillis, 224n16
Millingen, J. G., 51
Mill on the Floss, The (Eliot), 119–20, 146
mimesis. *See* realism
mirror: art as, 223n58; in camera obscura, 134–37; flaws in, 125–27, 156; in microscope, 148, 152–53; mind-as-mirror metaphor, 120–22, 125–30, 135–37; pier-glass metaphor, 148–51, 152; production of, 220n21; as vanity, deception, 223n1, 223n3
miscellany, 106–7
Mitchell, W. J., 65
Modern Domestic Cookery (Hammond), 112
Modern Painters (Ruskin), 125–26
Molineux, Dr., 36
Molyneux, William, 30–31
"monarch of all I survey" gaze, 194
Monro, John, 33
morality: in Eliot, 143; of the novel, 100, 107; in the novel, 108, 111, 122, 130, 141; of physician, 64–65, 85, 130; of the reader, 145–46; theories of, 89–93, 144–47
Morgagni, Giovanni, 58–61
Müller, Johannes, 123, 151
Myddelton, Starkey, 37
"Mystery of Inverted Vision" (Cooley), 77–78

narrative: case history as, 131; as cure, 179; death of, 117–18, 197; as psychoanalytic tool, 178–81; role in producing knowledge, 10, 31–32
narrative medicine, 2, 28, 201–2
Narrative of the Case of Miss Margaret McAvoy (Renwick), 212n56
narrator, 137, 164

INDEX

natural philosophy. *See* experimental philosophy
Negro, White, 41
Neilson, William: review of, 77
New Science, 33. *See* experimental philosophy
Newton, Isaac, 24
Nixon, Jude V., 216n2
Noble, Daniel, 75–77
normative, as a term, 51, 212n53
nostalgia, 106
novel of sensibility. *See* sensibility, novel of
Novum Organum (Bacon), 207n11
"numerical method," 66–67. *See* statistics
nurse. *See also* domestic medicine: death of, 109–10; in Gaskell, 110–11; suffering of, 111; training of, 80

objectivity, 58. *See also* "judgment against objectivity"; mechanical observation; "truth-to-nature"; aperspectivalist, 144–47, 154–56; revision of, 139
observation. *See also* depth of focus; perspective, visual: compared to experiment, 154; curious, 4. *See* curious observation; and discipline, 23; mechanical, 3. *See* mechanical observation; relation to representation, 3, 120–21, 136–37; training in, 121, 124, 220n17, 220–21n29
Old Curiosity Shop, The (Dickens), 88–89, 101–7
Oliphant, Margaret, 9–10
On Epidemic Diarrhea and Cholera (Johnson): review of, 76
"On Physical Pain" (Anstie), 82
On the Extent to which the received Theory of Vision requires, as to regard the Eye as a Camera Obscura (Wilson), 135
On the History of the Psycho-Analytic Movement (Freud), 171
On the Hygienic Management of Infants and Children (Baker): review of, 79
optical devices. *See* technology, visual
Origin of Species (Darwin): review of, 80
Osler, William, 109, 213n9
Otter, Chris, 3
Outlines of Physiology (Bennett): review of, 75

pain, 73, 82
Pargeter, William, 33, 37, 38
Park, Katherine, 35–36
Parsons, James, 40–41
passivity, of observer, 63–65, 126–29, 131, 137, 139. *See also* mechanical observation; subjectivity, suppression of
pathology, 55–56
patient: disappearance of, 214n46; emotion of, 46–49; narrative of, 56, 175, 178–79; physician's relation to, 58; resistance of, 192–95; role of, 48; suffering of, 174–75; suspicion of, 174
performance. *See* staging of medicine
periodicals, generalist, 80
periodicals, literary. *See also Athenaeum; Cornhill Magazine; Household Words; Macmillan's Magazine:* scientific content in, 55, 70–86, 204
periodicals, medical. *See* journals, medical
perspective, visual. *See also* objectivity, aperspectivalist: need for variety of, 145–46, 154–56, 224n22; of speculation, 159; and sympathy, 90–91, 144–47
Peterson, M. Jeanne, 24, 62, 74
Philosophical Transactions of the Royal Society, 36, 41, 43, 191
philosophy: experimental. *See* experimental philosophy; natural. *See* experimental philosophy
philosophy, experimental. *See* experimental philosophy
photograph, 145
phthisis. *See* consumption
physical examination, 57. *See also* case history
physician: as artist, 182–83; as author, 74, 80, 86, 204. *See also* "commons," literary; authority of, 9–10, 59, 191; empathy for, 99; as focus of case history, 200; as "man of letters," 25–26; as moral being, 64, 85, 98–99; as reader, 14, 25–26, 86, 204. *See also* "commons," literary; resistance to, 192–95; role of, 58, 161; suffering of, 175
physiology, 122–23
Physiology of the Senses, The (Johnson): review of, 75
"plain speech," 6, 7. *See also* curious observation; in 18th-century medicine,

· 256 ·

31–32, 48; and clinical voice, 58, 62, 69; and disinterestedness, 33–35; in Freud, 173–74; opposed to curious discourse, 32–35
pneumonia, 213n9
poetry, 2, 223n60; opposition to, 35, 64–65, 158, 185
point of view. *See* perspective, visual
Poovey, Mary, 12–13, 27
popularizers of science, 72–74, 81
popular science, 71, 75, 81, 87. *See also* domestic medicine; scholarship on, 215n48
Porter, Roy, 70–71
positivism, 6, 65, 123
Pratt, Mary Louise, 194
precision. *See* mechanical observation
Preliminary Discourse on the study of Natural Philosophy (Herschel), 6
Pritchard, Andrew, 224n12
professionalism: in 19th-century medicine, 46, 57, 61; attacks upon, in Freud, 171–73, 177, 200; attacks upon, in Lewes, 27; in case history, 27; difficulties in maintaining, 95–96; literary norms of, 23; and medical journals, 71; medical norms of, 23–24, 50–53, 74, 84
psychoanalysis: compared to clinical medicine, 169, 179–81, 182, 193; compared to curious observation, 179; compared to mechanical observation, 191; compared to speculation, 180, 182; as new science, 169–70
psychoanalytic case history: compared to clinical case history, 170–71; as narrative, 170–71; scientific markers in, 169–77
public health, 85–86, 108–10, 114; in case history, 27; in Hardy, 17–21; in novel, 27–28
puerperal fever, 96
putrid fever. *See* typhus
Pye-Smith, Philip Henry, 50, 70, 215n48
Pyle, Walter, 51

quackery. *See* sectarian medicine

Rai, Amit, 216n11, 216n12

Ramsbotham, Francis: review of, 78–79
reader: errors of, 137; expectations of, 204; relation to text, 92, 100–101; solicitation of, 35, 88–90, 93, 93–94, 100–101, 103, 107, 117, 141, 166, 185–86, 191, 198; suffering of, 92
readership: medical, 55; popular, 71; restricting, 55, 57, 74, 177, 185–86
reading. *See also* physician, as reader: importance in romance, 197; as psychoanalytic tool, 177–83, 181–82
realism: in 18th-century medicine, 32, 45–46; in 19th-century novel, 103–18; and authority, 122; classic, 120–21, 138, 149, 152, 154–55, 156; clinical. *See* clinical realism; criticism on, 2, 207n14; definition of, 7; in Dickens, 103–7; Dutch realist painters, 124–25, 140; in Eliot, 119–47, 148–52, 164; formal, 68; vs. "illusionism," 65; instrumental, 140; legal, 124–25; literary, 67–68; and mass production, 130, 221n37; medical (*see* clinical realism); opposed to egoism, 148–52; opposed to romance, 124–31, 164, 185, 198; revision of, 122, 149–50, 152; scientific (*see* clinical realism); and sentiment, 87–88, 118; social, 88–89, 103, 105–6, 107–16; and speculation, 163–67; of subject matter, 7, 125, 151; and sympathy, 89; theories of, 120–22, 125–26, 129–30; transcendence of, 108
reanimation, 58–59
"Recent Progress of the Theory of Vision, The" (Helmholtz), 134
Rector and the Doctor's Family, The (Oliphant), 9–10
recursive (nested) texts, 197
reform, medical, 10, 50–53, 56, 129, 211n49
reform, social: in 19th-century novel, 88–89, 103; in Dickens, 105–6; in Gaskell, 107–16
regular medicine. *See* clinical medicine
Reidel-Schrewe, Ursula, 174
"Relation Written ... Concerning an Aged Woman" (Robert), 211n43
"Remarkable Case of Deception" (Sayre), 52
"Remarkable Case of Euphoria" (Bramwell), 16–17

Remarks on Dr. Battie's Treatise (Monro), 33
Renwick, Thomas, 212n56
repetition, 67
Report on the Sanitary Condition of the Labouring Population of Great Britain (Chadwick), 11–13
representation: and discipline, 23; errors in, 137; relation to observation, 3, 120–21, 136–37
reproduction. *See also* "virtual witnessing": diseases of, 96; of scientific results, 67
research, medical: and rise of clinical medicine, 55–56
reviews, book, 1, 74–79
"Rhetorick," 32–35; in curious case, 45
Ridge, Joseph: review of, 77
Robert, Lord Bishop of Cork, 211n43
Roberts, Nancy, 216n12
roman à clef, 169, 185–86, 228n50
romance, 6, 35, 168–69; in 18th-century medicine, 31, 32; definition of, 7; in Dickens, 104; in Freud, 5, 178, 187–92, 189–90, 193–99; hero in, 187–92; imperial, 7, 169, 170, 187–99, 229n74; opposed to realism, 7, 164, 185, 198; opposed to true history, 21–22, 198; rejection of, 124–25, 131, 132–33, 164, 185; and sentiment, 89; and sympathy, 89
"Romantic materialism," 212n2
Ross, Sydney, 6
Rothfield, Lawrence, 2, 71, 224n22
Royal College of Physicians, 24, 76, 208n47
Royal College of Surgeons, 208n47
Royal Society for the Promotion of Natural Knowledge, 31–32, 33–35, 191. *See also* experimental philosophy
Ruskin, John, 125–26, 139–40, 150, 220n21
Russell, John Rutherford, 161
Ruth (Gaskell), 89–90, 107–16
Rylance, Rick, 212n59, 215n50

Sacks, Oliver, 201
Saint-Hilaire, Isodore Geoffroy, 51
Sandars, Joseph, 212n56
Sansom, Arthur, 95–96
satire, 103

Saturday Review, 130
Sayre, Lewis Albert, 52, 53
Scenes of Clerical Life (Eliot), 122
Schaffer, Simon, 31, 207n18
Schliemann, Heinrich, 190
Schott, Kaspar, 221–22n46
science: in medicine. *See* clinical medicine; opposed to art, 123–24, 158, 162–63, 178, 184. See also *ars medica;* role in culture, 26; as a term, 6
science, popular. *See* popular science
Science Index of the Athenaeum, 215n50
Science in the Nineteenth-Century Periodical index (SciPer), 79, 215n50
science wars, 24
scientific medicine. *See* clinical medicine
scientific method, 121, 225n24; in literary periodicals, 76–77
scientific realism. *See* clinical realism
scientific report, 207n12, 207n18
"Scientific Use of the Imagination, The" (Tyndall), 158
scientist: as a term, 6, 207n13
scopic regimes, 3, 202. *See also* clinical observation; curious observation; curious sight; mapping; mechanical observation; speculation; vision
secret, 189
"secret history," 176, 189
sectarian medicine, 211n49
self-restraint. *See* mechanical observation
sensationalism, 6, 35
sensibility, 32. *See also* emotion; insight; in 18th-century medicine, 36, 37–38, 210n28; in 19th-century medicine, 38, 68, 87–88, 92–93, 100; in 19th-century novel, 92–93; culture of, 47; in Freud, 174–75; novel of, 7, 46–50; of patient, 70; of physician, 70, 97; resistance to, 143; suppression of, 64–65, 70
sentiment, 6, 35. *See* insight; in 19th-century medicine, 38, 77, 87–88, 92, 117–18; in the case history, 46–49; causes of, 96; compared to grief, 102; compared to sympathy, 89; critique of, 93, 102; definition of, 89, 216n5, 216n7, 216n8; in Dickens, 100–107; in Freud, 174–75, 199–200; as insight, 93; at limits of medical knowledge, 94, 96; as link to 18th-century medicine,

93, 100; in the novel, 47, 88–89, 169; and realism, 87–88, 118; as violence, 117; and visuality, 217n18
Sexual Inversion (Ellis, Symonds), 183
sexuality: in case history, 28
sexuality, in case history, 173, 176–77, 183–86
Shapin, Steven, 31, 207n18
She (Haggard), 190, 196–99, 229n75
"shilling monthlies," 80. *See also Cornhill Magazine; Macmillan's Magazine*
Shuttleworth, Sally, 122, 219n9, 224n14, 225n25
sight: curious, 4. *See* curious sight
signs: in case history, 56
Sims, James, 62
singularity. *See also* "curious case"
skepticism, 43–44, 212n57; in 18th-century medicine, 36–37; in 19th-century medicine, 52, 121–22, 162–63; in Dickens, 87; in Eliot, 122, 132, 136–39, 147, 148, 150, 152–57, 167; and mechanical observation, 63–65, 128–31; of reader, 116–17, 177, 185–86, 198; and realism, 8
Smith, Adam, 90–93, 141, 216n8
Snow, C. P., 24
Snow, John, 27, 85
social realism. *See* realism, social
social reform. *See* reform, social
Society of Apothecaries, 208n47
Spalding, Douglas, 80
specialization. *See* professionalism
spectacle, 176, 186; in 18th-century medicine, 39–46; in 19th-century literary periodicals, 82–83; in 19th-century medicine, 53, 92–93; in 19th-century novel, 88, 92–93; in clinical realism, 128; in curious case, 45–46, 52; in sympathetic relation, 91–92
spectator: solicitation of, 93–94; suffering of, 92, 111
Spectator, The, 223n60
speculation, 7, 225n28 (*see* insight); in 19th-century medicine, 38, 121, 156–63; compared to mechanical observation, 149, 159–63; compared to psychoanalysis, 180, 182; in Eliot, 156, 163–67; opposition to, 64–65, 158–59; as realist, 163–67; rise of, 55

Spencer, Herbert, 123, 150
sphygmograph, 16, 27, 124
Sphygmography and Cardiography (Keyt), 94–95
Spiller, John, 135
Sprat, Thomas, 34, 40
Stack, Thomas, 42–45
Stafford, Barbara, 40, 210n19, 210n26, 212n57, 214n43
staging of medicine: in Dickens, 105–6; in Freud, 169, 187; in literary periodicals, 79–86
Stanley, Henry M., 193–94, 229n69, 229n71
statistics: in case history, 27, 57, 98, 208n45; in literary periodicals, 76–77, 85; and mechanical observation, 63; resistance to, 12–13, 70
Stephen, James Fitzjames, 93, 216n7
Stiebel, Lindy, 196
Stillé, Alfred, 63–68, 130–31, 139, 141–43, 158, 162
St. John, Horace Stebbing Roscoe, 75
St. Maur, Earl, 97–98, 118
Stoddart, Judith, 217n18
stomach, as metaphor, 119–20
Stones of Venice (Ruskin), 140, 220n21
"strange, therefore true," 37
"Stricture of the Oesophagus" (Bramwell), 16
stroke, 103, 111–12
Studies on Hysteria (Breuer and Freud), 170, 171–72, 173–76, 179, 181–83, 187–89
subjectivity. *See also* emotion; sensibility: inevitability of, 137; necessity of, 154; of patient, 69; of physician, 69–70, 81, 94, 175, 182; suppression of, 63–70, 69–70, 126–28, 139, 144–47, 221n31
suffering: of nurse, 111; of patient, 174–75; of physician, 175; of spectator, 92; and sympathy, 91–93, 174–75
Suggestions in Reference to the Means of Advancing Medical Science (Ramsbotham): review of, 78–79
Sully, James, 80
surgical report, 48–49, 81–82, 91
suspense, in case history, 16
Swain, William Paul, 100
Swift, Jonathan, 45
Sybil, 11–13

symbolization, 181. *See also* metaphor
Symonds, John Addington, 183
Sympathy (*see also* circulation of affect; insight; sentiment): in 18th-century novel, 7; compared to sentiment, 89; critiques of, 217n21; definition of, 89, 216n5; in Dickens, 89–90; in Eliot, 122, 138–44, 164–67; in Freud, 174–75; in Gaskell, 89–90, 108; as mode of transcendence, 117; of nurse, 111; obstacles to, 143; of physician, 15–16, 70, 94–100, 175; produced by realism, 120–21, 139–44; of reader, 89–90; and realism, 118, 143; from suffering, 91–93; as unrealized ideal, 147; as violence, 91, 117, 216n12; as visual process, 90–93, 138–44
symptoms: in case history, 56; of deathbed, 104; in Dickens, 101–5; in Disraeli, 11–12; in Eliot, 141; in Gaskell, 110–11, 115; guide to describing, 73; relation to language, 182
synecdoche, 194

tables, 27, 57
tabula rasa. *See* metaphor: mind-as-blank-page
"talking cure." *See* "cathartic method"
Taylor, Alexander: review of, 76
Taylor, Frederick, 104
technology, medical, 27, 57, 64, 213n13. *See also* microscope; sphygmograph; thermometer
technology, visual. *See also* camera obscura; lens, smoked glass; microscope; mirror; sphygmograph; transparency: in Bernard, 138–39; difficulty of using, 154–55; in Eliot, 131–38, 148–52, 163–67; and medical progress, 120–21, 124; problems with, 133–34, 152–57; resistance to, 124, 220n21
Thackeray, William Makepeace, 80, 100–101, 217n36
theories, medical, 61–63, 119–20; resistance to, 62, 121
Theory of Moral Sentiments (Smith), 90–93
thermometer, 214n46
Thomas, Lewis, 201
Thompson, Henry, 81–83

Through the Dark Continent (Stanley), 193–94, 229n71
Todd, Dennis, 210n26
tongue, lack of, 38
Topham, Jonathan, 74
Tougaw, Jason, 3
Traité de tératologie (Saint-Hilaire), 51
transcendence, 89, 108, 115–18, 117
transcription, 197
transfusion, 41–42
translation, 181–82, 191, 197
transparency (magic lantern slide), 132
Treatise of Human Nature (Hume), 90–93
Treatise of the Hypochondriack and Hysterick Diseases (Mandeville), 37
Treatise on Madness, 33
Trodd, Colin, 218n54
Trollope, Anthony, 130, 221n37
"true history," 21–22, 45, 198
truth: conflicting notions of, 1, 26, 144; difficulty of accessing, 131, 179; production of, 64, 67, 136; in recursive texts, 197; of sympathy, 117
"truth-to-nature," 59, 128
tuberculosis. *See* consumption
tumor, of skull, 14–15
"two cultures," 24
Tyndall, John, 156, 158, 225n24
typhoid fever, 68–70
typhus, 108–11, 113–16
typicality: and definition, 203; opposed to individuality, 9, 16, 21, 213n19; reference to a norm, 57, 59, 69, 208n37, 213n9

"Under Chloroform" (Thompson), 81–83
Under the Greenwood Tree (Hardy), 17–21
unknown. *See* limits of medicine

verisimilitude. *See* realism
"view from nowhere." *See* objectivity, aperspectivalist
virtue. *See* morality; sensibility
vision, 20, 170. *See also* observation; flaws in, 120–22, 125, 129–30, 133–38, 147, 148–52, 220–21n29, 221n45; importance in case history, 62; importance in sympathy, 90–93; and mastery, 91, 140;

as a mechanism, 134–46; modes of. *See* clinical observation; curious observation; curious sight; mapping; mechanical observation; speculation; theories of, 31, 134–37, 206n10
visuality, 26–27
visual technology. *See* technology, visual
voyeurism, 39–40, 45–46, 47, 176, 186
Vrettos, Athena, 108

Wakley, Thomas, 27, 50–51, 56
Ward, Mary, 135
Warner, John Harley, 51
Warter, John Southey, 66
Waterloo Directory, 204–5
water-newt, 38–39
Watson, Thomas, 124, 159, 225n31
Watt, Ian, 39–40, 68
Webster, Richard, 173
Westminster Review, 221n37
Whewell, William, 156, 207n13
Whitehead, Rev. H., 85–86
"White Negro" (Parsons), 41
Whytt, Robert, 32
Wikins, John, 183
Wilberforce, Samuel, 80
Wilkins, John, 209–10n14
Williams, Charles, 66, 97–99, 118, 123
Wilson, George: review of, 134–35
Winter, Sarah, 171, 178, 195–96, 229n84
witnessing, 40, 41; authority of, 31, 38; legal, 125–26, 147; virtual, 31, 33
Wood, Jane, 222n52
"working object," 59. *See also* typicality
Wormald, Mark, 152, 224n10, 224n12
"Worms Found in the Tongue" (Dent), 40
Wynter, Andrew, 80

Yeo, 225n24
Yonge, Charlotte, 116

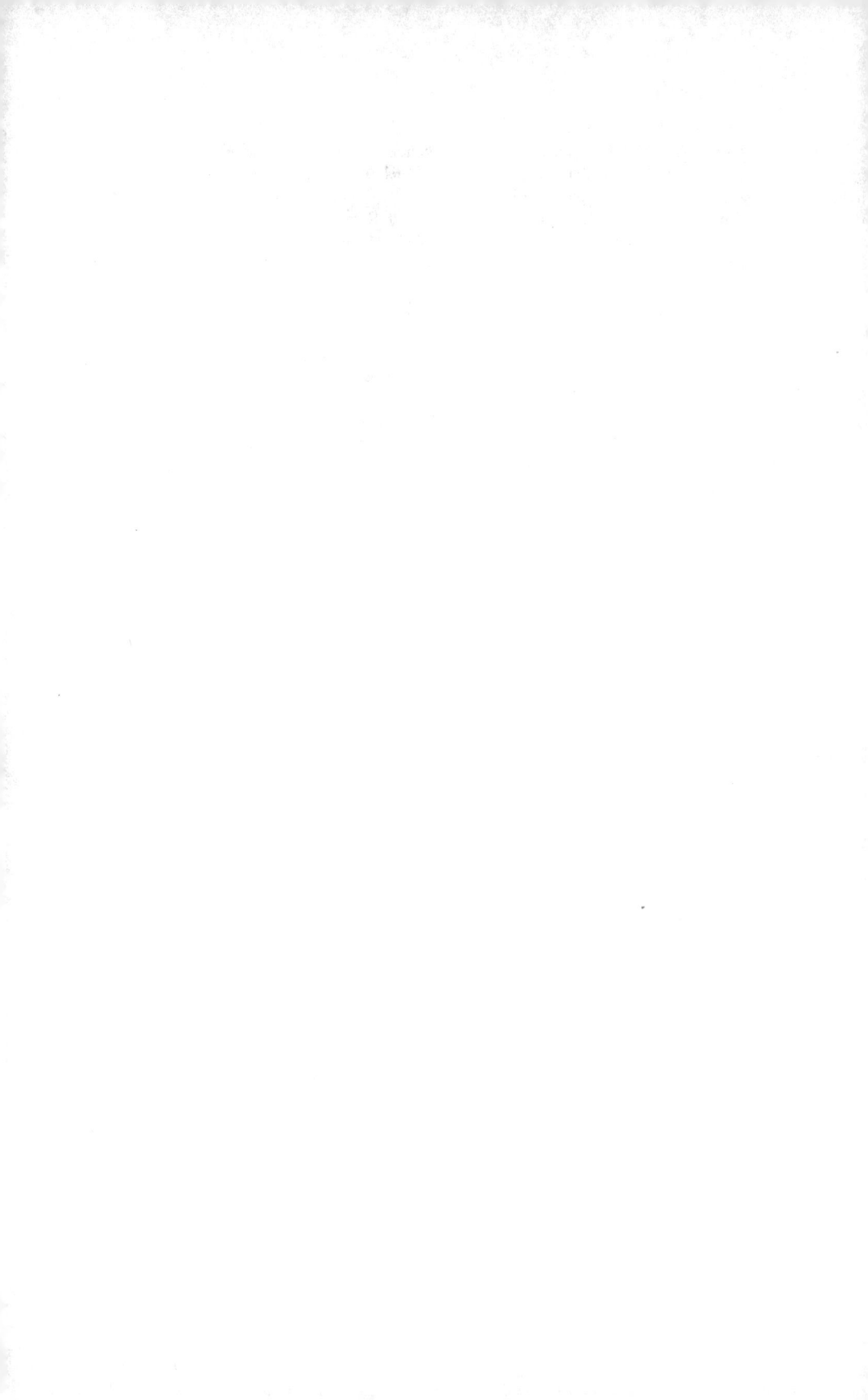

www.ingramcontent.com/pod-product-compliance
Lightning Source LLC
Chambersburg PA
CBHW021755230426
43669CB00006B/85